EXERCISE BENEFITS AND PRESCRIPTION

*Stephen Bird, Andy Smith
and Kate James*

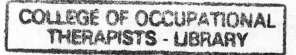
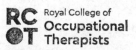

Stanley Thornes (Publishers) Ltd

First published as *Exercise Physiology for Health Professionals* in 1992 by Chapman and Hall.

This edition published in 1998 by
Stanley Thornes (Publishers) Ltd
Ellenborough House
Wellington Street
Cheltenham
GL50 1YW
UK

A catalogue record for this book is available from the British Library.

ISBN 0 7487 3315 9

98 99 00 01 02 / 10 9 8 7 6 5 4 3 2 1

Typeset by The Florence Group, Stoodleigh, Devon
Printed and bound in Great Britain by Redwood Books Ltd., Trowbridge

CONTENTS

ACKNOWLEDGMENTS

The authors and publishers are grateful to the following for permission to reproduce material:
Human Kinetics, Champaign, IL, USA for Table 5.1, reprinted from Bouchard, C., Shepherd R.J. and Stephens, T., *Physical Activity, Fitness and Health.*

EXERCISE AND PHYSICAL ACTIVITY: AN OVERVIEW OF THE BENEFITS

A general overview of the reasons for incorporating exercise into individuals' lifestyles

INTRODUCTION

Most people believe that exercise is good for them. However, despite this belief many also acknowledge that they do not take enough exercise. Furthermore, a considerable proportion of the population who perceive themselves to be 'fit and active' are in fact much less active than they think! In support of this, numerous surveys, such as the Allied Dunbar National Fitness Survey (1990), have reported low levels of activity, poor fitness throughout the population and an overestimation of exercise patterns. Given the many ascribed benefits of exercise upon an individual's physical and mental well-being, increasing the activity levels of the population has been identified as an important public health priority (Health of the Nation and More People, More Active, More Often). Therefore one of the challenges currently facing health professionals is to encourage individuals and communities to become habitually active. This may best be achieved by encouraging those who do least to do a little bit more. To meet this challenge health professionals will need to develop new professional practices based upon evidence from the growing field of exercise science.

When discussing the topic of physical activity, exercise, fitness and health some clarification of the commonly used terms is required. According to Bouchard *et al.* (1994) an active lifestyle is 'a way of life in which physical activity is valued and integrated into daily life', and physical activity may be defined as 'any body movement produced by skeletal muscles which results in a substantial increase in energy expenditure'. Exercise is a form of physical activity that is undertaken in a structured way for a specific purpose. It is often planned with the aim of improving some aspect(s) of physical fitness. Therefore an active lifestyle is one in which regular physical activity is included, possibly in the form of 'deliberate' exercise, but could involve less structured activities such as walking or cycling to work.

Physical fitness has been described as 'the capacity to meet successfully the present and potential physical challenges of life, and comprises of elements such as; flexibility, strength, anaerobic power, speed and aerobic endurance' (Lamb, 1984). Health is perhaps one of the most difficult terms to define. In the past it has been viewed as simply a condition of being 'free from disease' but more recently the definition has developed to incorporate a wider interpretation that includes the physical, mental, social, emotional and spiritual state of the individual on a continuum from near death to optimal functioning (Caspersen *et al.*, 1985; Bouchard *et al.*, 1994).

Exercise prescription, as the name implies, is the process of diagnosing, planning and advocating a form of exercise or exercise programme for an individual. Research that has investigated the responses and adaptations of participants to exercise has led to an understanding of how exercise may be used to convey various benefits to individuals. Effective exercise prescription involves determining whether an individual would benefit from participation in some form of exercise, the form of exercise that would convey most benefit, and the practical aspects of how often the individual should undertake the exercise, how hard it should be and how long it should last. A knowledge of these factors can then be applied by the health professional in the prescription of an exercise programme that will bring about the desired benefits to the individual.

It is argued by many authorities that 'exercise' is essential to the overall well-being of the individual. However, for many the technological developments of modern society have resulted in the exclusion of even basic levels of activity from their lifestyle. Consider, for example, the environment in which you live and work in terms of the opportunities it presents for active living: your activity levels might be constrained by town planning that favours the car over the pedestrian and architects who design wonderful lifts but hide stairs. Given the society in which we live exercise has to be reintroduced in the form of lifestyle changes, such as encouraging walking or specific exercise sessions. Bouchard and Shephard (1994) suggest that in most developed societies adults have an average of 3–4 hours discretionary leisure time per day, yet relatively few use any of this time in the pursuit of exercise or other physical activities.

Research has demonstrated that physical activity (in its many guises) can fulfil numerous physical, psychological and social needs of individuals and of society as a whole. However, since exercise is a complex phenomenon which can take on many forms including basic rehabilitation exercises, the physical work associated with everyday activities such as walking or climbing stairs, formal exercise classes, recreational games and competitive sport, not all forms of exercise fulfil these needs equally well. Therefore to meet the individual's requirements, any prescribed exercise must be tailored specifically. This why it is vital for a health professional working in the field of exercise to understand the basic principles of exercise and how to apply them. Prescribing the wrong exercise, or prescribing it in the wrong way, will not only reduce its effectiveness but could also have a detrimental effect on the participant. This could mean a physical injury or a negative experience which destroys the individual's motivation to become more active.

The diverse and complex nature of exercise is perhaps one of the reasons why the general population is confused as to what constitutes exercise, how they should go about it and what it will do for them. A misunderstanding of the effects of exercise that results in an individual participating in inappropriate exercise or expecting unrealistic outcomes can cause them to dismiss exercise as a 'waste of time'. For example, if a bout of exercise fails to produce the desired goals, a participant may be disillusioned and will almost certainly fail to persist with the activity. Unfortunately this problem is made worse by the portrayal of exercise as a means of achieving a 'model's figure' and suggestions of unrealistic 'get fit quick' routines. It is the responsibility of the health professional to guide and advise their clients, setting realistic targets and prescribing appropriate exercise programmes. Typically this advisory capacity falls upon the numerous health professionals whom the general public meet and expect to be knowledgeable in these matters: exercise specialists, physiotherapists, health promotion officers, nurses, osteopaths, occupational therapists and general practitioners. The needs of the individual clients will often differ very considerably, and to be effective the members of these professions must be able to prescribe exercise on an individual basis. This is important given the range of activities available and the diversity of perceptions of exercise. Simply telling an individual to 'take more exercise' is not sufficiently precise: the type, intensity, duration and the frequency of the exercise should be specified. To do this the professional must have a good understanding of what constitutes exercise, the benefits that can accrue from it and how to ensure that what is prescribed is appropriate for the individual. With time an individual's needs change, and therefore the professional must also be able to relate to other forms of exercise normally outside their usual field – for example, a patient with CHD could progress from basic rehabilitation exercises in a specialist unit to a more active lifestyle that incorporates regular exercises such as cycling and swimming.

In its widest context the general benefits of exercise include a reduction in the risk of physical disease, improvement or maintenance of physical capacity, recovery from illness or physical injury, promotion of mental health and the social interactions associated with activities. Each of these will be discussed separately and, whilst particular professions may have a specialised interest, the effectiveness of treatment can be enhanced only by an ability to relate to the full exercise spectrum. The role of this book is to provide health professionals with a basic understanding of exercise and how it may be applied in the context of their professional work. There is no magic formula that will ensure success, but certain guidelines can be followed when prescribing exercise. This knowledge should enable health professionals to use their judgement about individual clients and make appropriate, informed decisions about the incorporation of exercise into their treatment programme and/or lifestyle.

THE POTENTIAL BENEFITS OF EXERCISE

Regular participation in physical activity is reported to have implications for the general health and well-being of all members of the population, regardless of age, gender or whether they suffer from a recognised medical disorder or not. In summary, its effects include:

1. Promotion of good health
2. Prevention of 'ill health' via a reduction in the risk of various diseases throughout life
3. Enhancement of mental health and well-being
4. Maintenance and/or enhancement of physical capacity
5. Improvement of health and physical capacity following illness or an accident
6. Reduction in the severity of particular disorders
7. Growth, development and health of children
8. Minimisation of the effects of ageing
9. Provision of a social environment
10. Improvement in the capacity of an individual to cope with the physical demands of life – at whatever age.

The benefits of exercise should not be forgotten in any holistic approach to health and whilst research into its effects upon longevity remain inconclusive, there is no doubt that exercise can improve the quality of a person's life, regardless of age.

Exercise is therefore advocated as a means of promoting good health even for those who are apparently free from disease. Indeed, for the vast majority of the population exercise should be considered as a means of preventing ill health, especially because hypokinetic diseases (diseases associated with inactivity), such as coronary heart disease, are insidious, becoming apparent only at a fairly advanced stage. It should also be noted that physical activity is a relatively inexpensive intervention strategy and one that can help to prevent more costly treatments in the long term. These economic factors have been known for some time by large American corporations, who have established worksite exercise programmes to reduce their health insurance premiums.

For some individuals the assumption of a relatively sedentary lifestyle may be attributed to the increased availability of transport, a reduction in the physical demands of many jobs and the popularity of leisure pastimes involving a minimal amount of physical activity. For others it is enforced by a disability or condition that makes physical activity more difficult. However, for many a lack of exercise is simply due to other demands upon their time assuming a greater priority or an association of exercise with either boredom or physical discomfort. Once this stage has been reached, a sedentary lifestyle and general lack of physical fitness can result in a 'vicious circle' or 'downward spiral' in which the overall lack of physical activity causes a deterioration of physical capacity, which then makes physical activity more difficult and the individual less inclined to exercise; hence their condition continues to deteriorate. This physical decline is mirrored by a psychological downward spiral that can lead to a perceived loss of control, in which the patient does not even try to start a new exercise programme because they are convinced they will fail.

The consequences of a trend towards inactivity, coupled with dietary factors and the demands of modern society, are believed to be related to large increases in the incidence of certain diseases and unhappiness. This link has resulted in such diseases, which include coronary heart disease (CHD), hypertension, obesity, diabetes, some respiratory diseases, some digestive disorders and even some forms of cancer, being referred to as hypokinetic diseases.

THE ROLE OF EXERCISE IN THE PROMOTION OF GOOD HEALTH

There is much research to support the belief that appropriate forms of physical activity can reduce the risk and severity of many disorders (Hardman, 1996); in addition, exercise is reported to help control of related problems such as stress. Therefore, inactivity itself is considered to be a health risk by many authorities (Blair *et al.*, 1995), who recommend the participation in appropriate forms of exercise as a means of promoting or maintaining health (Åstrand and Grimby, 1986; Fentem *et al.*, 1988, 1990; Bouchard, 1989; Bouchard *et al.*, 1994).

In general, research into the topic of health and exercise aims to determine whether there is a definite relationship between the regular participation in physical activity and the development and maintenance of good health. However, as is often the case with research into human epidemiology, the complexities of disease and the human lifestyle make the reported benefits of exercise difficult to prove without exception. Therefore, whilst there is an undoubted relationship between exercise and health, the proof of the cause and effect is often open to debate. Critics of exercise suggest that, rather than regular exercise promoting good health, it is only those who are predisposed to good health that are inclined to exercise. In addition, many of the critics of exercise disparage its benefits by pointing to the incidence of exercise-induced injury (Solomon, 1985). In reality, significant exercise-induced injuries are relatively infrequent and, when they do occur, are often due to the individual either undertaking forms of exercise that are inappropriate for their physical condition or failing to adhere to certain safety aspects associated with the exercise. Thus the advocates of exercise would still suggest that most people are more at risk from underactivity than overactivity.

Although exercise may be prescribed as a means of promoting good health, it should also be remembered that inactivity is only *one* of the risk factors associated with disease, ill health and incapacity. Regular participation in vigorous physical exercise may indeed *reduce* a person's risk of suffering from disease or disability, but it cannot *guarantee* that person will not develop it. Thus, the beneficial effects of exercise must be considered in the context of other factors such as poor diet, stressful lifestyle, smoking and genetic predisposition to health or disease. Research findings also indicate that it is the current participation in exercise which conveys the benefits and a degree of protection against disease. This means that adults who were active ten years ago but have since assumed a sedentary lifestyle will have lost much of their previous advantage and appear to be almost as much at risk from hypokinetic diseases as those who have never participated in any form of regular physical activity. This is why the recent research and insights into exercise adherence (Chapter 4) is so important in helping health professionals to promote long-term compliance to an active lifestyle. It should also be noted that it is almost never too late to start exercising; benefits may be gained by individuals of all ages (Åstrand, 1994; Orban 1994).

EXERCISE FOR PHYSICAL HEALTH

Work by Blair *et al.* (1995) has highlighted exercise as one of the key factors in reducing all-cause mortality. This (and other) research reveals that exercise is an important component in reducing the risk of certain diseases. Consequently numerous local, regional and national initiatives have been launched to promote physical activity and to encourage a greater proportion of the population to become less sedentary. However, despite these campaigns, many surveys still indicate a low level of activity, which is described as being insufficient to maintain basic health amongst a large proportion of the population. This is despite the fact that most individuals believe that physical activity is good for them. Consequently, because knowledge of the benefits of exercise does not seem to be sufficient to change behaviour in its own right, exercise psychologists are developing ever more sophisticated models of participation (see Chapter 3).

The benefits of exercise to elderly people are similar to those to younger adults, although they tend to occur more slowly. Therefore, when prescribing an exercise programme for an elderly person the starting point will usu-

ally need to be at a very easy level and progression very gradual. Furthermore, as the maximum physical potential of an elderly participant is likely to be lower owing to the effects of ageing, the goals of the programme should also be set accordingly. However, the general content and type of exercises included should be very similar to those for younger adults and include activities such as walking, swimming, cycling, flexibility and strengthening exercises (MacHeath, 1984; Rikkers, 1986; Åstrand, 1994; Orban, 1994).

Research into the effects of exercise upon life expectancy are discussed later in this chapter. The potential increase may be 2–3 years, but what is generally perceived to be equally, if not more, important is the quality of life that retaining one's physical capacity can give to the later years, particularly in the retention of independence and ability to pursue a chosen lifestyle.

EXERCISE AND PHYSICAL CAPACITY

Appropriate exercise can be used to promote positive physical adaptations in the body such as improvements in cardiovascular capacity, muscle strength and joint mobility. The specific nature of such improvements depend upon the type of exercise undertaken, and therefore any exercise prescription must identify the specific goals it is trying to fulfil. Physical capacity is important to everyone, not just to elite athletes. A reduced or impaired physical capacity can have significant consequences upon lifestyle if it falls to a level where basic activities become difficult or impossible. For example, the Allied Dunbar National Fitness Survey (1990) revealed low levels of fitness amongst a large proportion of the population. The conclusions of this survey suggested that a significant proportion of the population would be unable to walk up a slight gradient, and many would be unable to open a jar or get out of a chair unaided. Deficiencies such as these are not only an inconvenience but, if severe, could cost a person their independence. Although such losses are primarily associated with increased age, the importance of maintaining physical capacity has specific implications for those suffering from a degenerative illness. Consequently, exercise that can ameliorate or improve any age-related declines in capacity can have major implications for a large proportion of society. In this context one of the roles of the exercise adviser is to optimise an individual's physical capacity to a realistic level that enables them to pursue the lifestyle of their choice.

Conversely, in the older age brackets there are a small number of individuals who, through participation in activities throughout life, have maintained a very impressive physical capacity. Notable amongst these are veteran cyclists, swimmers and athletes who continue to compete beyond the age of 60 and produce performances beyond the capacity of less active individuals 40 years younger. This further highlights the need to individualise exercise programmes and the potential problems of assuming that everyone in a particular age category will have similar needs and capabilities.

Physical fitness may be considered as a measure of a person's capacity to cope with the physical demands of his or her desired lifestyle – from simply moving around the home and doing basic household chores to coping adequately with the physical demands of an active lifestyle or (with more active individuals) participating in recognised forms of physical activity, including sports. Therefore precisely what is meant by 'physical fitness' depends on the individual. Factors such as age, inherent physical capabilities, acquired dysfunctions, injury, general aspirations and lifestyle all affect an individual's current and potential physical capabilities and hence their physical fitness.

If the physical capacity of an individual is impaired, so may their lifestyle be, or (on a more positive note) if physical capabilities can be improved (perhaps through participating

in an appropriate exercise programme) so can the lifestyle. This concept can be applied to virtually everyone – whether they are suffering from a major physical disability, are recovering from a disease or traumatic accident, or are generally 'well' but have fallen below their physical potential due to inactivity. In all cases an increase in physical capability will almost certainly improve self-esteem, satisfaction in achievements and the overall quality of life. This can be seen very clearly in physically disabled people, where an increase in physical capabilities may be realised as an improvement in the ability to move around the house and to perform basic household chores. In virtually everyone (disabled or not), any physical improvement is likely to make basic activities such as shopping or gardening less demanding and tiring. As a specific example, a client of one of the authors has recently commented how much easier they find it to turn the steering wheel of their car since they started resistance exercises for the upper body. Improved physical capacity is also likely to increase the overall feeling of 'well-being' and thus the mental ability to cope with the physical demands of the lifestyle. One of the functions of people involved in a health promotion, treatment or rehabilitation programme is to maximise the physical capacity of individual clients as appropriate to their needs. Although physical fitness is important for all, clearly the programme needed to achieve 'fitness' will be quite different for a coronary rehabilitation patient, a muscular dystrophy sufferer, an obese individual, an amputee, a currently sedentary 55-year-old man or a professional athlete who may have simply strained a muscle.

Physical fitness can be viewed as a spectrum. For some it may mean being free from disease, for others it may mean taking positive steps to avoid or reduce the debilitating effects of a disease, attaining a physical capacity within the restrictions of a disease or disability or reaching the peak of physical excellence.

EXERCISE PSYCHOLOGY AND MENTAL HEALTH

It is not surprising that, when some health professionals and their patients think about exercise, they focus on the physical benefits that can be achieved. After all, exercise has some very tangible physical effects – for example, it can increase your heart rate, make you breathe more deeply and in the long term change your body shape. However, exercise can also have some very significant psychological effects. These can occur at a very simple level – for example, the intrinsic enjoyment of a summer's walk – or at a much deeper level – as, for example, when a disabled child's self-esteem is enhanced by swimming a length of a pool for the first time. Indeed, it is not hard to find how the link between exercise and mental well-being has become embedded within our national psyche (consider phrases such as 'fun run' and 'a healthy body and a healthy mind'). What for many years has been a common-sense belief that exercise makes you feel good is finding increasing support from researchers in the developing field of exercise psychology. Just as exercise physiology is helping us to understand what type of exercises are best for different people so exercise psychology is helping to reveal the relationship between physical activity and mental health. Chapter 3 is devoted to exercise and mental health and Chapter 4 to exercise adherence. At this stage it is appropriate to consider questions that set the exercise psychology within this book in an appropriate context for health professionals.

WHAT IS EXERCISE PSYCHOLOGY?

Exercise psychology is a relatively new branch of psychology, which can trace its development from sports psychology to an emerging relationship with health psychology (Biddle and Fox, 1989; Biddle, 1997). Rejeski and Brawley (1988) have defined exercise psychology as 'the application of educational, scientific and professional contributions of psychology to the promotion, explanation, maintenance and enhancement of behaviours related to physical work capacity'. The growth of exercise psychology is demonstrated by the formal accreditation of sport and exercise psychologists by the British Association of Sport and Exercise Sciences (BASES) and by the work of the European Federation of Sports Psychology (FEPSAC).

Biddle (1997) has identified that the main topics and trends found in the current exercise psychology literature cluster around motivation, anxiety, imagery, self-efficacy, confidence, exercise and mental health and group dynamics. Here we will focus on mental health (Chapter 3) and exercise adherence (Chapter 4) and use insights from psychology to help develop an interdisciplinary approach to the principles of exercise prescription (Chapter 5), the assessment of patient and client groups (Chapter 6) and the role of the physiotherapist (Chapter 10).

The exercise psychology contained within this book is not intended to give you the skills to practise as an exercise psychologist. Those readers who are inspired by this text to seek a career in any of the exercise sciences are strongly recommended to contact BASES (address at the end of this chapter) to find out about professional accreditation. This book is intended to help you reflect upon your professional practice in the light of research and practical insights from exercise psychology. The material may also help you to work as part of an interdisciplinary team that includes an accredited exercise specialist. We hope that it will also help you to look at exercise from a different perspective.

IS IT REALLY IMPORTANT FOR HEALTH PROFESSIONALS TO UNDERSTAND EXERCISE PSYCHOLOGY?

As with any scientific discipline that claims to be relevant to the development of evidence-based practice it is important that health professionals adopt a critical and questioning perspective; this book should help you to develop these skills. We believe that insights from psychology have had a major effect on how health professionals are trained and on how they deliver services in a number of areas, including the approach to screening, pain relief and counselling. Given the contribution that psychology has made in these areas it would seem logical to assume that benefits will also accrue from applying insights from exercise psychology to the promotion and prescription of physical activity to both 'normal' and special populations.

As an illustration it would seem appropriate to demonstrate how exercise psychology can help you look at everyday situations in a different light. Consider, for example, the terms 'physical activity', 'exercise' and 'sport'. The definition of these words is more than a simple exercise in semantics because each is surrounded by cultural and social significance. For some people the word *sport* implies healthy competition, character-building hours on muddy playing fields and positive memories of childhood PE lessons; for others it brings back painful memories of cold showers and bossy PE teachers and may lead to barriers to participation – including the often-repeated statement 'I'm not the sporty type' (HEA, 1995). Calling a building a sports centre rather than a leisure centre, or a rehabilitation programme sports medicine rather than exercise therapy, may have unforeseen effects on the perception of potential users. Similarly, once we have agreed on the definition of the word *exercise* it is only natural that health professionals and researchers will begin to divide the world into exercisers and non-exercisers. Not surprisingly, as work by Smith and Biddle (1991) has shown, not all our patients will agree with the label we attach to them. Labelling may not only lead to misunderstandings but it may also be related to a process called 'actor–observer differences', which can cause motivational problems for both the client and the health professional. We

will look at this process in more detail in Chapter 3.

REHABILITATION EXERCISES FOLLOWING ILLNESS OR INJURY

For the health professional based in a hospital or private practice, a knowledge of exercise science and its practical application is important. Exercise is commonly used as a form of treatment and rehabilitation by physiotherapists, occupational therapists and other related practitioners. The desired effects of a prescribed exercise programme can be physiological, psychological and social. For some patients an exercise programme may be clinically based, with therapeutic or rehabilitative implications, for others it may occur in a wider social context. For many people the programme will involve a combination of the two, and perhaps a progression from the clinical to the social contexts.

In the clinical setting exercise may be used as a form of therapy in the treatment, prevention and rehabilitation of a wide range of disorders and problems, both physical and mental. When incorporated into a treatment programme for disorders such as hypertension and diabetes, exercise reduces the amount of medication required. Exercise also plays an important role in minimising the effects of degenerative diseases and in some cases may be used as a form of 'preventive medicine'. So, for many individuals exercise will be incorporated into a basic rehabilitation programme following injury or illness, or (in the case of degenerative diseases) may be used to minimise the decline in physical capability. The improvement or maintenance of a person's physical capacity may increase their ability to lead a more independent lifestyle, in which they can perform standard household tasks and daily activities more easily. In other situations exercise may provide the stimulus to develop physical, social and mental capabilities.

Terms such as 'exercise programmes' and 'training effects' often conjure up visions of competitive sporting individuals seeking physical excellence; however, exercise programmes and exercise science have a wider application, even within the sporting context.

Competitive performers form a specific group that often comes into contact with the health professional, especially when they have an exercise-related injury. For these individuals the inclusion of exercises in a rehabilitation programme has specific significance. However, to some extent they form a special case, requiring appropriate types of exercise that enable the injured part to recover while continuing to exercise and remain 'fit'. Some of the injuries in this group result from overuse caused by doing too much or inappropriate training; other examples of exercise-related injuries the therapist or doctor may encounter include those of a more traumatic nature such as pulled muscles, damaged ligaments and strained tendons. Such injuries are often treated by physiotherapists and sports doctors, who have to cope with the additional complication of a patient who wishes to return to sport as rapidly as possible. In such cases a gradual progressive exercise programme forms an essential component of treatment and must be designed in such a manner that the chances of the injury recurring are minimised: hence the early stages of a recovery programme may bear little resemblance to the strenuous levels of activity with which the athlete is familiar. However, it is essential that the programme commences at a level that the injured tissues can tolerate if they are to respond positively to the exercise. By doing so, the tissue's strength and tolerance will gradually increase, enabling progressive increases in loading, whereas resuming normal training loads while the injured part is still weak and vulnerable will increase the risk of recurrent injury and further complications. Any rehabilitation programme must therefore follow a planned and systematic approach, with a gradual transition to the form of training with which the athlete is familiar (Bird *et al.*, 1997). To achieve this smooth transition it may be necessary to discuss the situation with the individual's coach and establish how the training loads can be optimised, strengthening the tissues as they return to fitness and reducing the likelihood of further injury.

EXERCISE BENEFITS AND SPECIFIC SECTIONS OF THE POPULATION

EXERCISE AND THE HEALTH OF THE GROWING CHILD

The topic of exercise and the growing child is extremely broad, partly due to vast differences in the physical and mental capabilities of children of different ages and partly to the variation among children of the same age. There is no doubt that appropriate exercise can be of great benefit in the development and health of a child (Binkhorst *et al.*, 1985; Rutenfranz *et al.*, 1987). These benefits extend beyond the basic physical implications to include social and psychological aspects of health. They may have specific significance if the child has a disability. In addition to the specific problems associated with certain disorders, inactivity can result in general underdevelopment of physique and physiology, making the child relatively weak, prone to fatigue and susceptible to certain disorders throughout life. Inactivity during childhood might:

- limit physical capacity during childhood and later in adult life; and
- increase susceptibility to obesity, cardiovascular disorders and even osteoporosis.

Thus, for the young, exercise conveys numerous benefits, but inappropriate exercise also carries a slight risk of injury. Children undertaking too much exercise may be prone to a range of overuse injuries, as are adults. Young people are particularly susceptible to some overuse injuries because of their immature bodies.

Conversely, the vast majority of children are more at risk of the effects of underactivity than those of overactivity. It may therefore be the role of the health professional to prescribe exercise programmes to increase a child's participation in physical activity. Research indicates that exercise can help to promote a child's overall physical development, including skeletal, muscular, neuromuscular and cardiovascular aspects. Exercise may also help to develop a child's co-ordination, reduce the risk of obesity and help with social development. Various reports suggest that exercise is beneficial to children of all ages but that the greatest physical responses to exercise occur during or after the growth spurt (at 8–16 years in girls and 10–18 years in boys) and are associated with the various hormonal changes occurring at this time. The social, physiological and psychological benefits of exercise are therefore pertinent to all growing children, whether they are suffering from a specific disease or disorder, rehabilitating from an accident or illness or just developing normally. A general lack of physical activity can impair development; therefore any exercise programme should primarily be aimed at enhancing the physical and social development of the growing child, whilst taking into account the psychological issues.

It is particularly important to ensure that an exercise programme for a child is varied, and an element of fun should be included if possible. Variety will help to ensure a more comprehensive physical experience and development as well as reducing the chances of boredom. Similarly, if the child is to persist with them and get the most out of exercise sessions, the exercises or activities should be enjoyable. Appropriately designed forms of 'play' may be oriented towards the development of the cardiovascular system, strength, co-ordination and muscular control, with a combination of these effects being desirable.

Although diseases such as CHD are generally associated with mature adults, they do occur in children (Wilmore and McNamara, 1974; Gilliam *et al.*, 1977; Linder and DuRant, 1982). Of particular concern are reports that the initial stages of these diseases are present in a significant percentage of children. It has thus also been suggested that good health and activity in childhood can diminish the risk of these diseases occurring in later life. From a behavioural perspective, sedentary children tend to grow into sedentary adults, so it is important to establish positive exercise habits in childhood.

In this context, various authorities are concerned about the general lack of activity observed in many children (Armstrong and Welsman, 1997), including those who follow a normal school curriculum; hence the introduction of 'health-related fitness' into many schools. The aims of such innovations are to make children aware of the importance of exercise and to encourage their participation in physical activity up to a level beneficial for health. For a child with a specific physical or mental disability these concerns are magnified, particularly if they are unable to participate in the regular forms of physical activity that are available to most children.

The primary roles of exercise in childhood include the development of:

- the cardiovascular system;
- muscular strength;
- joint function;
- motor skills; and
- social and mental attributes.

The exercises used to develop these factors will vary, but can include games and activity sessions (both formal and informal) and in some cases specific exercise sessions with a specialist. A child's exercise programme is likely to include easier and less intensive exercises and be of shorter duration than that prescribed for most adults. When prescribing exercise for children the principles of specificity, duration and intensity must still be applied, but with some modifications. A number of other factors should also be considered – for example children do not possess the same aerobic or anaerobic capacities as adults, they tend to tire more rapidly and their bodies are not fully developed. Furthermore, it is important to make physical activity fun if at all possible, because a child will not be interested in pursuing an activity just because it is good for them. To achieve this, physical activities can be incorporated into games within groups or just between the child and their therapist. Specialised exercise programmes will be required to treat the particular aspects of specific disorders.

If attempting to put physical activity into the format of a game the health professional needs to carefully consider:

- the physical requirements of the game;
- the muscle groups that are being used;
- how the muscles are being used;
- the range of motion through which the joints are being moved;
- the demands that are being placed on the cardiovascular system;
- how additional overload could be applied to the activity.

When dealing with any child it is important to remember that the skeleton is not fully developed and that, although some running and jumping will promote bone strength, excessive stress on the bones should be avoided. An appropriate combination of activities which include running games, swimming or cycling, will have the desired strengthening effects on the musculature and cardiovascular function without unwarranted stress. If specific strengthening exercises are needed, body resistance or accommodating resistance exercises are likely to be most suitable, using light weights in certain circumstances. This is not to say that all impact should be avoided (indeed it is essential as a means of stimulating bone growth and developing bone strength), but excessive amounts of impact can cause injury.

The issue is that extreme forms of exercise can damage the immature skeleton. Of particular concern are the growth plates (epiphyseal plates) of the growing long bones. In the immature skeleton these are made of cartilage rather than bone, which makes them more susceptible to damage from excessive orrepeated stress. Epiphyseal injuries occur only when the exercise loads placed upon the child are too great and are therefore likely to occur only in children who undertake too much exercise or training in the pursuit of excellence in competitive sport – and even then they are relatively uncommon. The causes of such injuries include running too many miles every day on hard surfaces or repeated over-hyperextension of the back in gymnastic-type movements. However, these problems are unlikely to be caused by the type of exercise programmes prescribed by the health professional or by any other form of regular physical activity, and the risks are minimised by appropriate coaching when training for competitive sport. Only when that training is taken to an extreme in terms of intensity, duration or frequency, or if it is of an inappropriate type, may the child be vulnerable to injury.

EXERCISE AND THE HEALTH OF THE ADULT

For the adult, the reported health-related benefits of exercise are many and diverse. They are also often inter-related. These were listed earlier (p. 3) and will be reviewed in detail in later chapters.

EXERCISE, AGEING AND LONGEVITY

The variety and complexity of human lifestyles, and the natural genetic variation between individuals, makes the study of the relationship between exercise, ageing and longevity extremely difficult. A person's maximum physical capacity is generally considered to increase during childhood, reach a peak during the late teens to early 30s and then decline. There is no doubt that in the population as a whole general physical capacity gradually declines from middle age onwards. This decline involves all aspects of fitness, including aerobic capacity, strength and flexibility. It relates to many physiological parameters, including maximum heart rate, stroke volume, cardiac output, the ratio of blood capillaries to muscle fibre area, the speed of nerve impulse transmission and pulmonary factors. However, what is questionable is how much of the decline is due to an inevitable ageing process and how much is due to a change in lifestyle with age.

In many cases the observed ageing process can be attributed to a combination of the inevitable ageing phenomena, the presence of disease and a regression of physical capacity through inactivity. As people get older they tend to become less physically active. The reduction in physical activity may be due to their occupation, which often becomes less physically demanding, and other pressures such as family commitments, which can greatly reduce the amount of time a person spends in active leisure pursuits. Society has certain expectations about how physically active someone should be at a particular age. Therefore, we should consider whether the 'inevitable' reduction in physical capacity can be minimised by continuous participation in vigorous physical activity throughout life and, if so, to what extent the decline can be retarded. Whilst there may be much individual variation in the ageing process the findings of Bruce (1984) show that the decline in aerobic capacity of sedentary individuals is twice as rapid as in those who exercised regularly, suggesting that much of the observed reduction in physical capacity is premature.

The effects of exercise upon life expectancy are complex. There is a wealth of evidence supporting the notion that exercise reduces the risk of CHD and thus will increase life expectancy in that respect but the effects on the incidence of other diseases requires further research. Many of the animal studies that have been conducted under laboratory conditions indicate that regular exercise increases life expectancy. However, the relevance of these findings to humans remains to be seen. Human studies, including that of Karvonen *et al.* (1974) (who studied endurance skiers), indi-

cate that exercise increases life expectancy by 2–3 years. Since such increases in longevity are relatively small, most of the advocates of exercise emphasise its benefits in increasing physical capacity during life, and hence the quality and vitality of life, rather than the quantity in years. However, we are of the opinion that if on our deathbeds we were offered 3 extra years we would accept without hesitation!

Associated with the ageing process is a steady decline in aerobic capacity, maximum heart rate, flexibility and muscular strength and demineralization of the bones. However, regular participation in appropriate forms of exercise appears to reduce this decline. Indeed, improvements in cardiovascular function, strength and flexibility have all been observed in elderly people, although these adaptations tend to occur more slowly than in younger adults. Activities requiring exertion of muscular and/or gravitational forces on the bones, including almost all forms of physical activity, appear to reduce the demineralisation of the bones (osteoporosis) and thus reduce the risk of the individual developing weak bones that are liable to fracture. Exercise is also appropriate in reducing the decline in physical capacity in adults of all ages: research suggests that adults who exercise regularly throughout life are often physiologically younger than sedentary people of the same chronological age. This is evident from the many individuals over 70 who still participate in fairly vigorous forms of activity and even in competitive sport.

EXERCISE RISKS AND RELATED FATALITIES

According to Thompson and Farenbach (1994) 'The cardiovascular complications of vigorous physical activity include cerebrovascular accidents, symptomatic cardiac arrhythmias, aortic dissection, myocardial infarction, and sudden cardiac death.'

It is unfortunate that if a person collapses and dies during or after some form of physical activity it is often highly publicised, giving the impression that exercise is a major risk factor in causing sudden death and deterring many people from exercising. However, many people die in their sleep or from a heart attack whilst watching television but such deaths receive little or no publicity and there follows no media investigation into the 'dangers' of these more sedentary pastimes. Estimates of the incidence of sudden cardiac death during or immediately after exercise are difficult to compare due to the nature of the data and differences in methodology. Figures such as one death per 7500–15 000 joggers per year and one death per 396 000 jogging hours have been reported, with indications that the mortality rate is even lower during less vigorous exercise (Thompson *et al.*, 1980). Cardiac events also occur during or following 'non-sporting' activities, with 'snow shovelling' being a commonly referred to example, as it often involves relatively inactive individuals suddenly undertaking an activity which is far more physically demanding than they usually take. Work by Vuori *et al.* (1978) also suggests that when someone does experience an exercise-linked cardiac event, it was likely to happen anyway and perhaps the exercise only hastened the inevitable.

It is clear that for individuals suffering from certain cardiovascular disorders extremely vigorous exercise (such as very strenuous competitive sport) is neither advisable nor appropriate: the effects of the exercise, combined with the medical condition, may make participation in strenuous exercise 'risky'. However, this does not mean that these individuals should do no exercise; rather that it should be of appropriate intensity. Appropriate exercise is likely to convey substantial benefits to the individual without major risk. Problems usually occur only when individuals attempt strenuous activity for which they are not physically fit.

Indeed, as emphasised throughout this book, the vast majority of individuals are more at risk from underactivity than from overactivity. Prolonged underactivity will result

in reduced physical capacity and, perhaps, increased risk of hypokinetic disease. If the individual then attempts an inappropriately strenuous activity he or she may be at risk. Hence it is the combination of poor physical fitness, presence of disease and an inappropriate level of exercise that can cause problems, not just the exercise itself. In fact the incidence of sudden death in elite athletes and regular exercisers is very low (Zeppilli and Venerando, 1981; Kanel, 1982).

Death during exercise is usually a result of ventricular fibrillation caused by myocardial infarction and ischaemia (Cobb and Weaver, 1986). Post-mortem evidence following sudden death tends to reveal a recent myocardial infarction, fresh coronary artery thrombus and coronary plaque disruption (Thompson and Fahrenbach, 1994). One of the possible causes of sudden death during or just after exercise is an atherosclerotic thrombus that breaks off from an artery wall and blocks a cardiac blood vessel. Exercise may precipitate this occurrence because blood flow and blood pressure increase during physical activity. People who have not exercised for some time may be particularly vulnerable to this during the early stages of an exercise programme, so additional caution should be observed when prescribing intensity of exercise. Investigations suggest that the risk of sudden death increases with exercise intensity, age, a previously sedentary lifestyle and smoking (Siscovick *et al.*, 1984, 1985; Coplan *et al.*, 1988; Vuori, 1986).

A possible factor in the risk of sudden death in the early stages of an exercise programme is the clotting process; relative changes in plasminogen activator and plasminogen activator inhibitor may increase the risk of sudden death in the early stages of a programme but reduce it in the long term (Sellier *et al.*, 1988; Estelles *et al.*, 1989; Rydzewski *et al.*, 1990).

A cause of sudden death occasionally seen in young people is hypertrophic cardiomyopathy. This is a pathological enlargement of the heart, which should not be confused with the commonly observed (and beneficial) enlargement of the heart and thickening of the ventricular wall associated with endurance training (Shephard, 1996). Other conditions which have been identified as causing young people to die during exercise include congenital coronary artery anomalies, related disorders and myocarditis, all of which are, fortunately, relatively rare (Sharma *et al.*, 1997).

The use of cardiovascular testing and health screening for hypertrophic cardiomyopathies and other coronary risk factors has been suggested as a means of preventing exercise-related coronary events. However, the efficacy and practicalities of such procedures appears to be questionable because even extensive testing will not identify all individuals who are 'at risk' and the costs of large screening programmes would be prohibitively expensive. The work involved would be very great – and even if the facility were available it is likely that many people with potential problems would not use the service. Therefore, whilst individuals should not be discouraged from seeking health tests, which are extremely valuable, a national 'compulsory' screening programme is perhaps neither financially viable nor ethically feasible.

At a less extreme level, it is certainly true that the participation in exercise does carry the risk of exercise-related injuries, from minor aches and slight inflammations to strained muscles, all of which are due to the tissues being subjected to an unfamiliar amount of acute traumatic stress or chronic overuse. The implications of such problems are usually of minor inconvenience and can largely be avoided by following the general principles of exercise, which include starting at an easy level and progressing gradually.

There has also been some debate over the possible link between exercise and osteoarthritis, a degenerative joint disease characterised by pain when performing specific movements, joint stiffness and cartilaginous degeneration. Osteoarthritis primarily occurs in older adults, both sedentary and active.

A review by Panush (1994) suggests that research on the question of whether exercise increases the risk of osteoarthritis is often anecdotal and largely inconclusive, although some association has been found between the incidence of osteoarthritis and previous joint injuries, such as meniscal and ligament damage. Biomechanical malalignments may also contribute along with a genetic predisposition, environmental and immunological factors. However, the overall conclusions suggest that there is no evidence to conclusively demonstrate an increased incidence of osteoarthritis in active individuals, even in those who participate in intense athletic training; indeed, exercise may benefit the condition in some people.

A further area of research interest is the possible effects that fitness and an active lifestyle can have upon the risk of cancer. This was reviewed by Lee (1994), who concluded that there was some evidence to suggest that physical activity was associated with a reduced risk of colonic and breast cancer. However, the findings were contradictory for the incidence of prostatic cancer, studies variously showing a positive, inverse or no link with physical activity levels. The review also concluded that there was no apparent link (either positive or negative) between exercise and rectal or other forms of cancer.

In summary, the potential risks associated with exercise must be considered in context with the reported benefits. It is clear from the evidence that a lack of exercise and a sedentary lifestyle conveys serious health implications (Powell *et al.*, 1987), which are far more prevalent than the risks associated with exercise. However, if the exercise performed is inappropriate, these risks are real for certain sections of the population.

REFERENCES

Allied Dunbar National Fitness Survey (1990). *Summary report. Activity and Health Research*. London: Sports Council and Health Education Authority.

Armstrong, N. and Welsman, J. (1997). Physical activity and aerobic fitness. In *Young people and physical activity*. Oxford: Oxford University Press; 122–136.

Åstrand, P.O. (1994). Age is not a barrier: A personal experience. In *Toward Active Living*, Quinney, H.A., Gauvin, L. and Wall, A.E.T. (eds). Champaign, IL: Human Kinetics; 147–152.

Åstrand, P.O. and Grimby, G. (eds) (1986). Physical activity in health and disease. *Acta Medica Scandinavica (Supplement)*, **711**.

Biddle, S.J.H. (1997). Current trends in exercise and sports psychology research. *The Psychologist: Bulletin of The British Psychological Society* **10**(2), 63–69.

Biddle, S.J.H. and Fox, K. (1989). Exercise and health psychology: Emerging relationships. *British Journal of Medical Psychology*, **62**, 205–216.

Bird, S.R, Black, N and Newton, P. (1997). *Sports injuries; causes, diagnosis, treatment and prevention*. Cheltenham: Stanley Thornes.

Binkhorst, R.A., Kempter, H.C.G. and Saris, W.H.M. (eds) (1985). *Children and Exercise*, XI. Champaign, IL: Human Kinetics.

Blair, S.N., Kohl, H.W., Barlow, C.E., Paffenbarger, R.S., Gibbons, L.W. and Macera, C.A. (1995). Changes in physical fitness and all-cause mortality: a prospective study of healthy and unhealthy men. *Journal of the American Medical Association*, **273** (14), 1093–1098.

Bouchard, C. (ed.) (1989). *Exercise, Fitness and Health: A consensus of current knowledge*. Champaign, IL: Human Kinetics.

Bouchard, C. and Shephard, R.J. (1994). Physical activity, fitness, and health: The model and key concepts. In *Physical Activity, Fitness and Health. International Proceedings and Consensus Statement*, Bouchard, C., Shephard, R.J. and Stephens, T. (eds). Champaign, IL: Human Kinetics; 77–88.

Bouchard, C., Shephard, R.J. and Stephens, T. (eds) (1994). *Physical Activity, Fitness and Health. International Proceedings and Consensus Statement*. Champaign, IL: Human Kinetics.

Bruce, R.A. (1984). Exercise, functional aerobic capacity and aging: another viewpoint. *Medicine and Science in Sports and Exercise*, **16** (1), 8–13.

Caspersen, C.J., Powell, K.E. and Christenson, G.M. (1985) Physical activity, exercise and physical fitness: Definitions and distinctions for health related research. *Public Health Reports*, **100** (2), 126–131.

Cobb, L.A. and Weaver, W.D. (1986). A risk for sudden death in patients with coronary heart disease. *Journal of The American College of Cardiology*, **7**, 215–219.

Coplan, N.L., Gleim, G.W. and Nicholas, J.A. (1988). Exercise and sudden cardiac death. *American Heart Journal*, **115**, 207–212.

Estelles, A., Aznar, J., Tormo, G., Sapena, P., Tormo, V. and Espana, F. (1989). Influence of rehabilitation sports programme on the fibrinolytic activity of patients after myocardial infarction. *Thrombosis Research*, **55**, 203–212.

Fentem, P.H., Bassey, E.J. and Turnbull, N.B. (1988). *The New Case for Exercise*. London: The Sports Council and Health Education Authority.

Fentem, P.H., Turnbull, N.B. and Bassey, E.J. (1990). *Benefits of Exercise: the Evidence*. Manchester: Manchester University Press.

Gilliam, T.B., Katch, V.L., Thoriand, W. and Weitman, A. (1977). Prevalence of coronary heart disease risk factors in active children 7 to 12 years of age. *Medicine and Science in Sports*, **9** (1), 21–25.

Hardman, A.E. (1996). Exercise in the prevention of atherosclerotic, metabolic and hypertensive disease: a review. *Journal of Sports Sciences*, **14** (3), 201–218.

HEA (1995). *Health update 5: Physical activity*. Health Education Authority.

Health of the Nation (1993). *A Strategy for Health in England*. Presented to Parliament by the Secretary of State for Health (July 1992). London: HMSO.

Kanel, W.B. (1982). Exercise and sudden death. *Journal of the American Medical Association*, **248** (23), 3143.

Karvonen, M.J., Klemoia, H., Virkujarvi, J. and Kekkonen, A. (1974). Longevity of endurance skiers. *Medicine and Science in Sports*, **6**, 49–51.

Lamb, D.R. (1984). *Physiology of Exercise: Responses and Adaptation* (2nd ed.). New York: MacMillan.

Lee, I-Min (1994). Physical activity, fitness and cancer. In *Physical Activity, Fitness and Health. International Proceedings and Consensus Statement*, Bouchard, C., Shephard, R.J. and Stephens, T. (eds). Champaign, IL: Human Kinetics; 814–831.

Linder, C.W. and DuRant, R.H. (1982). Exercise, serum lipids and cardiovascular disease risk factors in children. *Pediatric Clinics of North America*, **29**, 1341–1354.

MacHeath, J. (1984). *Activity, Health and Fitness in Old Age*. London: St Martin's Press.

Orban, W.A.R. (1994). Active living for older adults: A model for optimal active living. In

Toward Active Living, Quinney, H.A., Gauvin, L. and Wall, A.E.T. (eds). Champaign, IL: Human Kinetics; 153–162.

Panush, R.S. (1994). Physical activity, fitness and osteoarthritis. In *Physical Activity, Fitness and Health. International Proceedings and Consensus Statement*, Bouchard, C., Shephard, R.J. and Stephens, T. (eds). Champaign, IL: Human Kinetics; 712–723.

Powell, K.E., Thompson, P.D., Caspersen, C.J. and Kendrick, J.S. (1987). Physical activity and the incidence of coronary heart disease. In *Annual Review of Public Health*, Breslow, L., Fielding, J.E. and Lave, L.B. (eds). Palo Alto, CA: Annual Reviews Inc; 253–287.

Rejeski, W.J. and Brawley, L.R. (1988). Defining the boundaries of sport psychology. *The Sports Psychologist*, **2**, 231–242.

Rikkers, R. (1986) *Seniors on the Move*. Champaign, IL: Human Kinetics.

Rutenfranz, J., Mocellin, R. and Klimit, F. (eds) (1987). *Children and Exercise, XII*. Champaign, IL: Human Kinetics.

Rydzewski, A., Sakakata, K., Kobayashi, A., Yamzaaki, N., Uramo, T., Takada, Y. and Takada, A. (1990). Changes in plasminogen activates inhibitor I and tissue type plasminogen activator during exercise in patients with coronary heart disease. *Haemostasis*, **20**, 305–312.

Sellier, P., Corona, P., Audouin, P., Payen, B., Plat, F. and Ourbak, P. (1988). Influence of training on blood lipids and coagulation. *European Heart Journal (Supplement M)*, **49**: 32–36.

Sharma, S., Whyte, G. and McKenna. W.J. (1997). Sudden death from cardiovascular disease in young athletes: fact or fiction? *British Journal of Sports Medicine*, **31**, 269–276.

Shephard, R.J. (1996). The athlete's heart: is big beautiful? *British Journal of Sports Medicine*, **30**, 5–10.

Siscovick, D.S., Laporte, R.E. and Newman, J.M. (1985). The disease specific benefits and risks of physical activity and exercise. *Public Health Report*, **100**, 180–188.

Siscovick, D.S., Weiss, N.S., Fletcher, R.H. and Lasky, T. (1984). The incidence of primary cardiac arrest during vigorous exercise. *New England Journal of Medicine*, **311**, 874–877.

Smith, R.A. and Biddle, S.J.H. (1991). Motivating adults for physical activity: towards a healthier present. *Journal of Physical Education, Recreation and Dance*, **62** (7), 39–43.

Solomon, H. (1985). *The Exercise Myth*. London: Angus & Robertson.

Thompson, P.D. and Farenbach, M.C. (1994). Risks of exercising: cardiovascular including sudden cardiac death. In *Physical Activity, Fitness and Health. International Proceedings and Consensus Statement*, Bouchard, C., Shephard, R.J. and Stephens, T. (eds). Champaign, IL: Human Kinetics; 1019–1028.

Thompson, P.D., Funk, E.J., Carleton, R.A. and Sturner, W.Q. (1980). Incidence of death during jogging in Rhode Island from 1975 through 1980. *Journal of the American Medical Association*, **247**, 2535–2538.

Vuori I (1986) The cardiovascular risks of physical activity. *Acta Medica Scandinavica (Supplement)*, **71**, 205–214.

Vuori, I., Makarainen, M. and Jaaskelainen, A. (1978). Sudden death and physical activity. *Cardiology*, **63**, 287–304.

Wilmore, J.H. and McNamara, J.J. (1974). The prevalence of coronary heart disease risk factors in boys 8 to 12 years. *Journal of Pediatrics*, **84,** 527.

Zepilli, P. and Venerando, A. (1981). Sudden death and physical exertion. *Journal of Sports Medicine.*, **21**, 299.

USEFUL ADDRESS

The British Association of Sport and Exercise Sciences, 114 Cardigan Road, Headingley, Leeds, LS6 3BJ. Telephone: 0113 289 1020, fax: 0113 231 9606.

THE PHYSIOLOGICAL BASIS OF HEALTH-RELATED EXERCISE AND FITNESS

A review of exercise metabolism, the different modes of exercise (aerobic and activity based, strength and mobility), their importance in the context of health, their physiological determinants, the responses and adaptations of the body to each mode of exercise, and the causes of fatigue during a bout of exercise.

INTRODUCTION

One of the aims of this chapter is to provide the reader with a basic understanding and a general appreciation of the biochemical processes involved in exercise metabolism. The content is therefore worded for those without a detailed biochemistry background, but the reader should be aware of the existence of greater biochemical complexities behind the processes described. In general the material is presented at a level commonly used for first-year undergraduate studies in exercise, health and related areas. Those wishing to pursue the topic in greater depth are invited to refer to the texts by Macleod *et al.* (1987), Hargreaves (1995), Shephard (1995), Brooks *et al.* (1996) and Maughan *et al.* (1997), and others specifically devoted to biochemistry.

The term 'exercise' covers a vast range of physical activities and movements. It includes mild rehabilitation work, strengthening exercises, gardening, walking, aerobics classes, swimming, playing football and running a marathon. All of these activities place very different demands upon the body. The mode of exercise dictates which muscle groups are used, the intensity determines which energy system(s) are used and the source of fuel, the duration influences how much energy is used, and the fitness of the individual reflects how they cope with the exercise. Altering any of these factors will change the stresses upon the body and consequently different adaptations/benefits will result. Therefore, since not all forms of exercise have the same effects, it is essential for the health professional to possess a good understanding of what is meant by 'exercise', the factors that can be manipulated and the type of adaptations that can be induced in order to prescribe an exercise regimen which is safe and effective for each individual.

OVERVIEW OF MUSCLE METABOLISM

All forms of physical activity are brought about by the actions of the muscles. Muscular action requires energy, which is ultimately derived from the energy stores contained within the body. These energy stores are utilised to produce adenosine triphosphate (ATP), which is essential in the process of muscular contraction (see p. 19 for details). As ATP is used up during muscular contraction it must be resynthesised immediately, or activity would cease: indeed, it is the slight drop in the ATP level in the muscles, in combination with an increase in the concentration of its breakdown products, which stimulates the muscles to generate more ATP.

To maintain the production of ATP the muscles are linked to other body systems via the cardiovascular system. This transports key energy sources used in metabolism, such as glucose and fats from the food digested in the intestine, oxygen to the muscles from the lungs and removes the waste products of muscle metabolism (e.g. carbon dioxide to the lungs, lactic acid to other tissues for oxidation and other metabolic breakdown products to the liver and kidneys). Excess heat is also removed from the muscle via the blood flowing through it. Some aspects of muscle metabolism are regulated by hormones, which are transported by the blood from the endocrine glands where they are secreted to their site of action.

Once a bout of exercise has ceased the muscles must replenish their depleted energy stores, adapt their structure and biochemistry, and repair any damage. These aspects of metabolism are again linked to other body systems via the blood which provides oxygen and other nutrients. The processes of maintenance and repair are partly regulated by hormones and involve individual blood components such as white blood cells. It can thus be appreciated that metabolism within the muscle is linked to numerous other systems and metabolic processes, all of which respond and adapt to activity. The acute responses to a single bout of exercise and the chronic adaptations to a sustained exercise programme will have profound effects on many systems of the body, not just the exercising muscles.

ENERGY AND EXERCISE

For muscles to work they need energy. This energy is obtained from the food consumed in the diet, principally carbohydrates and fats. Protein can also be used to provide energy, but its contribution is relatively small compared with the other two sources. The chemical energy contained within food is used by the body to generate specific high-energy molecules that can be used in processes such as muscle contraction. The most important high-energy molecule synthesised by the body is ATP. Millions of ATP molecules are used by the muscles during the process of muscular contraction. However, the body cannot store ATP in great amounts and it has been estimated that the muscles contain only enough ATP for approximately one second's worth of contraction. So, if the muscles are to work continuously and effectively this supply must be constantly replenished. This is achieved by the resynthesis of ATP as soon as it is used.

OVERVIEW OF THE ENERGY SYSTEMS

To maintain its level of activity the body must generate ATP at the rate required by the current activity being undertaken. The supply of ATP is achieved by a combined interaction of three energy systems or pathways:

1. The phosphocreatine system (anaerobic alactic).
2. Anaerobic glycolysis (anaerobic lactic system).
3. The aerobic system, which includes glycolysis or glycogenolysis if carbohydrates are the fuel source, or beta oxidation if fats are the fuel source, followed by the citric acid cycle (also called Krebs cycle) and the electron transport chain.

If these systems are unable to generate ATP at the rate required the body will experience the sensation of fatigue and the muscles will have to rest, or at least reduce the intensity of their activity.

The use of these systems and their relative contribution to the generation of ATP during muscular work depends upon a number of factors, including the condition of the muscles, the intensity of the exercise, the availability of the energy sources and the presence of metabolic waste products. Each system will be outlined separately before their integrated relative contribution during different forms of exercise is described.

Whilst this text will focus upon the production and use of ATP during exercise, ATP is actually used in a vast number of other metabolic processes within the body, not just muscle contraction: for example, to provide the energy required in synthesis of various biomolecules, in the ion pumps which help to maintain the appropriate concentration of ions both inside and outside cells, and in any body reaction that requires energy. For these energy-requiring activities ATP is synthesised in similar ways to those described here (primarily involving the aerobic system).

Since muscles require a lot of energy to perform their specialised function of contraction they need to be able to synthesise large amounts of ATP. This is achieved through various physiological adaptations including an extensive blood supply and the presence of large numbers of specialised organelles such as mitochondria, which are the site of much of the ATP synthesis.

ATP STRUCTURE AND UTILISATION

The breakdown of ATP provides the energy required for the process of muscular contraction. Without it muscular activity would not be possible and hence a constant supply of ATP is essential. ATP consists of an adenosine unit with three inorganic phosphate molecules attached to it – hence its name (Figure 2.1).

The bond between the second and third phosphate groups of an ATP molecule is relatively unstable and can be broken to produce adenosine diphosphate (ADP) and inorganic phosphate (Pi). The energy released when this bond is broken can be harnessed and used in various metabolic activities of the body, including muscle contraction. During muscular contractions high-energy ATP molecules are specifically linked to the process of cross-bridge cycling (Figure 2.2).

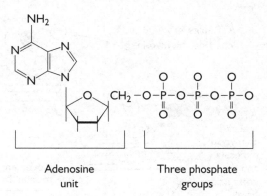

Figure 2.1 The structure of ATP

THE ROLE OF ATP IN THE PROCESS OF CROSS-BRIDGE CYCLING

This is summarised in Figure 2.2.

1. A molecule of ATP becomes associated with the head of each myosin molecule in the muscle (one ATP per myosin head), causing it to dissociate from the actin molecule.
2. The ATP is converted into ADP + Pi, and the energy released 'charges' the myosin head, causing it to change shape.
3. The ADP and Pi remain associated with the myosin head, which attaches to a binding site on the actin molecule.
4. Once the myosin binds to actin, the ADP leaves the myosin head, causing it to change shape and pulling the actin molecule past it.
5. Another ATP molecule becomes associated with the myosin, which breaks away from the actin and becomes ready to repeat the process.

Since one ATP molecule is used up by each myosin head each time a new cross bridge is formed, the need for its rapid synthesis in large amounts can be appreciated. Without ATP cross-bridge cycling could not continue and the muscle would not be able to contract.

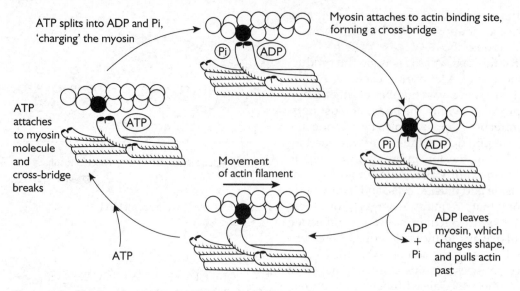

Figure 2.2   The involvement of ATP in cross-bridge cycling

ATP SYNTHESIS

The synthesis of ATP involves reforming the bond between the second and third phosphates. This is part of a cyclic process in which ATP is broken down into ADP + Pi and then resynthesised (Figure 2.3).

The energy for ATP synthesis is derived from the energy contained within the food eaten. The energy is released when the bond between the second and third phosphate groups is broken, and is used to drive various metabolic reactions such as muscular contraction. Therefore, ATP provides the link between the energy in food and the energy used in muscle contraction – in effect, it harnesses the energy stored within food in a way that can be used by muscles.

To understand ATP synthesis we need to study the metabolic processes and pathways that cause the recombination of ADP and Pi. These are:

1. The phosphocreatine system
2. Anaerobic glycolysis/glycogenolysis
3. The aerobic system (including glycolysis/ glycogenolysis or beta-oxidation, the citric acid cycle and the electron transport chain).

THE PHOSPHOCREATINE SYSTEM

The phosphocreatine system provides a process by which ATP can be generated very rapidly. Unfortunately the supplies of phosphocreatine are limited and therefore its contribution to the production of ATP tends to be constrained to the first few seconds of activity, after which alternative systems must assume the role of ATP synthesis.

Phosphocreatine consists of a creatine molecule to which an inorganic phosphate group (Pi) is attached via a high-energy bond. When a muscle contracts the process of cross-bridge cycling causes the level of ATP in the muscle to fall and the amount of ADP + Pi to rise. This activates the phosphocreatine system; the phosphocreatine molecules donate their phosphate groups and the energy associated with them to the ADP, producing ATP and creatine (Figure 2.4). The ATP generated from this reaction can then be used to continue to fuel the process of muscle contraction.

The phosphocreatine system is a fairly uncomplicated process that is relatively quick and simple in metabolic terms. It provides a very readily available and easily accessible means of generating ATP.

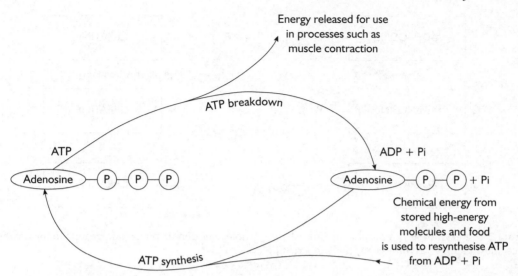

Figure 2.3 The cyclic process of ATP breakdown and synthesis

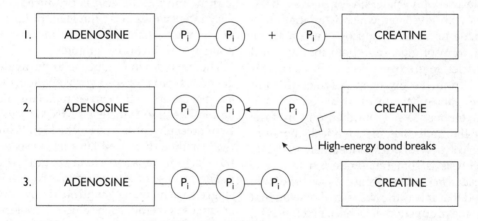

Figure 2.4 Summary of the phosphocreatine system

Following intensive muscular activity the phosphocreatine stores will need to be replenished. This is achieved during periods of low-intensity muscular work or rest by reversing the basic process. At this time the aerobic system produces additional ATP and some of the excess is used to react with the free creatine molecules (Figure 2.5). In this way the stores are rapidly replenished, ready for the next bout of intensive muscular work.

ANAEROBIC GLYCOLYSIS/GLYCOGENOLYSIS

Glycolysis uses a series of reactions to break down the sugar glucose, releasing energy, which is used in the formation of ATP.

Anaerobic glycolysis occurs in the fluid (cytoplasm) of the muscle cell. It involves the breakdown of glucose into pyruvate, some of which may then be converted into lactate (lactic acid). Glycogenolysis differs from glycolysis

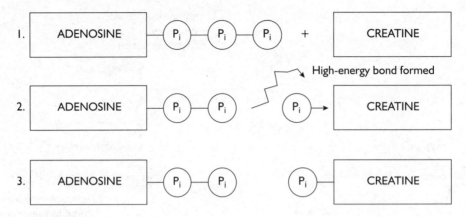

Figure 2.5   Resynthesis of phosphocreatine. The ATP molecules donate phosphate groups to the creatine molecules, thereby resynthesising phosphocreatine and ADP

only in its starting point: whereas the first stage of glycolysis involves the conversion of glucose into glucose-6-phospate, glycogenolysis commences with glycogen, which is a large polymer made up of many glucose units and the storage form of glucose in both the liver and the muscles. In glycogenolysis a glucose unit is cleaved from the glycogen polymer to form glucose-1-phosphate; this is then converted to glucose-6-phosphate. From then onwards the fate of the molecules are identical; therefore only glycolysis will be described here in detail.

Glycolysis is sometimes referred to as the *anaerobic lactic system* because it was originally believed that it was the absence of oxygen that caused the production of lactic acid. However, this is now known to be not entirely correct as even fully aerobic muscle produces a small amount of lactic acid (Spurway, 1992). The reason for its production is now thought to be related to the chemical kinetics of the system and the relative abundance of some of the reactants involved.

Glycolysis yields a total of two molecules of ATP for every molecule of glucose used. The starting point of glycolysis is *taken* to be glucose, although it could be a 'glucose unit' that has been derived from the breakdown of glycogen – in which case the process yields three ATP because breakdown of glycogen

yields one further ATP. The more intensive the exercise the faster this system has to work and the more lactic acid is produced. During very intensive exercise the level of lactic acid in the muscle (and blood) can increase to the point where it causes fatigue.

The breakdown of glucose to pyruvate also generates two pairs of hydrogen atoms which are picked up by the carrier molecule nicotinamide adenine dinucleotide (NAD^+) to form two molecules of NADH – the significance of these will be discussed later in the section on the electron transport chain (p. 28).

The process of glycolysis involves nine key stages, each being controlled by specific enzymes. Overall each glucose molecule is eventually broken down into two molecules of pyruvate. During the process two molecules of ATP are used up but four are synthesised, resulting in a net production of two ATP molecules. A more detailed description of glycolysis is shown in Figure 2.6.

If the metabolic conditions permit, the process of glycolysis also forms the first phase for the *aerobic* production of ATP. Both systems (anaerobic and aerobic) may operate concurrently but their relative contribution towards the production of ATP will depend upon the intensity of the muscular work being performed and the availability of oxygen

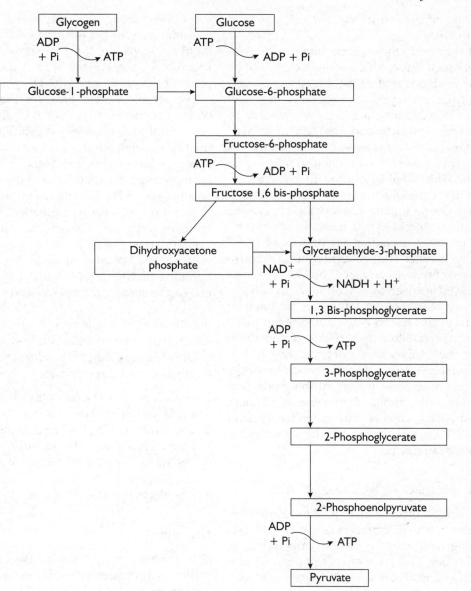

Figure 2.6 Glycolysis

within the muscle. The rate at which glycolysis operates depends upon the exercise intensity and hence the muscle's demand for ATP.

If the exercise intensity is low to moderate, of the sort which can be maintained comfortably for many minutes, then glycolysis will operate at a moderate rate, the products going into the citric acid cycle and electron transport chain (see pp. 25 and 28). This is preferable because it does not produce fatiguing levels of lactic acid and enables more of the available energy to be converted into usable ATP. It is therefore more economical energetically. Such exercise is described as *aerobic* because of the use of oxygen in the electron transport chain.

If, however, the exercise intensity is relatively high the products of glycolysis will be generated too rapidly for them all to pass into the citric acid cycle. Consequently they will begin to accumulate and the pyruvate will be converted into lactic acid. The build up of lactic acid makes the muscle more acidic (i.e. the pH falls) and if there is sufficient acid fatigue will ensue. This is felt as a burning, aching sensation in the muscles during intensive muscular work. Owing to the increased acidity, various functions associated with muscular contraction are inhibited, including the process of cross-bridge cycling. The production of ATP is also slowed because of some of the enzymes involved in anaerobic glycolysis, especially the enzyme phosphofructokinase, are inhibited by acid. For this reason ATP cannot be produced by glycolysis alone for prolonged periods of time; the primary means of generating ATP is the aerobic system. Glycolysis is used to supply the pyruvate and supplement the production of ATP only during shorter bursts of more intensive muscular activity, when the demand for ATP exceeds the rate at which the aerobic process can function.

THE 'AEROBIC' PRODUCTION OF ATP

The aerobic production of ATP is a multistage process which commences with glucose, glycogen or fat and ends with carbon dioxide and water. This releases energy for ATP production and, because the breakdown to carbon dioxide and water is far more complete than the breakdown achieved in glycolysis it releases considerably more energy (and hence produces far more ATP) for each glucose used. In the long term the aerobic system is thus capable of providing considerably more energy than either of the anaerobic systems and is therefore the preferred energy system of the body, being used continuously both at rest and during exercise. However, it is sometimes unable to generate ATP fast enough for short bursts of high-intensity exercise such as a sudden run for the bus or climbing a steep flight of steps. In these circumstances the anaerobic energy systems are recruited to supplement the production of ATP.

The aerobic system provides the muscles with a continuous supply of ATP and, as the name implies, it requires oxygen. The system uses both carbohydrate and fat as a source of energy, which means that its fuel reserves are far more extensive than those of the phosphocreatine system. Unlike anaerobic glycolysis it does not result in the accumulation of fatigue-inducing lactic acid. The aerobic system is the primary source of ATP during low-intensity exercise and, because it does not generate fatiguing products, means that aerobic exercise can be sustained for prolonged periods. It is also a significant contributor to the supply of ATP in more intensive activities, in combination with the two anaerobic systems.

The aerobic system for producing ATP may be divided into three phases:

1. Glycolysis (in the case of glucose) or beta-oxidation (in the case of fats)
2. The citric acid cycle – also known as the Krebs cycle (after the scientist who first described it) or the tricarboxylic acid cycle (TCA cycle).
3. The electron transport chain.

Glycolysis

The process of glycolysis was discussed earlier as a separate anaerobic system for the generation of ATP (Figure 2.6). During low or moderate-intensity exercise most of the pyruvate generated from this system is transported with the aid of a carrier into specialised organelles called the mitochondria. Here it loses a carbon dioxide molecule in a reaction with coenzyme A to form acetyl coenzyme A. Consequently, because most of the pyruvate is used up in the process, only small amounts of lactic acid are generated and fatiguing concentrations do not build up. An additional and very significant advantage of the aerobic system is that the resultant acetyl coenzyme A is further metabolised to produce considerably more ATP, far more than via glycolysis alone. Overall this means that far more energy is made available from the aerobic breakdown of glucose than via its anaerobic breakdown.

Key aspects of 'glycolysis' and its role within the aerobic system are as follows:

- Glycolysis uses carbohydrate in the form of glucose or 'glucose units', which are derived from the breakdown of glycogen.
- The first stage of carbohydrate metabolism is identical to that already discussed for anaerobic glycolysis. However, during low and moderate-intensity exercise lactic acid does not accumulate to the high levels that cause fatigue.
- Instead, the pyruvate generated in glycolysis is transported into the mitochondria where it reacts with molecules of coenzyme A to form acetyl coenzyme A. These combine with oxaloacetate to form citrate (citric acid) (Figure 2.7). This is the starting molecule for the citric acid cycle, the second stage of the aerobic system.

Therefore it can be seen that the reliance upon the anaerobic pathway depends upon the intensity of the exercise, and hence the demand for ATP, which dictates the rate at which glycolysis takes place. The aerobic use of the products from glycolysis in the citric acid cycle is preferable to the anaerobic system because it generates more ATP per glucose unit and does not result in the accumulation of lactic acid. In fact a major determinant of an individual's capacity to perform prolonged forms of low-intensity activity depends upon their ability to use the products of glycolysis in the citric acid cycle and to supply the muscles with oxygen. Therefore it is not surprising that major adaptations of the muscle to aerobic exercise include an increase in the muscles' ability to use the oxygen supplied to them by an enhanced cardiovascular system.

In summary, glycolysis results in the conversion of glucose into pyruvate (two molecules for each glucose used) with a net gain of two ATP for each glucose used. The pyruvate is then transported into the mitochondria where it is broken down further and incorporated into the citric acid cycle in a process that will ultimately produce more ATP. Glycolysis also results in the generation of two NADH molecules, which are ultimately used to produce more ATP via the electron transport chain (p. 28).

At this point it may be noted by those concerned with biochemical accuracy that in the glycolytic process, and in the citric acid cycle described later in the chapter, each NADH produced is associated with a H^+ ion. These H^+ ions have been included in the figures for accuracy but have been omitted from the text to prevent unnecessary complications in the discussion.

Beta-oxidation

Fat can also be metabolised aerobically to produce ATP, although its initial metabolism is very different to that of glucose. Fatty acids (a major group of fats) are a major energy source for the body, both at rest and during exercise. Fatty acids are long chains of carbon atoms, each with a number of hydrogen atoms attached (hydrocarbons). In order for fats to be used as an energy source they must be broken down, first to their constituent fatty acids and then into small acetyl groups via a process called beta-oxidation. The acetyl groups then react with coenzyme A to produce acetyl coenzyme A, which enters the citric acid cycle in the same way as the acetyl coenzyme A formed from glycolysis.

The citric acid cycle

This cycle was first described by Hans Krebs, and it is still sometimes known as the Krebs cycle. It is also called the tricarboxylic acid (TCA) cycle. The citric acid cycle occurs

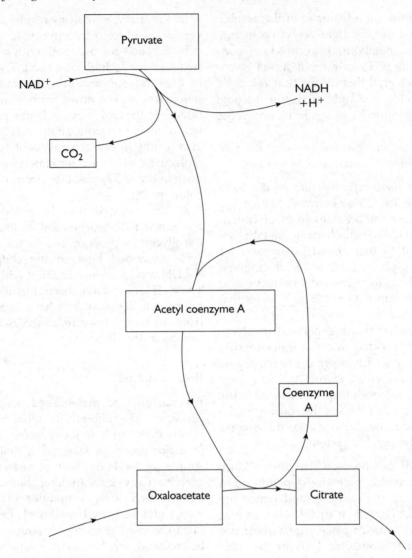

Figure 2.7   Conversion of pyruvate into acetyl coenzyme A and its entry into the citric acid cycle

within the matrix of the mitochondria (Figure 2.8). Mitochondria were originally thought to be discrete individual organelles but recent evidence suggests that an interconnected set of tubes forms a *mitochondrial network* or *reticulum* (Brooks *et al.*, 1996).

The citric acid cycle follows on from glycolysis or beta-oxidation, both of which result in acetyl units combining with oxaloacetate to form citric acid. Citrate is sequentially broken down into oxaloacetate. This breakdown process involves numerous enzyme-mediated steps (summarised in Figure 2.9) and at various stages energy is released that can be gainfully used to synthesise ATP either directly or at a later stage. Upon completion of the cycle the oxaloacetate recombines with another acetyl group to once again form citrate – hence (as the name implies) the process is repeated in a cyclic manner.

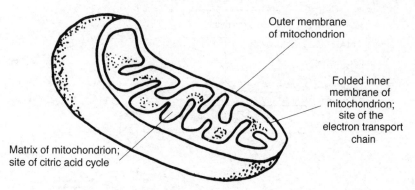

Outer membrane
of mitochondrion

Folded inner
membrane of
mitochondrion;
site of the
electron transport
chain

Matrix of mitochondrion;
site of citric acid cycle

Figure 2.8 A mitochondrion

During the cycle various products are formed, including ATP, carbon dioxide, hydrogen atoms and guanosine triphosphate (GTP). The carbon dioxide produced by this aerobic system diffuses out of the muscle fibre and into the blood, which transports it to the lungs where it is exhaled. For each acetyl group (whether produced from glycolysis or beta-oxidation), two carbon dioxide molecules are produced in the citric acid cycle. For each pyruvate produced from glycolysis, one carbon dioxide molecule is produced in its conversion into an acetyl group and two are produced during the citric acid cycle. Since two pyruvate molecules are produced from each glucose molecule, a total of six carbon dioxide molecules are produced for each glucose molecule used.

This cycle also results in the production of pairs of hydrogen atoms. These are picked up by two kinds of carrier molecules: nicotinamide adenine dinucleotide (NAD^+) and flavine adenine dinucleotide (FAD). These coenzymes transport the hydrogen atoms to the next stage in the process (the electron transport chain, see p. 28). Hydrogen atoms are also produced during glycolysis; these are also picked up by the NAD^+, two NADH molecules being produced for each glucose molecule entering glycolysis. During its conversion into an acetyl group, pyruvate loses a further two hydrogen atoms and as a result two more NADH molecules are

produced for each initial glucose molecule. In each pass of the cycle four more pairs of hydrogen atoms are produced, resulting in three molecules of NADH and one of $FADH_2$. Since two molecules of acetyl coenzyme A are produced from each glucose molecule the cycle is repeated twice for each initial glucose molecule and the citric acid cycle produces six NADH and two $FADH_2$ molecules for each glucose. Therefore the breakdown of each glucose molecule through glycolysis, the conversion of pyruvate into acetyl coenzyme A and the citric acid cycle produces a total of ten NADH and two $FADH_2$ molecules.

Each cycle also produces one molecule of GTP, which reacts with ADP to produce ATP and GDP. So, for each glucose molecule, the cycle produces two ATP molecules (one per cycle). Thus, the breakdown of each glucose molecule results in the net production of four molecules of ATP, ten of NADH two of $FADH_2$ and six of carbon dioxide.

Each acetyl group produced from the breakdown of fatty acid will go through the citric acid cycle and hence will produce three NADH and one $FADH_2$.

The hydrogen atoms produced are transported by their carriers to the next stage of the process, the electron transport chain, during which some of the energy they contain is used to produce more ATP. Indeed, most of the ATP molecules produced during the aerobic breakdown of glucose or fat are

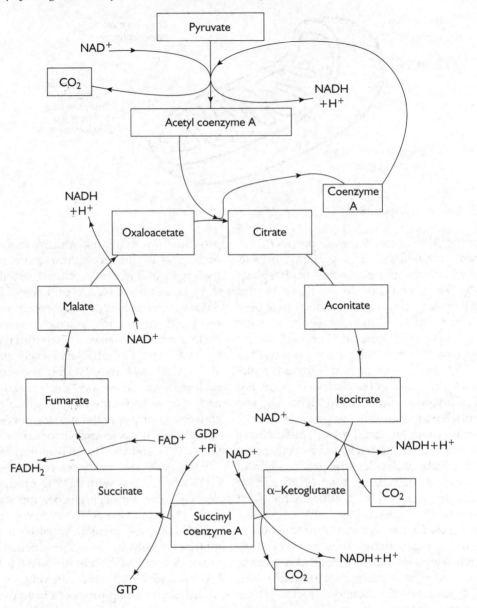

Figure 2.9   The citric acid cycle

produced during this third and final phase of the aerobic system.

The electron transport chain

This consists of a series of carrier molecules which are situated in the inner membrane of the mitochondrion (Figure 2.8). They are strategically organised to facilitate the passage of hydrogen atoms or electrons from one carrier to the next. At various stages in the transfer of the hydrogen atoms and electrons down the system energy becomes 'available' and may be used to synthesise ATP from ADP and Pi (Figure 2.10).

During the electron transport chain the

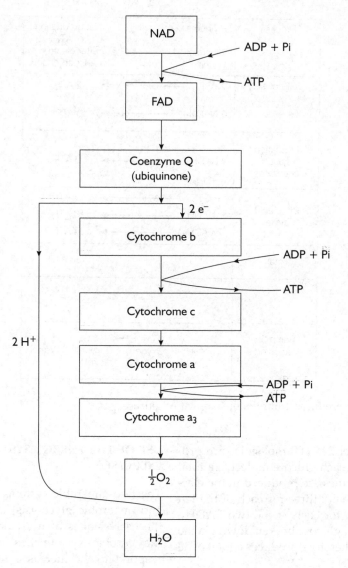

Figure 2.10 The electron transport chain

hydrogen atoms are initially passed from NAD to FAD (except those that were directly picked up by FAD from the citric acid cycle). This transfer produces one ATP molecule and, since each glucose unit produced ten NADH, a total of ten ATP molecules are produced per glucose at this stage. Next the hydrogen atoms are passed from FAD to coenzyme Q (also known as ubiquinone). At this point the hydrogen atoms dissociate into two hydrogen ions ($2H^+$) and two electrons ($2e^-$). The electrons are passed along a series of cytochrome carriers (cytochrome *b*, cytochrome *c*, cytochrome *a* and cytochrome a_3). During the transfer from cytochrome *b* to cytochrome *c* and from cytochrome *a* to cytochrome a_3, ATP is produced. So for each glucose unit (which produced ten NADH molecules and two

Process	Products per glucose unit	Net production of ATP after electron transport chain
Glycolysis	2 ATP $\longrightarrow$	2 ATP
	2 NADH $\longrightarrow$	6 ATP
Formation of acetyl coenzyme	2 NADH $\longrightarrow$	6 ATP
Citric acid cycle	2 GTP $\longrightarrow$	2 ATP
	6 NADH $\longrightarrow$	18 ATP
	2 FADH$_2$ $\longrightarrow$	4 ATP
Total		38 ATP
Summary equation	$C_6H_{12}O_6$ + 6 O_2 $\longrightarrow$ 6 CO_2 + 6 H_2O Glucose Oxygen Carbon Water dioxide	

Figure 2.11   ATP produced from the breakdown of glucose

FADH$_2$) a further 24 ATP molecules are produced. Thus for each glucose molecule a total of 34 ATP molecules are produced in the electron transport chain: three for each of the ten NADH and two for each of the two FADH$_2$. Each molecule of glucose broken down via the aerobic system therefore produces a total of 38 ATP (Figure 2.11).

The final electron acceptor in the electron transport chain is oxygen, which reacts with the electrons and hydrogen ions to produce water. The rate at which the whole system can work largely depends upon the availability of oxygen.

The exact details of the processes by which NADH and FADH$_2$ are formed, and their progress through the electron transport chain, are complex. Further details of the biochemistry and reaction kinetics may be attained from texts such as that by Brooks *et al.* (1996).

USE OF THE ENERGY SYSTEMS DURING EXERCISE

The two anaerobic systems (phosphocreatine and anaerobic glycolysis) are used either in the early stages of muscular activity, before the aerobic system has had a chance to respond to the increased demands for ATP, or during very intensive periods of muscular activity when the aerobic system is unable to generate ATP quickly enough to meet the demands of the muscles. The anaerobic systems supplement the supply of ATP that is constantly produced by the aerobic system. In reality, therefore, it is not just a matter of turning the systems on or off or switching from one to the another, but of using them together, phasing the relevant pathways and metabolic reactions in and out as necessary.

During exercise the relative contribution of each pathway towards the production of ATP depends on:

- the intensity of the exercise;
- the state of various physiological factors; and
- the body's capacity to cope with the demands of the activity.

In terms of ATP production per litre of oxygen used, glucose is a more economical energy store than fat; however, in terms of ATP production, 1 g of fat produces more ATP than 1 g of glucose (Table 2.1). Hence, in terms of weight, fat may be considered to be more economical than glucose. The body's stores of glycogen are more limited than those of fat because of the relative calorific values. The body's fat stores of about 7–15 kg can furnish about 4000 minutes of exercise, but to obtain a similar value somewhere between 15 and 30 kg of glycogen would be needed. Fat, although it is a more energy efficient storage medium, cannot be metabolised quickly enough to provide the energy needed in acute exercise. The use of two energy sources is thus both advantageous and a compromise because it enables the body to use a source which is most efficient in terms of weight (fat) and oxygen cost (glucose), when needed.

During strenuous muscular activity the aerobic system is unable to synthesise ATP rapidly enough and its production is supplemented by an increased rate of glycolysis, resulting in the accumulation of lactate. The phosphocreatine system is also used in the initial stages of muscular activity because there may be a slight delay between the commencement of more strenuous muscular activity and an increase in the activity of the aerobic system. The phosphocreatine system is thus used to provide additional ATP until the aerobic system has increased to cope with the new increased demand (if it can).

MAINTAINING AND REDUCING THE ENERGY STORES

The body's stores of fat and glycogen/glucose are provided by food. Starch, glucose and glycogen in the food are broken down into glucose. That which is not required immediately is stored, primarily as glycogen in the muscle and liver. Fats that are eaten, or produced by the body from other excess nutrients, are stored as fat in specific sites around the body.

These stores of energy are used to sustain metabolism. A bout of exercise represents a large increase in metabolism and thus use of these stores. During exercise the increased production of ATP will use up the glycogen and fat stored. The extent to which each of these is reduced will depend upon the intensity of the exercise, its duration and frequency. The more intense the exercise the greater the demands upon the glycogen stores and the more likely they are to become depleted. During prolonged exercise, such as in running a marathon, the muscle's glycogen stores can fall so low as to cause fatigue and inhibit further exercise. This depletion of glycogen means that the remaining energy stores of fat must furnish the production of the ATP needed by the muscles instead of glycogen. Since the muscles cannot generate ATP from fat quickly enough to sustain this intensity of exercise the runner must slow down from a running to a jogging or walking speed.

The fat stores are also used during exercise, which is one of the reasons why exercise is recommended for fat reduction. A pound of fat contains approximately 3500 kilocalories. In terms of exercise this is the equivalent of approximately 35 miles of walking or 7–10 hours of aerobics. However, even though fat

Table 2.1 The ATP yields from glucose and fat

Substrate	Energy yield per litre of oxygen (kcal)	Energy yield per gram substrate (kcal)
Glucose	5.05	4.02
Fat	4.74	8.98

stores can be reduced by exercise their depletion is a gradual process and in all but extreme cases the stores are unlikely to fall to levels which adversely affect exercise performance.

To maintain health and the capacity to exercise it is important to maintain and replenish the body's glycogen stores by eating a diet rich in starch – foods such as bread, pasta, rice and potatoes. Eating a diet which is low in these foods can cause the muscle's glycogen stores to become depleted over a period of days. Glycogen depletion causes a feeling of fatigue, lethargy and an inability to exercise. Unfortunately the rapid initial weight loss observed in some diets is often attributable to glycogen depletion rather than reduction in fat, which tends to occur very gradually over a period of weeks. This can elevate an individual's expectations during the first few weeks of a diet – their weight rapidly declines, but then disillusionment occurs in the following weeks as the weight loss slows down. Continuation of an exercise regime could be made more difficult through the fatigue experienced due to low levels of muscle glycogen. It is important for the health professional to be aware of these issues – when designing a programme for fat reduction through an appropriate combination of exercise and dietary advice, he or she should try to ensure that it promotes long-term fat loss whilst maintaining the important glycogen stores.

THE CAUSES OF FATIGUE DURING EXERCISE

Physiological fatigue may be considered as a state in which the maintenance of a certain intensity of exercise is inhibited or prevented. There are many causes of fatigue, several of which can act simultaneously to produce the overall sensation and inhibit further muscular work. It should be stressed at this point that severe fatigue or exhaustion is usually unnecessary during an exercise session that is oriented towards health: in many cases an exercise intensity that induces mild fatigue will be sufficient to stimulate the desired benefits. The state of exhaustion witnessed by those training for sporting excellence is associated with trying to attain the peak of physical fitness and is specific to the demands of that sport; it is not a prerequisite for the development of health. The causes of fatigue can be considered under four headings:

- Depletion of energy stores
- Accumulation of inhibitory metabolic waste products
- Dehydration, and the elevation of body core temperature above the homeostatically permitted level
- Neurological fatigue.

DEPLETION OF ENERGY STORES

During physical activity that is sustained for several minutes it is usual for both fat and carbohydrate (in the form of glucose or glycogen) to be used as an energy source. If the duration of the activity is in excess of 90 minutes it is possible for the glycogen stores of the body to be significantly reduced. This 'glycogen depletion', with its consequent lowering of blood glucose levels, will result in the muscles being deprived of this important energy source and thus making them more dependent upon fat. Unfortunately, fat cannot be used to generate ATP at a very rapid rate which means that the rate of supply of ATP to the muscles slows down, greatly inhibiting their capacity to contract and inducing a situation commonly experienced by marathon runners near the end of a race, referred to as 'hitting the wall'. Whilst glycogen depletion is less likely during more moderate exercise of shorter duration, a diet that is deficient in carbohydrate can result in a steady depletion of the glycogen stores over a period of days and consequently this form of fatigue *can* occur in an exercise programme that is designed for health-related fitness.

During extremely intensive short-duration muscular activity, such as weight training and sprinting, the muscle's stores of ATP and phosphocreatine can become depleted. However, they are rapidly replenished, enabling the exercise to be repeated at or close to the previous level within a few minutes. In more sustained forms of activity the depletion of ATP and phosphocreatine are generally considered to be of secondary importance to the effects of accumulated metabolic waste products such as lactic acid in causing fatigue.

ACCUMULATION OF INHIBITORY METABOLIC WASTE PRODUCTS

During very strenuous muscular activity the rate of demand for ATP will be high, and may exceed the rate at which the citric acid cycle can operate. However, glycolysis will accelerate to supplement the production of ATP, and will generate pyruvate at a rate above that which can be dealt with by the citric acid cycle; consequently lactic acid will accumulate, making the muscle more acidic. The increase in acidity has a number of effects on the processes involved in muscle contraction.

1. Inhibition of glycolysis. This also inhibits further production of ATP. The increase in acidity is thought to specifically inhibit the enzyme phosphofructokinase which controls one of the key stages of glycolysis.
2. The contractile process of cross-bridge cycling can be inhibited. The increase in acidity may inhibit the release of calcium ions from the sarcoplasmic reticulum and/ or their binding to the troponin molecule.
3. The increase in acidity will also be detected as a burning sensation or pain within the muscles.

This is a relatively short-term form of fatigue as the level of lactic acid will fall rapidly upon cessation of the exercise and will return almost to resting levels after 10–15 minutes.

DEHYDRATION AND TEMPERATURE CONTROL

During prolonged forms of exercise the body may sweat profusely in order to regulate its temperature. The hotter and more humid the environment the greater the potential for sweat loss. If fluid is not replaced during the exercise the participant will dehydrate rapidly. This reduction in fluid volume will reduce the efficiency of the cardiovascular system to supply the muscles with oxygen, which can contribute towards other forms of fatigue. If the state of dehydration persists then the participant may stop sweating in order to conserve body fluids. This will reduce the body's ability to lose heat and may rapidly lead to overheating (hyperthermia). If the body temperature rises to a few degrees above its optimum, many metabolic reactions will be impaired because enzymes are very sensitive to temperature. In extreme cases dehydration can lead to collapse – which, if not treated, may be fatal. A state of semi-dehydration will thus reduce the capacity of the body to exercise and cause a form of general fatigue. Dehydration may be prevented or reduced by regular intake of fluid before, during and after exercise: small doses (such as 150 ml every quarter of an hour when exercising in hot conditions) are recommended by many authorities.

NEUROLOGICAL CAUSES

Possible neurological causes of fatigue include the depletion of acetylcholine and/ or other neurotransmitters at the neuromuscular junction (synapse). In this context it has also been suggested that fatigue could occur within the central nervous system. The precise physiological nature of central nervous system failure is complex but may be significant in prolonged forms of exercise. Repeated use of the joints may also contribute towards a general feeling of fatigue during sustained activity.

PERSISTENT FATIGUE

The previous sections outlined a number of transient causes of fatigue, which are experienced by the participants of exercise programmes and are normal phenomena. How-ever, there are factors that may cause a more persistent feeling of fatigue, which, if encountered, require some attention. For example, a general feeling of fatigue is associated with certain disorders such as post-viral fatigue and anaemia. Fatigue may also occur when the body is combating a minor disease such as a cold or flu and in these circumstances it is unwise to exercise. Therefore, although certain types of fatigue (normally short term) are naturally associated with strenuous exercise, participants and their supervisors should be wary of other types that are of a more general nature and could indicate a disorder or illness.

THE COMPONENTS OF HEALTH-RELATED FITNESS AND PHYSICAL CAPACITY

In order to fully understand the concept of an individual's 'physical capacity' or health-related fitness it is first necessary to describe the components in some detail. Furthermore, an understanding of the different modes of exercise will provide the basis for tailoring an exercise programme to meet the specific health and fitness aims of the individual. A good comprehension of these factors should enable the exercise specialist to appreciate the specific implications of particular forms of exercise and how they may be manipulated to achieve fitness objectives.

An individual's physical fitness and/or physical capacity is determined by a large number of factors, including the following:

- The condition of the heart and lungs
- The condition of the blood and blood vessels
- Muscular strength
- The physiological and biochemical properties of the muscles and other organs
- Nutritional state
- Muscular endurance
- Mobility and flexibility of the joints
- Co-ordination
- The general condition of numerous body systems, including those related to endocrine and immunological function
- Motivation and empowerment to be physically active.

All these factors are important in determining someone's capacity to perform basic movements and/or exercise. Although these factors are often considered under separate headings they are often interrelated, and all are required to a greater or lesser extent in any form of physical movement. A lifting activity (such as lifting a bag) may require a greater strength contribution than a stretching activity (such as reaching up into a cupboard), which will require more mobility. However, an element of strength and mobility are needed in both. The relative importance of each aspect will depend upon the type of movement being performed. For the health professional it is important to identify which factor(s) may be constraining a person's ability to perform a physical movement or activity and hence the type of exercise most likely to improve the limiting factor(s). Undertaking the appropriate form of exercise should increase the participant's ability to perform the desired movement or activity. Likewise, an awareness of the impact of different modes of exercise upon health-related factors will enable effective exercise regimens to be prescribed. For example, an exercise prescriber must know which forms of exercise will improve muscle strength, which will increase bone density and which will reduce the risk of CHD. Failure to incorporate this knowledge into an exercise programme may render it ineffective in achieving the stated goals and consequently the participant may commit time, effort and resources to a programme from which they receive no benefit (in terms of the factors important to them). He or she may then become disillusioned and dismiss exercise as a waste of time.

The components of physical capacity, their importance, their determinants, the exercises that can be used to develop them, the responses and adaptations to the exercises, and their impact upon health will be outlined under the following headings and discussed further in specific chapters.

1. Cardiorespiratory capacity and aerobic fitness
2. Muscle strength
3. Joint mobility and flexibility.

CARDIORESPIRATORY CAPACITY AND AEROBIC FITNESS

Aerobic fitness refers to an individual's capacity to perform prolonged forms of physical activity. It is therefore an integral part of an individual's endurance capabilities. It is a complex phenomenon, depending upon the capacity of the cardiovascular system to deliver oxygen to the working muscles and on the capacity of the muscles to use that oxygen. It therefore relates to the condition of the heart, lungs, blood, blood vessels and muscles. The oxygen supply to the muscles of an individual with a poor cardiovascular system and little endurance will be impaired and, as a result, that individual will tire quite rapidly even when undertaking tasks that would normally be considered as relatively undemanding – activities such as walking, cycling, climbing stairs and almost any activity that requires repetitive muscular contractions over a prolonged period of time. A clear link can therefore be made between the enhancement of an individual's aerobic capacity and their overall ability to cope with the physical demands of their lifestyle. Participation in aerobic activities can also provide a social activity, enhancing the overall quality of life. In addition to these general benefits, regular participation in aerobic exercise and the level of aerobic fitness that results are also associated with a number of positive health benefits including reduction in the risk of certain diseases such as hypertension, CHD, diabetes, obesity and a number of stress-related disorders. The details of these are discussed more fully in Chapter 11.

EXERCISE AND ACTIVITIES FOR INCREASING AEROBIC FITNESS

Exercise for aerobic fitness tends to be of a relatively low to moderately high intensity and can be maintained for a prolonged period of time. Examples include walking, steady cycling, gentle jogging, steady swimming and aerobic classes. The term 'aerobic' is applied to these activities because of the way in which the energy needed to perform them is obtained. During aerobic exercise the muscles are supplied with the ATP required for contraction via the aerobic system (see p. 24). With this system, oxygen is used up during the final stage of the electron transfer chain and therefore the individual's oxygen consumption increases while performing such activities. This is why, during these activities, the participant breathes harder and their heart rate increases.

The aerobic system, unlike the anaerobic system, does not produce waste products that result in the rapid onset of fatigue. Thus, an activity that uses the aerobic system as the major energy source may be continued for a prolonged period. Conversely, if the intensity of the activity were to be substantially increased so as to result in a significant accumulation of lactic acid, the muscles would rapidly fatigue (this occurs when a person rapidly climbs stairs, lifts heavy weights, runs, cycles or swims fast). Fatigue can eventually occur in aerobic activities as a result of dehydration or when the activity is so prolonged that the glycogen stores become depleted, but in practice fuel depletion and dehydration usually occur only after hours of exercise, as in the case of marathon running. Whilst the health professional should be aware of the possibility, it is not likely to occur in individuals pursuing moderate forms of activity, provided that their nutrition is adequate and they drink plenty of non-alcoholic and non-caffeinated fluids.

Like all other components of physical fitness the aerobic aspects cannot be completely isolated: any activity that may be considered as 'aerobic' will require a certain amount of muscular strength, flexibility and co-ordination. For instance, swimming, cycling and walking all require a certain amount of muscular strength in order to pull the body through the water, push down on the pedals or push against the ground.

Aerobic activities that are performed at a low or moderate intensity can be considered as being 'steady-state' activities; the intensity of the activity will remain fairly constant throughout the exercise session and, after taking a few minutes to adjust the body's physiological responses such as heart rate and ventilation, will be maintained at a fairly constant level.

Other forms of activity, such as many racquet and team games, are classified as 'intermittent', since the level of activity may be quite high at times but then fall to a relatively low level when the shuttlecock or ball is not in play. These 'intermittent' or 'repetitive sprint' activities will have a major aerobic requirement along with the other aspects of physical fitness. Both the anaerobic and aerobic systems will be used during intensive phases of the activity; the aerobic system will continue to be used in the recovery phases of lower intensity activity in order to maintain the body's level of basic activity, to repay any oxygen deficit and to get rid of any metabolic waste products which accumulated during the intensive play. (The oxygen deficit is the amount of oxygen that needs to be taken up to return the body to its resting state – including replenishment of oxygen stores and oxygen that is used to oxidise metabolic waste products. Repayment of the oxygen deficit is one of the reasons why a person continues to breathe heavily for some time after a bout of strenuous exercise.) It is thus used to help the body to recover from the intensive activity. Intermittent activities include badminton, tennis, squash, basketball, volleyball, soccer and hockey.

Exercises and games are often used as part of the rehabilitation and recovery process of many individuals, including those who have suffered heart attack, major illness or amputation. However, as with all forms of physical exercise, the intensity must be appropriate. The 'intermittent' activities vary considerably in intensity, depending on the skill of the players and the competitiveness of the situation. Therefore, care must be taken to ensure that such activities are not too demanding for the physical condition of the individual. Owing to their aerobic requirement, these activities may be used to enhance a person's aerobic capacity (and, hence, physical fitness) but they cannot be prescribed with the same degree of precision as steady-state activities.

Activities that may convey social as well as aerobic benefits include golf, which requires a considerable amount of walking, and exercise to music, such as low-impact aerobics. These activities can provide a major means of therapy for many individuals, bringing social and psychological as well as physiological benefits.

IMMEDIATE PHYSIOLOGICAL RESPONSES TO ACUTE AEROBIC EXERCISE

It is important to clarify that an 'acute response' is that occurring during a single (acute) bout of exercise, which induces temporary responses that return to the pre-exercise level very soon after the exercise stops. Conversely long-term adaptations to health and fitness are observed after repeated bouts of exercise (chronic) and are maintained for days, weeks or months. These chronic adaptations are discussed in later chapters. When moving from a state of rest to a state of exercise there is an increase in the energy requirements of muscles proportional to the intensity of the exercise. In response to increased energy needs, a number of pulmonary, cardiovascular and hormonal changes occur within the body to increase the supply of oxygen and nutrients to the muscle and to facilitate the removal of metabolic products such as carbon dioxide, lactic acid and heat (the accumulation of which causes premature fatigue). Since these responses take time to come into full effect the intensity of the exercise should be gradually increased at the beginning of the activity and gradually reduced at the end of the session. These considerations are discussed more fully on p. 97

To continue a bout of exercise beyond a few seconds the supply of oxygen to the muscles must increase. This is achieved via a number of responses and adjustments to the cardio-respiratory and hormonal systems. The magnitude of these responses will depend upon the intensity of the exercise, the fitness of the participant and individual variations. The responses are driven by disturbances in the body's homeostasis such as a decrease in the oxygen content or increase in the carbon dioxide content of the blood, a decrease in the pH of the blood and cerebro-spinal fluid (increase in acidity), joint movement and anticipation of the exercise. In summary:

- The rate and depth of breathing increase to enhance the supply of oxygen into and exhalation of carbon dioxide from, the lungs.
- An increase in cardiac output (Q) results from an increase in both stroke volume and heart rate.
- The distribution of blood around the body is adjusted, with a greater proportion being diverted to the exercising muscles. This is achieved via the selective vasodilation of blood vessels supplying the exercising muscles and vasoconstriction of those supplying other organs such as the gut.

The above cardiovascular and pulmonary responses are partly caused by an increased secretion of the hormones adrenaline (epinephrine) and noradrenaline (norepineph-rine). These hormones also stimulate the release of glucose from the liver and fatty acids from adipose tissue. They therefore enhance the supply of energy to the muscles as well as promoting its use and the removal of waste products. The levels of circulating adrenaline and noradrenaline depend on many factors but are generally in proportion to the demands of the exercise, higher levels occurring during maximal exercise and lesser responses being noted during submaximal work. It is also common for the circulating levels of these hormones to increase just before a bout of exercise in an anticipatory response which prepares the body for the forthcoming activity.

All of these responses are temporary and the body will return to its resting levels soon after the exercise ceases, although not imme-diately because an elevated ventilation and cardiac output are needed for some minutes after the exercise has finished to repay any oxygen deficit which has built up. The dura-tion of elevated metabolism after exercise will depend upon the intensity and duration of the exercise.

If the intensity of the activity is quite stren-uous a significant amount of lactic acid will be produced. Some will diffuse out of the mus-cles into the blood and will be transported to the liver, where it will be converted back into glucose. This glucose can then be transported back to the exercising muscles for further use. The overall process of producing lactic acid from glucose and then converting it back into glucose is called the Cori cycle (this is sum-marised in Figure 2.12). The Cori cycle is of significant importance during prolonged peri-ods of exercise as it helps to prevent fatigue, firstly by reducing the amount of lactic acid and secondly by sustaining the body's glyco-gen stores.

Following strenuous muscular activity, dur-ing which the anaerobic systems have been used, the aerobic system operates to facilitate recovery from the exercise. After a bout of exercise the aerobic system will produce

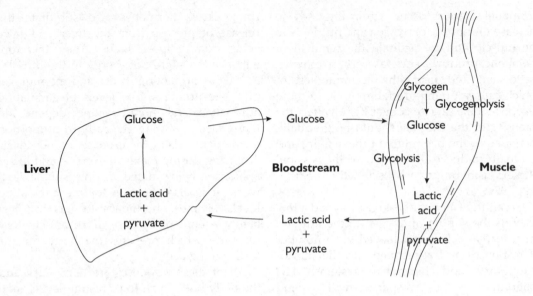

Figure 2.12   Summary of the Cori cycle

excess ATP that can be used to resynthesise the phosphocreatine stores and remove the lactic acid that will have accumulated. The magnitude of the oxygen deficit that needs to be repaid will depend upon the intensity and duration of the preceding exercise.

Quite often slight adjustments to physiological processes will occur even before exercise has commenced, in anticipation of a bout of exercise. For example, the thought of exercise will cause a rise in sympathetic nervous activity and the secretion of sympathetic hormones such as adrenaline and noradrenaline. This will result in a rise in the heart rate, breathing rate and the mobilisation of energy fuels such as liver glycogen and free fatty acids. It may also initiate changes in the circulation of the blood, including the vasodilation of blood vessels to the working muscles and vasoconstriction of blood vessels which supply other organs such as the kidneys and gut, preparing the body for the exercise. For this reason adrenaline is sometimes termed the 'fright, fight or flight hormone'. Physiologically the initial responses to the anticipation of exercise appear to result from

increased activity of the cerebral cortex; however, once the activity has commenced the major area for controlling respiratory and cardiovascular response is the brainstem, of which the medulla oblongata appears to be the most important.

As the body exercises, the immediate changes that occur act as stimuli, and are detected by receptors or sensors in the muscles, cardiovascular system and nervous system. Information from these sensors may then cause intrinsic reflex responses within the muscles, or the information may be sent via sensory neurones to the cardiorespiratory control centres of the brain. Here the information is processed and a number of responses (including changes in hormonal secretions and cardiac and muscular activity) may result. The overall effects of these changes include:

- an increase in heart rate;
- an increase in the stroke volume of the heart;
- an increase in cardiac output;
- an increase in the rate and depth of breathing, which will increase the amount

of air ventilated by the lungs each minute (minute ventilation);

- circulatory changes; and
- changes in blood pressure.

The physiological responses occurring before, during and after exercise may be considered under the following headings:

- pulmonary responses;
- cardiovascular responses;
- hormonal responses.

PULMONARY RESPONSES

The lungs are the site of gaseous exchange between the air and the blood. Within the alveoli oxygen diffuses into the blood and carbon dioxide diffuses out of the blood. Inhaled air contains approximately 79% nitrogen, 21% oxygen and small traces of other gases such as carbon dioxide. Exhaled air typically contains approximately 16% oxygen, 4% carbon dioxide, 79% nitrogen and small traces of other gases. Whilst the precise proportions of oxygen and carbon dioxide in expired air will vary depending upon the individual and their state of activity, the important points to note are the decrease in oxygen and a corresponding, although not always exact, increase in carbon dioxide. Oxygen consumption and carbon dioxide production are a direct result of the activity of the aerobic energy system.

The energy demands of most forms of exercise will result in an increase in the activity of the aerobic system. This will therefore increase the muscle's need for oxygen and production of carbon dioxide. During strenuous forms of exercise a person's oxygen consumption can rise to over 3.5 litres per minute – and in excess of 5 litres per minute in elite endurance athletes. To supply the demand for more oxygen, both the rate and depth of breathing are increased. At rest a person's breathing rate may be 12 cycles a minute. The volume of each breath is approximately 0.5 l so this results in a 'pulmonary ventilation' of 12 × 0.5 = 6.0 l per minute.

During strenuous exercise these respiratory parameters increase significantly: the rate can increase to 45 breaths per minute and the volume of air inhaled with each breath to 3 l, producing a pulmonary ventilation of 135 l min⁻¹. Again, precise values will depend upon the individual, his or her lung capacity and the intensity of the exercise. This increase in pulmonary ventilation substantially increases the amount of oxygen getting into the lungs and the amount of carbon dioxide that is removed. This therefore facilitates oxygenation of the blood (and thus the muscles) and removal of the carbon dioxide from the blood (and thus from the muscles).

An increase in pulmonary ventilation may be observed before, during and after exercise. The slight increase that can occur before exercise is an 'anticipatory response', which helps to prepare the body for the exercise. Preparatory changes in pulmonary ventilation are stimulated by the activity of the sympathetic nervous system and sympathetic hormones such as adrenaline. Once physical activity has commenced these neural and hormonal inputs will continue to promote pulmonary ventilation, with the strength of their stimulation depending upon:

- the acidity of the blood and cerebrospinal fluid;
- carbon dioxide production;
- oxygen consumption;
- heat production; and
- joint movement.

All these factors are related to an increase in muscular activity, which increases oxygen consumption, carbon dioxide production and heat production. Increased carbon dioxide production will also cause an increase in the acidity of the blood and cerebrospinal fluid because carbon dioxide dissolves in the water of the body fluids to produce carbonic acid:

$$CO_2 + H_2O \rightarrow H_2CO_3$$

Strenuous exercise will also result in the production of lactic acid, which will make the blood and cerebrospinal fluid even more acidic. The main stimulus for the rate and depth of breathing is the acidity of cerebrospinal fluid (also the partial pressures of carbon dioxide and oxygen). An increase in acidity stimulates sensors in the brain to signal to the respiratory control centre to increase pulmonary ventilation. The pulmonary response to exercise is therefore in proportion to its intensity. Other factors, such as heat production and joint movement, which also influence pulmonary ventilation, are also likely to occur in proportion to the exercise intensity.

CARDIOVASCULAR RESPONSES

The function of the cardiovascular system is to transport the blood around the body. The contraction of the heart moves the blood through the blood vessels. The heart is made of cardiac muscle and consists of four chambers: two atria, which receive blood from either the body or the lungs, and two ventricles, which pump blood either to the body or to the lungs. In a normal heart the blood cannot pass directly from one side of the heart to the other and the two sides contract together in synchrony. At rest the heart beats approximately 72 times per minute, each side ejecting approximately 70 ml of blood with each beat. Blood ejected from the right side of the heart is transported via the pulmonary arteries to the lungs, where it is oxygenated and gives up its carbon dioxide. It returns to the left side of the heart via the pulmonary veins. The left side of the heart then pumps the oxygenated blood to the rest of the body. As the blood passes through tissues and organs it gives up its oxygen and collects waste products such as carbon dioxide. This 'deoxygenated' blood is returned to the right side of the heart to be pumped back to the lungs and the cycle is repeated (Figure 2.13).

The frequency with which the heart contracts is known as the heart rate (HR) in beats per minute (beats min^{-1}). The amount of blood ejected by each side of the heart with each beat

is called the stroke volume (SV). Together these parameters determine the amount of blood that is ejected by each side of the heart each minute; the cardiac output (Q): HR × SV = Q. The cardiac output of an individual will depend upon their age, gender, size and current state of activity. Typical resting values for an adult are given below.

$$\text{HR (beats min}^{-1}) \times \text{SV (ml beat}^{-1})$$
$$= \text{Q (ml min}^{-1})$$
$$72 \times 70 = 5040$$

For an adult a typical resting cardiac output would thus be in the region of $5\,l\,min^{-1}$. To supply the muscles with more oxygen during exercise the cardiovascular system has to increase its delivery of oxygenated blood. This will also facilitate the removal of waste products and assist with the process of thermoregulation, as the blood takes heat away from the active muscles. An overall increase in the supply of blood (and hence oxygen) to the muscles is achieved via an increase in cardiac output and changes in the circulation of blood around the body.

Cardiac output is increased by a combination of an increase in heart rate and stroke volume, both of which increase in proportion to the intensity of the exercise. During intensive forms of exercise the heart rate may increase to around 170 beats min^{-1} and the stroke volume may increase to 120 ml beat^{-1}. This will give a cardiac output of approximately $20\,l\,min^{-1}$. These increases are caused by

- increased stimulation from the sympathetic neurones, increasing the rate of discharge of the pacemaker region (sinuatrial node) of the heart
- a decrease in the level of parasympathetic nervous activity to the heart (parasympathetic innervation reduces heart rate)
- an increase in the secretion of the sympathetic hormones adrenaline and noradrenaline, which increase the heart rate.

The observed increase in stroke volume during exercise is also thought to be caused

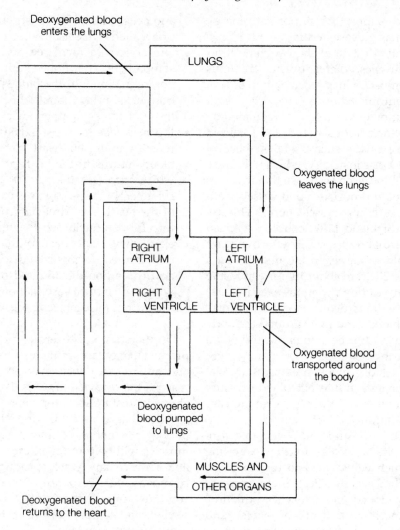

Deoxygenated blood
enters the lungs

LUNGS

Oxygenated blood
leaves the lungs

RIGHT
ATRIUM

LEFT
ATRIUM

RIGHT
VENTRICLE

LEFT
VENTRICLE

Oxygenated blood
transported around
the body

Deoxygenated
blood pumped
to lungs

MUSCLES AND
OTHER ORGANS

Deoxygenated blood
returns to the heart

Figure 2.13 The cardiorespiratory system

by an increase in the amount of blood returning to the heart. The additional amount of blood returning to the heart results in an increase in the filling of the ventricles; this causes an additional stretch on the walls of the ventricles which, in response, contracts more forcefully. The relationship between an increase in venous return and an increase in stroke volume is known as Starling's Law. However, the exact mechanism for increasing stroke volume is subject to some debate.

The distribution of blood around the body can also be adjusted during exercise via vasodilation of blood vessels that supply the exercising muscles and vasoconstriction of blood vessels that lead to other areas such as the gut. This results in an increased proportion of the blood going to the muscles, which are a priority area during exercise, whilst organs that are not very active during exercise receive a smaller proportion. The increased supply of blood to the muscles will also increase the supply of important energy sources such as glucose and fat.

At rest only 15–20% of the cardiac output goes to the muscles, whereas during strenuous exercise the muscles may receive up to 85% of the cardiac output.

Redistribution of blood flow is regulated by the sympathetic nervous system and localised changes in the muscle, such as a fall in the level of oxygen or a rise in acidity, which will cause an additional localised response that involves the dilation of appropriate blood vessels leading to the exercising muscle fibres. This redistribution of blood flow, coupled with an increased cardiac output, can effectively increase the blood supply to the muscles by a factor of over 20, from about $1\,l\,min^{-1}$ at rest to over $16\,l\,min^{-1}$ during strenuous exercise.

Blood pressure is determined by the force with which blood is pumped around the body and the resistance it encounters in the blood vessels. During exercise there is a slight increase in systolic blood pressure but relatively little change in diastolic blood pressure due to the combined influences of an increase in cardiac output, which would tend to increase blood pressure and a general vasodilation of the arterioles to the exercising muscles, which would tend to reduce blood pressure. The overall effect is to increase cardiac output and circulatory vasodilation, which enhances the delivery of oxygen and nutrients to the working muscles without causing a substantial rise in blood pressure that could damage the blood vessels and other organs.

An anticipatory rise in heart rate and slight changes in the circulation may occur before exercise. More substantial changes in cardiac output and circulation occur during exercise, brought about by

- Neural influences: an increase in the activity of the sympathetic nervous system along with a decrease in the activity of the parasympathetic nervous system. These increase the heart rate and stroke volume and cause dilation or constriction of appropriate blood vessels.
- Hormones: an increased secretion of the sympathetic hormones adrenaline and noradrenaline into the bloodstream. These hormones bring about effects similar to those of the sympathetic nervous system.
- Intrinsic factors: these relate to a stretch reflex within the heart. During exercise blood returns to the heart at a faster rate, which increases the rate of filling of the chambers of the heart and stretches the walls of the heart. This stretching prompts more forceful contraction so that more blood is ejected with each beat. Within the circulation, intrinsic factors include changes in the acidity, carbon dioxide and oxygen levels, which will induce vasodilation of blood vessels within the exercising muscles.

During strenuous exercise metabolic waste products may accumulate within the body and an oxygen deficit may occur. For these reasons the cardiac output is likely to remain above its resting level for some time after the exercise has ceased. During this 'recovery period' the enhanced blood supply to the muscles will help to repay the oxygen deficit and remove any waste products. Thus the cardiovascular responses to exercise will continue until the acidity, carbon dioxide, oxygen and temperature have been restored to an appropriate level.

Since the most significant influences on cardiac output and circulation are the acidity of the blood and cerebrospinal fluid, carbon dioxide production, oxygen consumption and heat production, it can be seen that the pulmonary and cardiovascular responses to exercise increase the supply of blood, oxygen and other nutrients to the exercising muscles and enhance the removal of metabolic waste products that would induce premature fatigue. The factors that stimulate the pulmonary and cardiovascular responses are similar, and the extent of their responses are in proportion to the intensity of the exercise.

HORMONAL RESPONSES

The hormonal changes observed before, during and after exercise are generally associated with:

- increasing the supply of nutrients and oxygen to the muscle;
- removing metabolic waste products; and
- promoting the repair and growth of tissue after the exercise.

Almost all hormones affect (or are affected by) exercise in some way. Very often their actions are interrelated, making the topic of exercise endocrinology complex. Therefore only a very brief overview of a few selected hormones will be given.

Adrenaline and *noradrenaline* stimulate a number of pulmonary and cardiovascular responses to increase the supply of blood, oxygen and nutrients to the exercising muscles. *Growth hormone* promotes the release of fat for use as an energy source – but is perhaps most noted for its role in the repair/growth of tissues after exercise. *Testosterone* is an anabolic (growth-promoting) hormone which, in the context of exercise, has a primary role in the growth and repair of tissues following exercise. It is produced by both males and females, but males generally possess higher levels as it is also androgenic (promotes the male secondary sexual characteristics). *Erythropoietin* promotes the production of erythrocytes (red blood cells). Its secretion is increased in response to exercise and enhances the oxygen-carrying capacity of the blood. *Cortisol* is generally considered to be a 'stress' hormone, produced under conditions of physical and mental stress. During sustained strenuous exercise cortisol promotes the production of glucose from other metabolites via a process called gluconeogenesis. On a long-term basis excessive overtraining can result in the overproduction of cortisol, producing an imbalance between it and other hormones. The suggested effects of such an imbalance include suppression of the immune system, which makes those who overtrain more vulnerable to minor infections such as colds and flu. Cortisol imbalance has also been linked to disruption of the menstrual cycle.

EXERCISE AND MUSCULAR STRENGTH

Muscular strength refers to the capacity of a muscle or group of muscles to exert force. Everyday examples include lifting an object or moving the body or a limb against a force (often gravity). Lower than desirable muscular strength can occur if a muscle or group of muscles is not used regularly. Underuse can result in a reduction in the size of the muscle (muscular atrophy), which may be extreme if a limb has been immobilised for some time – for example when a broken bone has been put in a cast. Lack of use of the muscle due to failure of the nervous system to stimulate it adequately can also result in atrophy and reduced muscular strength. The reasons for lack of regular neuromuscular stimulation may vary from a serious medical condition to a simple lack of use brought on by a more sedentary lifestyle. Regardless of the cause, the effect of reduced muscle strength can inhibit an individual's capacity to perform basic activities. Exercise programmes designed to improve muscular strength should improve the muscle condition, increase muscle strength and generally increase the individual's capacity to perform activities that require muscular strength. In many cases muscular strength exercises will reverse the process of atrophy and increase the size of the muscles (through hypertrophy) as well as increase strength. However, some medical conditions may limit the amount of 'improvement' that is possible and it may be necessary to aim exercises primarily at minimising a degenerative process rather than seeking to produce specific increases in strength.

For most individuals, muscular strengthening exercises are prescribed with the intention of maintaining or developing the strength required to cope with the physical demands of their lifestyle such as normal household tasks, gardening and DIY. Muscle strengthening can help elderly people by reducing the risk of falls and helping them to open jars, climb onto buses, get out of a chair unaided and generally to maintain their independence. The muscular strengthening exercises that are prescribed on a therapeutic or general conditioning basis are not likely to result in the participant developing excessively large muscles even if weights, pulleys and multigyms are used. Any patient who is concerned about developing such a physique through a basic therapeutically oriented exercise programme should be reassured that this will not happen: the large muscles possessed by powerful athletes are obtained only through considerable amounts of training with very heavy weights. It takes much effort to increase muscle mass and women, who are often more concerned about developing large muscles than men, need not worry, especially because they tend to have significantly lower levels of anabolic hormones than men.

THE IMPORTANCE OF MUSCULAR STRENGTH

The skeletal muscles of the body fulfil many functions. They initiate the movement of the body and body parts; they regulate movements being caused by external forces; they prevent unwanted movements; they help to maintain the posture.

Muscular strength is a complex aspect of a person's physical capacity – which, like all other 'fitness components', is not isolated but is intimately related to other aspects of a person's physical capacity. Muscular strength can be described as a continuum. At one extreme muscles have the property of 'maximal strength', the maximum amount of force a muscle or group of muscles can generate in a single maximal contraction. This determines whether an individual is capable of lifting or moving a heavy object. At the other end of the spectrum there is what is often referred to as 'muscular endurance', an individual's capac-

ity to repeat or sustain muscular contractions over a prolonged period. If this is put into the context of daily activities it will be a factor in determining a person's capacity to perform household chores such as cleaning, gardening or even carrying shopping. A good level of muscular endurance will enhance the capacity to perform these activities without becoming unduly fatigued.

In some prolonged activities, such as walking, local muscular endurance is linked to a person's capacity to provide their muscles with oxygen (their aerobic capacity). To have a good level of muscular endurance the muscles must be strong enough to perform the movement but must also be able to repeat the movement for the desired duration without waste products accumulating. The strengthening exercises incorporated into a programme should thus develop a balance between maximal strength and muscular endurance because both are important to the individual. Although the exercises used to develop maximal strength and muscular endurance are similar, the number of repetitions and the intensity of the exercise will vary considerably. The development of maximal strength will require relatively few repetitions of high-intensity exercises; muscular endurance requires a relatively high number of repetitions of lower intensity exercises.

The strength requirements of a sports performer will often exceed those required for everyday activities. When a therapist treats an injured athlete he or she should be aware of the specific demands of the individual's sport. If a muscle is weak following an injury, the stresses placed upon it by a particular sport could increase the likelihood of the injury recurring; therefore it is important for the therapist to ensure that the muscle is strong enough to cope before the individual returns to full training or competition.

MUSCULAR POWER

Muscular power is related to muscular strength and is determined by the maximal strength of the muscle(s) and the speed with which they contract. Any dynamic muscular movement requires a certain amount of power, and improvement in the maximal strength of a muscle is likely to increase its power. However, power itself is only usually specifically 'trained for' in the sporting context, where it is important in activities such as sprinting, throwing, jumping and acceleration. Therefore, in the context of exercise programmes associated with the development of a person's physical capacity for 'normal' everyday activities, the specific development of power is not usually a major concern.

When involved with the treatment of injured athletes the specific development of power becomes important. The principles of training must be applied, with the progressive introduction of power-related exercises once the muscles have regained the required strength. Failure to do this will return the individual to sport in a condition where they are unable to cope with the physical demands of the activity and are vulnerable to further injury. Incor-poration of these exercises into their rehabilitation programme should be discussed with all those concerned, including the trainer and coach.

JOINT MOBILITY AND FLEXIBILITY

The terms mobility and flexibility are used interchangeably by some authorities and yet convey different meanings to others. In this book we use joint mobility, flexibility and suppleness to refer to the amount of movement attainable at a joint or over a number of joints (as in the case of the spine).

ACTIVE MOBILITY

Active mobility refers to the amount of movement an individual is capable of when using their own muscular contractions – for example, how far he or she can bend to the side unaided or how high they can raise their arms unaided.

PASSIVE MOBILITY

Passive mobility is the range of movement possible at a joint or over a series of joints when the joint or limb movement is aided by an external force, such as help from a therapist or assistant. The assisted nature of passive mobility means that more movement is usually possible under passive conditions than through active contractions alone. However, both are important in terms of physical capacity (fitness) and as a means of therapy or physical training. Quite clearly a reduced amount of active mobility could impede an individual's ability to perform a number of basic tasks. Improving mobility can produce a number of benefits in the type and range of movement possible as well as the ease with which those movements can be performed.

THE IMPORTANCE OF JOINT MOBILITY

In general the joints of young children are extremely flexible but mobility can be lost through the ageing process, lack of use, injury and medical disorders. Throughout life even the most basic body movements require a degree of joint mobility and if it is diminished (for whatever reason) the range of movement possible at that joint will be restricted. Such restriction can make certain movements or activities more difficult and, in some cases, beyond the capabilities of the individual. This will impede an individual's capacity to be independent, to undertake activities such as housework and gardening or even to perform basic reaching movements. Lack of joint mobility can also make an individual more vulnerable to injury during physical exertion and more prone to 'stiffness' following household activities as well as exercise sessions. Therefore, the development and maintenance of joint mobility is important if the individual is to be able to perform many basic movements and activities with ease and without discomfort (either during or after the activity). The amount of mobility needed will depend upon the intended lifestyle. Some individuals will desire basic levels of joint mobility that will permit them to move freely and accomplish basic household tasks. At an extreme level some sports, such as gymnastics, require far greater flexibility and regaining this after injury is an essential part of their rehabilitation programme. So, whilst the development of sports-related mobility may primarily be the role of the coach, it is often the therapist who initiates stretching activities to improve flexibility after an injury.

For many adults joint mobility is diminished due to underuse, as occurs when a joint is not regularly exercised through its full range of movement. In such cases joint mobility can be enhanced by basic stretching routines that help to restore a fuller range of movement at the joint. This will make movement of the joint easier and less likely to cause discomfort. In other instances an injury, or the effects of a disease, may complicate the situation and a programme of stretching exercises must take such complicating factors into consideration. In basic terms, when trying to develop joint mobility the exercise adviser should be wary of any exercise that causes pain. Pain is a warning of potential damage and movements that cause excess discomfort should be avoided – unless they are specifically prescribed by a medical specialist as an integral part of a rehabilitation programme.

CO-ORDINATION

Co-ordination refers to the integrated working and movement of body systems and body parts. Lack of co-ordination, at whatever level, will impair movement and hence reduce the ability to perform physical tasks. The development of co-ordination is physiologically complex but through practice (training) improvements can occur, producing more 'economical' movements and thereby improving physical functioning.

The use of exercises which mimic a particular movement, or component of a complex movement, are important in any rehabilitation programme, particularly one associated with the recovery from injury. In such a programme the therapist will need to consider not only the muscle groups involved in the movement and their particular functions (including those of fixators as well as movers) but also the rate at which the movement takes place, and hence the aspects of muscle recruitment and co-ordination. Such a programme may progress from working on the isolated functions of each muscle through to their co-ordinated response in producing the desired movement, and from a relatively slow speed up to the rate at which the movement takes place in normal circumstances. This form of progression is relevant to all activities – from the simple lifting action used to put a jar into a cupboard up to the extremely rapid throwing action of the javelin thrower.

PSYCHOLOGICAL AND MENTAL HEALTH ASPECTS OF EXERCISE PROGRAMMES

Given the many physiological adaptations to exercise detailed in this chapter it will not surprise the reader to find that psychological adaptations to exercise also occur. Some of these may directly result from the physiological adaptations to exercise (for example, weight loss is often accompanied by an increased sense of well-being), although some psychological adaptations may be independent of physiological processes. For example, attending an exercise class for the first time may increase self-confidence as a result of overcoming the nervousness of joining a new group of people in a strange environment. However, the psychological adaptations to exercise are less well researched and understood than the physiological adaptations. Despite this comparative lack of knowledge we may postulate the following adaptations to exercise without inferring a causal relationship.

FUN

Taking part in some forms of physical activity may be akin to childhood play in that it leads to spontaneous enjoyment and happiness. The importance of this response should not be underestimated, despite the lack of scientific research – which may have something to do with academic snobbery! Most health professionals working on physical activity programmes can recount stories of patients having so much fun during a session that 'their face lit up' and that 'they forgot all their worries for a few minutes'.

MENTAL HEALTH

As we will discuss in the next chapter, there is no accepted definition of mental health. However, research suggests that exercise is positively associated with good mental health in terms of reduced levels of anxiety and depression.

SOCIAL SUPPORT

Taking part in physical activity may not only lead to social approval from significant others; it may also bring the patient into contact with new people and groups. In this way sport, exercise and physical activity can help keep people in touch with their neighbours and local community in a society which appears to be moving to the use of information technology as a means of communicating.

ATTITUDES

Taking part in exercise can change attitudes to health-promoting behaviours and a patient's level of confidence in being able to take control over their own lives. If you succeed at sticking with an exercise programme you may feel that you can reclaim control over other areas of your life such as diet or stress management.

MENTAL ILLNESS

It has been suggested that a very small number of the population have developed (or are in danger of developing) exercise addiction. This may take the form of an excessive frequency and duration of exercise – to the extent that physical activity dominates the individual's life. This narrowing of behavioural patterns may also be accompanied by a restricted energy intake. The condition can become so severe that the patient will continue to exercise despite injury and illness and neglect family and work responsibilities. However, it should be noted that the reported instances of this condition are very small, although undoubtedly more research and professional attention are needed.

REFERENCES

Brooks, G.A., Fahey, T.D. and White, T.P. (1996). *Exercise Physiology, Human Bioenergetics and its Applications* (2nd ed.). London: Mayfield Publishing Co.

Hargreaves, M. (ed.) (1995). *Exercise Metabolism*. Champaign, IL: Human Kinetics.

Maughan, R., Gleeson, M. and Greenhaff P.L. (1997). *The Biochemistry of Exercise and Training*. Oxford: Oxford University Press.

Macleod, D., Maughan, R., Nimmo, M., Reilly, T. and Williams, C. (1987). *Exercise: Benefits, Limitations and Adaptations*. London: E. & F.N. Spon.

Shephard, R.J. (1994). *Aerobic Fitness and Health*. Champaign, IL: Human Kinetics.

Spurway, N.C. (1992). Aerobic exercise, anaerobic exercise and the lactate threshold. *British Medical Bulletin*, **48**, 569–591.

WHAT IS MENTAL HEALTH AND WHY IS IT IMPORTANT?

It is not so long ago that 'health' was defined merely as the absence of disease. Today health professionals are increasingly likely to subscribe to a more complete and dynamic definition of the term health, such as that of the World Health Organization (1985):

> a conception of health as the extent to which an individual or group is able, on the one hand, to realise aspirations and satisfy needs and on the other hand, to change or cope with the environment. Health is therefore seen as a resource for everyday life, not the object of living; it is a positive concept emphasising social and personal resource as well as physical capacities.

Implicit within this holistic view of health is the importance of the mental and social well-being of the individual and group. When things go wrong mental health problems become a major challenge for the individual and our health and social care systems. Goldberg and Huxley (1992) estimated that each year between 260 and 315 people per 1000 suffer an episode of mental disorder lasting at least two weeks. Many of these individuals do not seek help from their general practitioner (GP) but of those that do some are cared for through the primary healthcare team, others by a specific mental illness service or (very rarely) as inpatients in psychiatric units. Those who do seek professional help are included within Department of Health figures (Table 3.1).

Table 3.1 Number of patients referred to mental health services 1990–1991 (Department of Health, 1991)

Age range (years)	Number treated
Children up to the age of 19	2 800
20–34	47 600
35–54	52 900
55–74	41 700

The importance attached to tackling mental illness is illustrated by its inclusion as a key area within the Health of the Nation Survey (Department of Health, 1992), in which the stated objective is to 'reduce ill-health and death caused by mental illness'. Within this strategy, targets are set in relation to both the health and the social functioning of mentally ill people and significantly reducing the suicide rate. It is suggested that this will be achieved by improving information and understanding, developing comprehensive local services and further developments in good practice.

Unlike physical diseases, which often have clear and measurable biological indicators, mental health is difficult to categorise and describe. Society's view on what is normal helps to define 'abnormal' behaviour and those who will be labelled mentally ill. Goldberg and Huxley (1992) argue that our definition of mental illness should not be limited to symptoms but should adopt a triaxial approach that also incorporates personality and social function. Whilst being aware of the difficulties in defining mental illness health professionals should be familiar with the following:

- *Depression* is the term used to describe when someone feels bad about themselves and their lives; at times they may feel complete despair.
- *Manic depression* is characterised by mood swings. Periods of deep depression are followed by mania in the form of over-activity and excited behaviour.
- *Anxiety* is a natural reaction to external pressures. However, anxiety can become severe and affect the individual both physically and mentally.
- *Schizophrenia* is a physical condition that results in a dramatic disturbance in the individual's thoughts and feelings.

As well as understanding the conditions associated with mental illness it is important to reflect upon both the risk factors for these conditions and how they affect people's lives. Factors that predispose an individual to mental illness include the genetic inheritance of the individual, the environment in which they live and work, their exposure to stressful events and the value systems and beliefs held by the broader community. In most cases the determinants of mental illness are multifaceted, the lines between genetic and environmental influences being intertwined in a complex thread of causality.

Having a mental health problem affects a person's feelings (the *affective* dimension), their thoughts (*cognitions*) and behaviour. It may also be the case that, unlike the position with physical illness, both patients and their families find it difficult to understand and talk about the condition. Whilst most of us feel comfortable telling people that 'we have a touch of the flu' (and would expect this revelation to elicit some sympathy and support), admitting that we 'have a touch of depression' may take some courage – we could be labelled 'weak' or 'unable to cope'. By not being open

and able to communicate about our mental health we may cut ourselves off from the support of significant others, therefore heightening feelings of depression and anxiety, and may also not seek the professional help we may need.

Despite the importance of mental health to both the individual and the broader community, exercise interventions have tended to focus on physiological rather than psychological outcomes. Most public health campaigns have used the media to promote physical activity as a means of reducing the risk of coronary heart disease (CHD) or obesity, and little mention has been made of psychological well-being. The emphasis on CHD is also seen in many GP referrals to exercise programmes, in which both the health professional and the exercise leader appear to underestimate the importance of exercise and mental health. This may simply be a result of lack of awareness or training in exercise science, which some agencies have tried to address through the development of specific courses (see Case Study 1).

What, then, is the role of exercise within the prevention and treatment of mental health problems? Is it a possible intervention that health professionals could adopt to meet the needs of their patients with depression, anxiety or dementia? Historically there has been a widely held belief that a healthy body and a healthy mind are linked, and reflecting on your own experience may lead you to conclude that this view holds some truth. Consider how you felt when you were at 'your fittest' and compare that with when you had 'let yourself go'. Although personal experiences may give us a starting point to discuss physical activity with our patients they do not constitute scientific evidence. Indeed, despite there being a large body of research on the relationship between exercise and mental health there are few examples of good practice that can be used to guide the interventions of health professionals. There is a clear need to build and disseminate examples of good practice.

Case Study 1: Professional development in exercise and mental health

The North Yorkshire Specialist Health Promotion Service facilitates a GP referral scheme to leisure centre-based exercise programmes that work with a large number of patients every year. A training needs analysis of the programme identified that both health professionals and exercise leaders required staff training in the physiological and psychological processes underpinning the scheme. To meet this need an interdisciplinary team from the Health Promotion Unit and the University College of Ripon and York St John wrote and validated a ten-credit module on exercise prescription. The psychology component of this course covered both the social psychological determinants of exercise adherence and the mental health outcomes from participation. Students were also given the opportunity to reflect upon their own experience of working with patients with mental health problems. The psychology aspect of the module was assessed through an hour-long examination. This illustrates that some GP referral schemes are concerned with both psychological and physiological outcomes and that structured learning environments can be created in which health professionals can work together with exercise leaders to improve their understanding of exercise psychology.

Acknowledgement: Fiona Bell and Andrew Buckton.

MENTAL HEALTH AS A MOTIVATION TO EXERCISE

It is important to recognise that mental health is not just an outcome to be achieved through exercise: it is also a motivational element that encourages people to be active. For example, which of the following stories corresponds with your own experience or that of your patients?

A Ron Tooby woke up and stretched. As he swung slowly out of bed he contemplated his cholesterol count, which his doctor had explained was too high. Determined to improve his HDL/LDL ratio he put on his jogging shoes and headed for the park.

B Ron Tooby woke up and yawned. He looked at his alarm clock and was surprised to see he had woken up an hour early. As his brain slipped more firmly into consciousness he realised he had woken because the sun was shining brightly through the curtain and the dawn chorus was in full song. 'What a great day for an early morning walk' he thought as he gently got out of bed.

C Ron Tooby woke an hour early. 'Oh blast', he says, as he pulls the covers over his head and goes back to sleep!

Although story **C** is probably the most realistic, story **B** tells us more about the factors that affect the decisions of those who decide to be active in real life. Although most people are concerned about their health the concern does not trigger them to be physically active in their day-to-day lives. When people decide to exercise it is often because of a spontaneous motivation to take advantage of a pleasant situation or the desire to feel good and have fun.

The importance of mental health as a motivation for people to be more active is supported by research findings showing that psychological variables are just as important as physical factors such as weight loss.

1. The Canadian Fitness Survey (1983) found that people exercised to:
   - feel better
   - have fun and excitement
   - control their weight
   - improve their flexibility
   - relax and reduce their stress levels.

2. The Heartbeat Wales Study (1987) found that people are more likely to exercise if:
   - their friend comes too
   - they have free time
   - their doctor tells them to
   - they want to lose weight
   - they want to maintain health.
3. The Allied Dunbar National Fitness Survey (1992) identified the following reasons for exercising:
   - to feel in good physical shape
   - to improve or maintain health
   - to feel a sense of achievement
   - to get out of doors
   - to have fun
   - to relax.

As health professionals, we can use the results from studies like these to inform our practice. If you are working with patients and want to use enhanced well-being and mental health as a means of promoting physical activity:

1. Ensure that all your health-promotion material related to physical activity emphasises fun and enjoyment.
2. Encourage your patients to keep exercise kits in their car and place of work so that they can take advantage of a sudden rush of motivation, a long lunch-break or a sunny day.
3. Incorporate fun into an exercise class by the use of appropriate music, games, partner and group work; combine indoor and outdoor work and lead by example, by enjoying the sessions yourself. This last point is very important, and exercise leaders should ensure that they avoid 'burnout' by not taking too many classes and by balancing the needs of the group with their own motivational and health levels. Remember: fun is infectious, but so is depression!
4. Work with agencies in your community to promote good pedestrian and cycle ways and safe accessible parks. Link with local schools to promote traditional games such as Hopscotch, Cat's-cradle and Rounders.
5. Buy colourful balls, skipping ropes, kites, Frisbees, exercise bands, softballs, bean bags and hoops.

EXERCISE AND MENTAL HEALTH IN THE GENERAL POPULATION

A major theme in modern healthcare is that prevention is not only better for the patient but is also more cost-effective. Since up to 20% of the population may suffer from some form of mental illness (Scottish Home and Health Department, 1980; Kurtz, 1992) it is important that health professionals consider how to prevent these problems. Unfortunately, very little research has been conducted into the preventive effect of physical activity on mental illness (Martinsen and Stephens, 1994). However, the work that has been conducted seems to hold some promise: for example, Gotestam and Stiles (1990) found that physically active Norwegian soldiers were less depressed 12 weeks after a real-life stressor than a group of sedentary soldiers. Obviously this, and similar studies, must be viewed with some caution as it can be argued that no one single factor such as physical activity can explain the incidence of mental illness. It seems more likely that good mental health is determined by a number of interrelated factors, of which physical activity is one.

It would be inappropriate to view mental health purely from a negative dimension. Physical activity not only helps in the prevention and treatment of specific problems but also helps everyone within the community to achieve a quality of life that brings with it a sense of well-being and the 'feel good' factor. A considerable amount of research has been conducted in this area, some of it using the Profile of Mood States (POMS; McNair *et al.*, 1971). This well established psychological tool estimates a subject's mood in terms of tension, depression, anger, vigour, fatigue and confusion. For a number of years investigators using POMS have shown that runners and other athletes have more positive mood states than less active subjects (for example see the early work of Wilson, 1980). Other methods of measuring good mental health support these findings. Significant among these is the analysis conducted by Stephens (1988) on the results of major lifestyle surveys of a sample of 56 000 people in the USA and Canada: he found a positive association between physical activity and good mental health. In their study of 5661 British subjects, Steptoe and Butler (1996) showed that using the GHQ: Malaise inventory it was possible to find a positive association between physical activity and emotional well-being. In another large-scale study, of 1634 schoolchildren, Gordan and Grant (1997) showed that around 25% of the sample reported that sport made them feel happy and good about themselves.

Impressive as these finding are, we must view the research using POMS and the descriptive studies of Stephens and others with caution. Simply because two variables, in this case physical activity and mental health, are related it does not mean that one causes the other. It may be that a third variable, for example level of disposable income, causes the effect. Caution must also be expressed in terms of the direction of the relationship: one could, for example, argue that you are more likely to be active if you feel good about yourself, rather than that being active makes you feel good.

An interesting perspective on how exercise may affect mental health comes from applying the three questions that Thompson and Mathias (1994) have suggested help us to understand specific mental health conditions. These questions are 'What do you do?' 'What do you think?' 'What do you feel?' Applying these questions to exercise, rather than (as Thompson and Mathias intended) to conditions such as depression, it may be possible to develop a greater understanding of how exercise affects mood state. Informal dialogue with exercise leaders and health professionals produced the responses shown in Table 3.2.

Table 3.2   Thoughts and feelings associated with exercise

What do you do when you exercise?	*What do you think when you exercise?*	*What do you feel when you exercise?*
Move purposely	Concentrate on moving	Warm
Move rhythmically	Focus on the body	Awake
Be with others	Problem solve	Happy
Socialise	Let thoughts float	Sense of achievement

Although the ideas in Table 3.2 are speculative it may be that, by asking clients these three questions, health professionals will be able to identify any mental health benefits that the individual may achieve.

It is important to conclude by asking ourselves what we know about the relationship between physical activity and mental health in children. This is an important question, as the answer may help us to build a healthier tomorrow and prevent some of the problems caused by mental illness in adult populations. The Health Education Authority 'Young and Active Symposium' (Biddle *et al.*, 1998) strongly supported the connection between the volume of physical activity amongst children and their level of mental health, based on both published literature and expert opinion. Indeed, a significant proportion of the researchers present argued that the evidence for mental health outcomes in children was more robust than the evidence relating to the physical benefits that accrue from physical activity. What appeared less certain was whether these benefits track into adulthood and whether active children with good mental health become active adults with good mental health.

Two particularly significant papers within the literature on children, activity and mental health are those by Biddle (1993) and Kurtz (1992). Biddle argued that the mental health benefits from school physical education (PE)

may be determined by the level of training and understanding of the PE teacher and the kind of experience they provide. The contribution of Kurtz was to point out that children suffering from chronic illness such as diabetes may be at more risk from developing mental health problems than other children. These are, of course, those children who may be least likely to take part in physical activity unless targeted with well designed and managed programmes of physical education and activity.

EXERCISE AND MENTAL HEALTH IN ELDERLY PEOPLE

It would be wrong to imply that mental health problems are part of the ageing process: many people maintain a positive outlook and a sense of fun into their later years. However, some mental illnesses – for example dementia and depression – can develop in older people and, as the following figures (Greengross, 1997) show, the challenge of caring for this section of the population is likely to grow into the new millennium:

- By 2012 the number of people over the age of 75 will increase by 20%.
- By the year 2006 people aged over 50 will account for 34% of the total population.
- The Institute of Actuaries estimates that by the year 2011 there will be 725 000 people aged 60 and over requiring full-time care.

Within our current elderly population 15–20% suffer from depression (Blanchard, 1997). This may be partly due to the increased exposure to stressful events (e.g. bereavement of significant others) as we age and the effect of reduced independence. Loss of mobility and social functioning mean that large numbers of our community spend their later years in residential and nursing homes. The physical move from the 'family home' to the 'centre' may be stressful in itself; it may also cause isolation, and resulting depression. This malaise is symbolised for many by images of rows of old people propped up in chairs starring blankly at a television screen. However, it does not have to be like that – in many residential and nursing homes new and innovative ideas are being explored to promote what the Health Education Authority has called 'Active for Later Life'. Projects like that described in Case Study 2 reinforce the point that depression is not an inevitable part of the ageing process and can be tackled by a range of interventions. Even if exercise does not have a direct effect on mood state improvement in muscular endurance and cardiovascular function may improve independence and so indirectly improve the quality of life for both elderly people and their carers.

Although depression may not be the sole preserve of old people the likelihood of suffering from dementia does increase significantly with age. It is estimated that 20% of those who live beyond the age of 80 succumb to its ravages. Dementia is characterised by failing intellect and memory, leading to confusion and an inability to function independently. It would be inappropriate to suggest that physical activity can have anything but a marginal effect on the progress of this condition. However, physical activity may add something to the quality of life of both the patient and their carer – even if this simply means getting outdoors for some fresh air and breaking the claustrophobic spell of the home.

Physical activity may have a preventive effect on one specific type of dementia: multi-infarct dementia. This is caused by a hardening of the arteries that carry oxygen and glucose to the brain. The process is the same as that which occurs in the blood supply to the heart and which can lead to myocardial infarction. The narrowing of the arteries to the brain leads the patient to suffer a series of small stokes, the culminative effect of which is dementia. Multi-infarct dementia is most common in men and, like myocardial infarction, has as risk factors lifestyle factors including diet and exercise (Thompson and Mathias, 1994).

Case Study 2: Exercise and the elderly in residential care

In 1992 Mendip District Council ran a pilot study in two towns to promote physical activity to elderly people living in residential care. The pilot study was so successful that by 1996 the 'Flex-exercise For Fun' programme covered all five main towns in Mendip and the surrounding villages and hamlets. The scheme is based around qualified and experienced exercise leaders who train and support staff in residential, nursing and sheltered homes to run physical activity sessions for their clients. The staff from the homes attend a course on basic exercise physiology and psychology and are given set routines to use in the homes. At first the sessions are led by the exercise leader, with the home's staff assisting but over time the sessions move to being team taught and finally the staff at the home run their own programme. Mendip District Council loans the centres equipment with which to carry out the 'Flex-exercise For Fun' programme and also advises on how to apply for grant aid to support this type of work. To date 40 homes have been involved in the scheme, with 82 home-based staff having been trained and supported by 12 exercise leaders.

Acknowledgements to Glen Crocker and Diane Crone-Grant.

EXERCISE AND MENTAL HEALTH IN CLINICAL POPULATIONS

Physical activity for patients with severe psychosis or neurosis who require long-term care can be justified on three main grounds.

1. It provides 'time out' from the normal therapeutic regimen and provides patients and carers alike with a leisure opportunity. Programmes that adopt this perspective are characterised by group sessions at leisure centres and swimming pools and often adopt an informal recreational approach.
2. Some patients need to exercise to control secondary health problems, such as obesity, which may affect both their physical health and mental well-being. Sometimes this approach is used on an individual basis and combined with dietary advice.
3. Structured and supervised exercise programmes can be used as an adjunct to other treatments for anxiety and depression. Such programmes are rare in the UK. However, just as cardiac rehabilitation programmes are carefully structured and supervised on the basis of frequency, intensity and dura-

tion, so exercise programmes targeted at mental illness may require both structure and direction if they are to produce results. See Chapter 5 for the principles of exercise prescription.

Whilst many clinicians would not dispute that patients with mental health problems benefit from leisure opportunities and that their general physical well-being can be improved through exercise, the contention that exercise may have a direct effect on the patient's mental condition is more likely to be contested. Mental illness is predominately treated by pharmacological, psychotherapy or counselling-based interventions and little emphasis is placed on physical activity. Although it would be inappropriate to suggest that exercise-based therapies could replace any of these approaches there is some evidence to suggest that physical activity could be used as an adjunct. This approach first came to prominence when a panel of experts were bought together by the US National Institute of Mental Health to produce a consensus statement on the relationship between exercise and mental health. The group's position was published by

Morgan and Goldston (1987), who reported that evidence was available to support a positive association between physical fitness and mental well-being. Furthermore the panel went on to recognise that, whilst severe depression requires treatment by appropriately qualified professionals using medication and psychotherapy, exercise could be used as an 'adjunct'. More recently, Biddle (1995) reviewed the literature in this area and concluded that exercise has:

- a small beneficial effect on self-reported anxiety;
- a moderate beneficial effect on psycho-physiological indicators of anxiety;
- a moderate-to-large beneficial effect on depression;
- a positive relationship with general psychological well-being;
- an association with selected aspects of personality adjustment;
- a small effect on cognitive functioning;
- a very small risk that some individuals can become compulsive about exercise;
- both positive and negative effects on prosocial behaviour.

Running parallel to the research into the use of exercise as an intervention strategy for patients with mental health problems a number of pilot studies have been established to explore the practical issues raised by providing such services in the UK. One such was conducted by Crone-Grant and Smith (1996) in Somerset. By bringing together Mendip District Council and the Avalon and Somerset NHS Trust the project was able to work with patients from a semi-secure unit for people suffering severe periods of mental illness. A major lesson learned from the project was the need for exercise leaders and health professionals (in this case occupational therapists) to work together as a team. This requires not only a mutual understanding of each other's skills and competencies but also the time to develop trust and mutual respect. One of the most interesting parts of the study

was the way in which the qualified and experienced exercise leader working on the project reviewed and restructured her exercise routines to meet the needs of the patients. She developed a number of strategies to maintain the concentration and attention of the patients, who often had trouble concentrating for even short periods of time. Given the important role played by the exercise leader the pilot study reported that the following skills were needed to facilitate physical activity within this population:

- knowledge of mental health problems;
- knowledge of exercise prescription;
- wide repertoire of movement skills;
- caring attitude;
- adaptability;
- confidence;
- quick thinking;
- awareness of individual needs;
- patience;
- a sense of humour.

Although it would be unwise to make too many generalisations from one study, this and other work in the UK demonstrates that, if sensitively handled, exercise can be built into the daily routines of even the most severely mentally ill patient.

EXERCISE AND DRUG ABUSE

The abuse of alcohol, drugs, glue and nicotine (which may be viewed as a symptom of poor mental health) can lead to severe mental illness, characterised by dependence and addiction. It would be inappropriate to talk about the positive effect exercise can have on substance abusers without first acknowledging the problems that exist in some sports and exercise environments with both drugs and alcoholism. Whilst it is hard to estimate how many competitive sportspeople take performance-enhancing drugs it is clear from high-profile incidences, such as that of Ben Johnson at the Seoul Olympics in 1988, that a subculture exists in some sports. The use of drugs such as anabolic steroids is considered immoral and has been banned by the governing bodies of sport, and their use can have extremely negative effects on both the physical and psychological health of the performer. The phenomenon of 'steroid rage' and its association with domestic violence has been reported within the media and investigated by sports scientists.

The use of steroids may be confined to a small group of elite athletes who are prepared to cheat their way to the top and to those involved in subcultures surrounding body building but the link between alcohol abuse and sport may be more common. Alcohol-related problems within the national game of football are never far away from the headlines; in recent years well known players have been convicted for drink–driving offences and drink-related violence is common on the terraces.

Some sports, and some sports clubs, have built customs and social rituals on alcohol. Whilst not wishing to adopt too puritanical a stance on this issue, particularly given the new, more lenient guidelines on alcohol intake, it is clear that more research is needed on the links between alcohol abuse and sports participation. Any such work should consider the use of alcohol not only by the participants but also by the sedentary spectators!

Arguably more damaging than the alcohol–sport link is the tobacco–sport association. Banned from advertising on television cigarette manufactures have targeted sports such as snooker, cricket and motor racing to market their products. This not only raises serious questions about how sports administrators view the importance of *health sport* but it also raises concerns about the effect on young fans. Thankfully the British government is taking steps to ban tobacco advertising, leaving future historians to ponder why it was ever felt appropriate or ethical for cigarettes to be promoted through sport to young people.

Looking now at the positive effect that physical activity can have for individuals with substance problems, Martinsen and Stephens (1995) report that in the USA exercise is often used as part of 'comprehensive treatment programs of substance abuse and dependence'. Although only limited evidence exists to support the use of exercise within such interventions, a logical argument can be made for its use if one agrees with Sinclar's definition of a problem drinker as 'a person who, through an interplay of genetic and environmental factors, has had the alcohol-drinking response so often reinforced that it becomes too strong for the individual to continue functioning in society.' Exercise might not be able to alter a personality-based disposition to addiction but it may affect the patient's environment by providing:

- 'time out' from the day-to-day stress of living;
- an opportunity for contact time with counselling staff;
- an opportunity to socialise with others having a similar problem or with a common interest in exercise;
- a boost to self-esteem through meeting exercise-related goals;
- a distraction from cravings.

It is important that any exercise programme for substance abusers is carefully designed and discussed by the carers and takes into account the physiological effects of the substance being abused. For example, it is important to recognise that alcohol is a diuretic and that exercising while dehydrated could put additional stresses on already damaged liver and kidneys. Substance abusers often have poor nutritional status, and the intensity and duration of any exercise should reflect this problem.

EXERCISE ADDICTION

Whilst the vast majority of people do not do enough physical activity (see Chapter 4) a very small number may have become obsessive or addicted to aerobic exercise. Despite the media's interest in this phenomenon there has been only limited research into the subject and there is some confusion over the most appropriate terminology – some authors talk about 'positive addiction' (for example Glasser, 1976), which would appear to be a contradiction in terms. de Coverley Veales' (1987) concept of exercise dependence, in which he draws parallels with those dependent on alcohol, gambling or drugs, is more appealing. In short, the individual who is dependent upon exercise demonstrates behavioural patterns that are controlled and dominated by the need to train and stick to a rigid routine. Individuals suffering from this problem will exercise with muscular or skeletal injuries and will even suffer withdrawal symptoms if forced to stop training. Runners appear particularly prone to this problem (Benyo, 1990). Concern has also been expressed that exercise addiction may be associated with eating disorders such as anorexia nervosa through processes linked to obsessive concern with body weight and altered body image. Clinicians working with anorexics should be aware of both the shared and distinguishing features of exercise dependence and eating disorders; they are directed to McSherry (1984), Dishman (1988) and Biddle and Mutrie (1992) for more details.

EXERCISE AND MENTAL HEALTH: SUGGESTED MECHANISMS FOR THE LINK

Throughout this chapter evidence from both scientific studies and 'grass roots' work has been presented to show that mental health is affected by physical activity. However, a major topic that has not yet been addressed is the mechanism by which this effect occurs: what happens in the brain, the mind or the body to enable participation in, for example, a jog around the park to alter emotional and mental well-being? We need to understand this mechanism to be able to clarify if the relationship is causal. It may also be possible that, by understanding the mechanism, we will be able to develop more effective and reliable interventions.

Morgan and O'Connor (1988) suggested four possible mechanisms that may explain the relationship between exercise and mental health.

1. The *monoamine hypothesis*. This suggests that exercise adherence may alter the level or balance of dopamine, serotonin or noradrenaline within the brain. Much of the experimental work in this area has investigated the role of noradrenaline by measuring 3-methoxy-4-hydroxphenol-glycol (MHPG), which is its urinary marker. Whilst urine-based studies are a non-invasive method of exploring brain biochemistry some concern has been expressed as to their accuracy (Schildkraut *et al.*, 1983). The evidence to date suggests that, although this is still an interesting line of inquiry, the hypothesis has not been proven.

2. The *thermogenic hypothesis*. How do you feel after you have had a warm bath or sauna? For many of us, exposure to heat leads to a pleasant and relaxed frame of mind – and may even lead to sleep. Anecdotal evidence suggests that participants in aerobics classes and jogging report similar feelings. This is perhaps not surprising, given that physical activity will raise core and peripheral body temperatures. Whilst this mechanism may explain a short-term sense of well-being in exercisers it is less likely to account for longer term changes in those suffering from depression and anxiety. However, work by Avery *et al.* (1982) has shown that patients with depression suffer from disturbance in thermoregulation – which would suggest that the thermogenic hypothesis requires further investigation.

3. The *endorphin hypothesis*. Since the jogging boom began there have been reports of a 'runner's high', described as a sense of euphoria and mastery. Researchers have suggested that this phenomenon may be caused by endorphins and both the 'runner's high' and the 'endorphin hypothesis'

have entered runners' folklore. Since endorphins are naturally occurring morphine-like substances which help to control pain and create a sense of euphoria, this hypothesis would at first appear to have some merit. The argument may be expressed in terms of our evolutionary heritage, when humans ran to find food or to avoid being eaten. In this wild environment it made sense for the body to develop a system by which aerobic exercise is associated with the release of an opiate-like substance (endorphins) to help regulate pain and discomfort. However, whilst these arguments may sound persuasive, a series of research reviews in the early 1980s (see Steinberg and Sykes, 1985) have cast doubt on the validity of the endocrine hypothesis by raising methodological concerns about work in this area and the nature of the biochemical mechanism concerned. On a personal note the authors have a combined running experience of 40 years and are still waiting for an endorphin rush!

4. The *distraction hypothesis*. Unlike the three other hypotheses, the distraction hypothesis does not depend upon a physiological or biochemical explanation. Quite simply, it states that exercise leads to an improvement in mental health because it gives participants 'time out' from their day-to-day problems. At first this may seem too simplistic – and indeed Morgan and O'Connor (1988) themselves state that 'the idea that exercise is no better than a quiet rest in reducing anxiety and blood pressure could potentially discomfort many exercise enthusiasts' – but this view may underestimate the importance of 'quality time out' for patients who suffer from anxiety and depression. It may be that, in severe cases, resting in a quiet place simply gives the patient the time to dwell on negative thoughts and emotions. For these patients the only break from the condition may be through the distraction of the exertion or the concentration needed to play sport or to exercise (see Table 3.2). More work is needed within this area.

Biddle and Mutrie (1992) also acknowledge the importance of understanding the mechanism that underpins the relationship between exercise and mental health. However, they adopt a slightly different perspective from that of Morgan and O'Connor and begin their work by acknowledging that 'human beings are complex organisms, and it is unlikely that any one of the mechanisms will provide a complete explanation of a particular behaviour.' This multifaceted approach has implications, not only for how research in this area needs to develop an interdisciplinary approach but also for the way we work with our patients. It is clear that within groups of patients classified as depressed or anxious some will respond positively to exercise-based interventions and others will not. Unfortunately, identifying those who will benefit is still largely a matter of common sense and intuition.

Biddle and Mutrie also conceptualised the possible mechanisms from a more social psychology perspective. Like Morgan and O'Connor, they discuss the possible role of distraction but they move beyond this to consider the effects of self-esteem and mastery experiences. Since depression is interwoven with doubts about individual self-worth, exercise may provide an opportunity to experience positive emotions and achievements – simply through the exercise process itself ('I can jog a mile') or as a result of exercise-related outcomes ('I have lost weight and toned up'). Self-esteem may also be related to the importance others place on the behaviour pattern of the patient with depression. Taking part in exercise often elicits spontaneous positive reinforcement – for example, praise for completion of an exercise class or saying admiringly 'I don't know how you do it'. Although we should not discount the importance of the monoamine, thermogenic or endorphin hypotheses it would appear that adopting a social psychological perspective may promote a more direct and relevant understanding of the relation between exercise and mental health. This may lead to a position in which exercise-based therapies are not seen as having any unique effects but, like music or art-based therapies, are seen as suitable simply for some patients who have a particular interest in that particular activity. This motivation may stem from a desire to lose weight, tone up or simply to be outdoors and active.

CONCLUSION

When many people think about exercise they think about its physiological benefits, especially related to conditions such as coronary heart disease, obesity and hypertension. However, there is also a considerable amount of evidence to support its role as an adjunct to treatment for people with anxiety and depression. Although it would be inappropriate to portray exercise as a panacea, this wide range of benefits can be supported from an evolutionary perspective: since Australopithecines first stood upright on the plains of Africa four million years ago our bodies have evolved to hunt and gather (or, put another way, to walk briskly). Our modern society, which puts lifts before stairs and confines many of us to sedentary occupations and leisure pursuits, is a very new environment in which to place a body designed for movement. Just as we are not surprised to find that animals kept in small cages suffer behavioural problems we should not be surprised to find that being active makes humans feel good about themselves.

As Steptoe (1991) stated: 'It can now be said with much more confidence that aerobic and anaerobic exercise have valuable effects on the mood both of normal individuals and those with stress-related problems'. If exercise can be developed into an effective intervention strategy to help prevent or treat mental health problems the public health and financial benefits could be significant. At present around 8% of the UK National Health Service budget is spent on mental health problems, with each mental health bed costing £30 000 per annum (Department of Health, 1992). The

challenge, as we shall explore in Chapter 4, is to ensure that a nation that is habitually sedentary becomes 'more active, more often'.

REFERENCES

Allied Dunbar National Fitness Survey (1992). London: Sports Council and Health Education Authority.

Avery, D.H. *et al.* (1982). Nocturnal temperature in affective disorders. *Journal of Affective Disorders,* **4**, 61–71.

Benyo, R. (1990). *The Exercise Fix.* Champaign, IL: Leisure Press.

Biddle, S.J.H. (1993). Children, exercise and mental health. *International Journal of Sports Psychology,* **24**, 200–216.

Biddle, S.J.H. (1995). Exercise and psychosocial health. *Research Quarterly for Exercise and Sport,* **66**, 292–297.

Biddle, S.J.H. and Mutrie, N. (1992). *Psychology of Physical Activity and Exercise.* London: Springer-Verlag.

Biddle, S.J.H., Sallis, J. and Cavill, N. (1998). *Young and Active?* London: Health Education Authority.

Blanchard, M. (1997). Working with people with mental illness. *Active for Later Life Conference Booklet.* London: Health Education Authority.

Canadian Fitness Survey (1983). *Fitness and Lifestyle in Canada.* Ottawa: Canada Fitness Survey.

Crone-Grant, D. and Smith, A. (1996). Pilot study exploring links between leisure operators and mental health units. *Sports Industry.* Aug/Sept.

de Coverley Veale, D.M.W. (1987). Exercise dependence. *British Journal of Addiction,* **82**, 735–740.

Department of Health (1991). *Health and Personal Social Services, England.* London: HMSO.

Department of Health (1992). *The Health Of The Nation.* London: HMSO.

Dishman, R.K. (1988). *Exercise Adherence: Its Impact On Public Health.* Champaign, IL: Human Kinetics.

Glasser, D.L. (1976). *Positive Addictions.* New York: Harper and Row.

Goldberg, D. and Huxley, P. (1992). *Common Mental Disorders – A Bio-Social Model.* Routledge: London.

Gordan, J. and Grant, G. (eds) (1997). *How We Feel.* London: Jessica Kingsley.

Gotestam, J.H. and Stiles, T.C. (1990). Physical exercise and cognitive vulnerability: A longitudinal study. Presented at the Association for the

Advancement of Behavioural Therapy. San Francisco.

Greengross, Lady (1997). Healthy ageing – who and what are we talking about? *Active for Later Life Conference, 18–20 February 1997*. London: HEA.

Heartbeat Wales (1987). *Exercise for Health: Health Related Fitness in Wales*. Heartbeat Report 23. Cardiff: Heartbeat Wales.

Kurtz, Z. (ed.) (1992). *With Health in Mind*. London: Action for Sick Children.

Martinsen, E. and Stephens, T. (1994). Exercise and mental health in clinical populations. In *Advances in Exercise Adherence,* Dishman, R.K. (ed.). Champaign, IL: Human Kinetics; 55–72.

McNair, D.M. *et al.* (1971). *Manual for the Profile of Mood States*. San Diego, CA: Educational and Industry Testing Service.

McSherry, J.A. (1984). The diagnostic challenge of anorexia nervosa. *American Family Physician*, **29**, 141–145.

Morgan, W.P. and Goldston, S.E. (eds) (1987). *Exercise and Mental Health*. Washington, DC: Hemisphere.

Morgan, W.P. and O'Connor, P.J. (1988). Exercise and mental health. *Exercise Adherence: Its Impact on Public Health,* Dishman, R.K. (ed.). Champaign, IL: Human Kinetics; 91–123.

Schildkraut, J.J., Orsulak, P.J., Schatzberg, A.F. and Rosenbaum, A.H. (1983). Relationship between psychiatric diagnostic groups of depressive disorders and MHPG. In *MHPG: Basic Mechanisms and Psychopathology,* Maas, J.W. (ed.). New York.

Scottish Home and Health Department. (1980). *Mental Health in Focus*. Edinburgh: HMSO.

Steinberg, H. and Sykes, E.A. (1985). Introduction to symposium on endorphins and behavioural processes: Review of literature on endorphins and exercise. *Pharmacology, Biochemistry and Behaviour*, **23**, 857–862.

Stephens, T. (1988). Physical activity and mental health in the United States Canada: evidence from four population surveys. *Preventative Medicine*, **17**, 35–47.

Steptoe, A. (1991). Aerobic exercise, stress and health. *Proceedings of the VIII European Congress of Sports Psychology*, Vol. 4. Cologne: Academia.

Steptoe, A. and Butler, N. (1996). Sports participation and emotional well-being in adolescents. *Lancet*, **347**, 1789–1792.

Thompson, T. and Mathias, P. (1994). *Mental Health and Disorder*. W.B. Saunders.

Wilson, V.E. (1980). Mood profile of marathon runners, joggers and non-exercisers. *Perceptual and Motor Skills*, **50**, 117–118.

World Health Organization (1985). Health Promotion: a WHO Discussion Document on the Concepts and Principles. *Journal of the Institute of Health Education*, **23**(1), 1985.

ADHERENCE AND COMPLIANCE TO EXERCISE AND REHABILITATION PROGRAMMES

4

This chapter will explore the reasons why so many people find it hard to stick to an exercise prescription, rehabilitation programme or an active lifestyle. As well as looking at the research into exercise adherence we will consider practical intervention measures to promote active living and encourage the reader to reflect upon their own exercise behaviour.

A useful starting point to the content of this chapter is to consider the following:

1. In an average week (a full 7 days) how many times do you usually exercise at a moderate level (e.g. brisk walking) for more than 30 minutes? If it is less than the Active for Life guidelines of five times a week what support would you need to do a little bit more?
2. How would you feel if you suffered from insomnia and visited your GP only to be advised to 'get some more sleep'? Some patients receive similarly unhelpful advice, when they are told to 'take more exercise' without any help on how to make this major lifestyle change.
3. Counterintuitively, self-motivation (as measured by the SMI scale; Dishman and Gettman, 1980) has failed to explain why some people exercise and others do not (see, for example, Roberston and Mutrie, 1989).

THE SCALE OF THE PROBLEM

Despite the impression created by mass-participation events like the London Marathon and the use of sports apparel in fashion, very few people actually start and stick to an exercise programme. The Allied Dunbar National Fitness Survey (1992) estimated that seven out of ten men and eight out of ten women do not take enough physical activity to promote good health. This low uptake is compounded by the large number of drop outs from exercise programmes. Dishman (1988) estimates that in the typical supervised exercise setting, about 50% of the clients or patients will drop out of the program within six months or a year. A number of health authorities have conducted research into the physical activity patterns of their own communities. For example, the Somerset Health Authority Lifestyle Survey (1992) found that only 6% of the population of Somerset took part in vigorous activity at least three times a week. A similar study in the Avon Health Authority area in 1989 reported that 75% of those in the lower socioeconomic groups never participated in health-promoting physical activity. This scientific evidence is reflected in the classified ads of most local newspapers, selling exercise bikes and other equipment that has been 'hardly used'!

The scale of non-adherence to physical activity within the American population lead to the publication in 1997 of the first Surgeon General's report on physical activity and health. As many as 60% of American adults do not take part in regular physical activity and 25% are completely sedentary. To add to these concerns, daily physical activity amongst children is low. Indeed, between 1991 and 1995 enrolment in physical education classes in the USA dropped from 42% to 25%.

Non-adherence to exercise programmes causes a number of problems:

1. The potential public-health benefits of physical activity are limited by poor uptake and low compliance. As a public-health strategy physical activity will make a significant impact on the incidence of coronary heart disease and mental illness only if people start and stick to a lifetime of exercise.
2. At an individual level many people fail to meet their own goals of weight loss, toning or rehabilitation because they drop out of the programme. Most, if not all, of the readers of this book will have started a new exercise regime full of good intentions, only to find that their new-found commitment and lifestyle disappeared after a few weeks.
3. Non-adherence also makes it difficult for researchers to conduct research into exercise science. Not only do they sometimes find it difficult to recruit volunteers but also those who do sign up may drop out before the end of the investigation.

It has been suggested that the problem of non-adherence to exercise is a specifically British problem and even that it is related to our 'bad weather', which makes an outdoor lifestyle less attractive than in more temperate climates. However, evidence suggests that a sedentary lifestyle is endemic within many Western countries, irrespective of climate (see Dishman, 1988, 1995 for excellent reviews). Non-compliance is also a common problem across a range of medical and health interventions, pharmacological prescriptions and attendance to many forms of health-screening programmes.

It is also clear that research into levels of physical activity is hindered by the lack of a standardised, reliable and valid measurement tool. Despite their sophistication, heart-rate telemetry systems and advanced pedometers are not always appropriate and their relative expense prohibits their use by many health professionals in the evaluation of physical activity interventions. The questionnaire-based formats for estimating physical activity are prone to problems of poor recall and over-estimation of activity levels, as are interview-based techniques. To help health professionals find better ways of measuring the physical activity patterns of their subjects and patients Medicine and Science in Sport and Exercise (1997) have published a collection of physical activity questionnaires which readers will find an invaluable resource.

ADHERENCE TO EXERCISE AS A BEHAVIOURAL PROCESS

Being physically active throughout your life is a very complex behavioural process at both the macro and micro level. For a person living to 75 years, to follow a recommended exercise prescription of three times a week after the age of 18 an active lifestyle may be translated into 8892 sessions! In addition these discrete bouts of exercise will take place against the backdrop of the individual's developing life-history, from teenager to young adult to parent and grandparent. The sports we play as teenagers may be replaced by exercise classes in our twenties and thirties and move toward brisk walking and other activities in our middle to later years. Sticking to an active lifestyle over this period of time calls for motivation, habitual behavioural patterns and the ability to adapt our lifestyle to new circumstances bought about by ageing and our changing role in society.

At the micro level we may consider that each exercise session is made up of a number of behavioural steps. For a visit to the gym we have to pack our kit, travel to the centre, warm up, exercise, cool down, shower, change and travel home. Given both the complexity of this behaviour and the individual differences that occur within in it the reader should not be surprised to learn that exercise scientists conducting research into exercise adherence have encountered many challenges. For example, during one study in which scientists were attempting to find the variables that discriminated adherers from non-adherers to an exercise programme one of the subjects said 'I really don't agree with your chosen criteria, who can possibly consider themselves active or sedentary? These are merely labels' (Smith and Biddle, 1991). As we consider why so many people do not exercise and how we should intervene to help them we should not forget the voice of this subject. Whilst the health professional may consider a patient to be inactive their own perception of their activity levels may be very different.

Our understanding of exercise as a behavioural process has been helped by a number of researchers – including Sallis and Hovell (1990), who suggested that people adopt, maintain, drop out of (and sometimes resume) exercise programmes. Prochaska and Marcus (1994) have proposed a 'stages of change' model, which will be discussed later in this chapter.

WHY DO PEOPLE FIND IT DIFFICULT TO LIVE AN ACTIVE LIFESTYLE OR ADHERE TO EXERCISE PRESCRIPTIONS?

When considering why many people do not exercise it may be helpful to relate the material that follows to two specific questions.

1. Why do so few people actually start an exercise programme in the first place?
2. Why do so many of those who start then drop out?

By considering both adoption and maintenance of active lifestyles we should obtain a more complete understanding of exercise adherence than if we consider only one of these processes.

Research into exercise adherence is still developing. Biddle (1996) identified three trends that characterised this growth.

1. Much of the early research looked at supervised and structured exercise programmes (e.g. in gyms) although more recent work has looked at free living activity. When considering some of the research presented in this section readers should be aware that the finding may be very specific to the situation in which the information was collected (e.g. an aerobics class) and may not transfer to their own working environment (e.g. a walking programme).
2. Early work in this area was atheoretical, which in some cases lead to poor methodologies and descriptive results. Today most work is based on sound theoretical approaches, often from social psychology.
3. Exercise adherence is no longer viewed as a dichotomous variable but as a behavioural process.

From this developing research the following seven factors can be associated with the physical activity levels of communities and individuals:

- gender and age;
- genetic factors;
- the environment;
- barriers;
- knowledge;
- attitudes;
- confidence.

GENDER AND AGE

A number of studies, including the Allied Dunbar National Fitness Survey (1992), have indicated that women do less exercise than men. Work by Sallis (1993) indicates that these gender differences can also be observed among children, with boys doing 14% more physical activity than girls. A number of reasons can be put forward to account for these findings, including the proposal that females are more reliable at recalling their activity levels and less likely than males to overestimate their exercise patterns. An alternative explanation is the continued discrimination against women in relation to sport, exercise and physical activity, evidence for which can be seen in sports clubs that are *still* 'men only', and the time demands placed upon women who juggle family and work commitments. Wigmore (1996) argues that women's participation in physical activity and involvement in sport is limited by factors related to societal attitudes, media representation, lack of women in coaching and administrative roles and stereotypical views on body image and shape. Sexist comments that 'women do not take part in sport and exercise because of an inferior physical make up' have no foundation in science, which continues to show that women can develop high levels of aerobic and muscular fitness. It should also be noted that a number of scholars, notably Messner and Sabo (1990), are beginning to explore the position of men in sport and exercise using perspectives normally associated with the study of women in sport. By investigating the complex area of masculinity and male body image new insights may be revealed into how best to develop exercise programmes that promote participation equally to both genders.

Research, including the Allied Dunbar National Fitness Survey (1992), also indicates that physical activity declines with age. It is unclear whether this is a natural part of the ageing process or is determined by cultural and social norms. Again, this trend appears to begin early in life; Sallis (1993) reports that between the ages of 10 and 16 the activity of boys declines at a rate of 1.8% and that of girls at a rate of 2.6%.

The Surgeon General's Report (1997) on physical activity and health succinctly summarises current understanding of the effect of demographic influences on physical activity: 'physical inactivity is more prevalent among women than men, among blacks and Hispanics than white, among older than younger adults, and among less affluent than the more affluent.' Health professionals need to be aware of these inequalities when they develop policies and intervention programmes to deliver physical activity to the public.

GENETIC FACTORS

Work by Dishman and Gettman (1980) and day-to-day observation tell us that people who are overweight are less likely to exercise than those who are thin. An obvious conclusion is that exercise makes you lose weight. However, an alternative interpretation of these observations argues that those who are thin are attracted to physical activity and those who are obese avoid it. Since our somatotype is largely determined by genetics we may all be born with a specific disposition to be active or sedentary. If genetics does explain some behavioural patterns we may have to revisit some of our basic ideas of health promotion, which often assume that the individual has the freedom to choose between different behavioural patterns.

THE ENVIRONMENT

Most research into exercise adherence has focused on the decisions and actions of the individual and has assumed that they have complete control over whether to adopt either health-promoting or health-damaging behaviours. A major critic of this perspective, particularly in relation to health-related fitness within the National Curriculum, is Professor Andrew Sparkes. In 1989 he stated that 'there is a strong tendency within the health related fitness movement to assume that a homogenous culture exists in which we are all free to choose our lifestyles. But this is simply not the case.' In short, whilst some individuals within our community have the resources to prioritise membership to exercise centres others have to target their limited incomes to more pressing concerns such as housing and basic nutrition. Promoting physical activity to some sections of the community who have more significant and fundamental health needs may not only lead to social alienation but could also be an ineffective use of limited health resources. The effect of town planning, transport policy and architectural design upon exercise behaviour requires more attention and research.

BARRIERS

A frequently used word within the exercise adherence literature is 'barriers'. Although this area of work has much merit and continues to make a significant contribution to our understanding of why many people do not exercise, it also has a number of limitations. For example, it would seem logical to argue that a barrier can stop an individual from exercising only if that individual intended to exercise in the first place – put another way, you can only have a barrier if you first have an intention. This means that the effect of barriers on actual participation depends on the number of people in the society who intend to exercise but are stopped by insurmountable barriers! Research into barriers also carries the risk of finding *post hoc* attributions for existing behavioural patterns – excuses. I may say 'I do not exercise because time is a barrier' but this may not be the real reason.

Despite these criticisms it is important that health professionals are aware of the main studies investigating barriers to exercise. Not only will this knowledge be helpful in the planning of appropriate interventions but it will also help guide and inform our conversations with our patients and clients. The Health Education Authority has been instrumental in commissioning a number of research projects to investigate the barriers encountered by adults (aged 16–69). One such study, conducted by Kiloran *et al.* (1995), identified that both males and females perceived similar constraints on their exercise behaviour:

- 'I am not the sporty type' was reported by 24% of men and 37% of women

- 'I need to rest and relax in my spare time' was reported by 24% of men and 25% of women
- 'I don't enjoy it' was reported by 9% of men and 13% of women
- 'I haven't got the time' was reported by 41% of men and 44% of women.

As in a number of other studies, 'not having enough time' was the most frequently reported barrier. Further research is needed to see if those who are most active have more free time than those who are sedentary or, conversely, if both groups have the same amount of free time but have different priorities. Research is also needed to see if giving people more free time actually leads to an increase in their levels of physical activity. Clearly health professionals must reflect upon how they will deal with the time barrier when it is raised by their patients. Intervention measures can include help with time management skills and advice on types of activity that take very little time – for example, taking the stairs instead of the lift.

Research that looks at specific types of exercise tends to identify more detailed and context-specific barriers than the more general work of Killoran. For example, a range of studies (Finch and Morgan, 1985; Joshi and Smith, 1992; British Medical Association, 1992) reported the following barriers related to cycling:

- concern over road accidents;
- worry about air pollution from traffic;
- the time and effort involved in riding and storing a bike at work;
- the difficulties related to clothes storage if cycling to work;
- the weather;
- concerns related to bike theft;
- social attitudes in general to cycling.

General barriers and barriers to specific activities may have important implications in helping clients to become more active. Whilst information leaflets can tackle the generic barriers that relate to most views on exercise (e.g. ' I'm not the sporty type') when working on a one-to-one basis with clients it may be more valuable to concentrate on specific issues (e.g. 'what should I do with the bike when I arrive at work?').

From an academic and research perspective the work on barriers can be criticised for being too descriptive and atheoretical. However, some researchers have attempted to develop specific measurement scales and to locate barriers within the broader social-psychological literature. If this trend continues we may see some significant breakthroughs in our understanding of the exercise adherence process in the first years of the new millennium.

KNOWLEDGE

It might at first seem common sense to argue that knowledge of the relationship between physical activity and good health would lead to behavioural change. Unfortunately, it has been known for some time that simply giving people knowledge about health outcomes does not always prompt them to adopt health-promoting behaviours (Biddle and Mutrie, 1992) – consider how many people smoke despite being aware of the risks of lung cancer! The Allied Dunbar National Fitness Survey (1992) showed that 80% of the population think that exercise is good for health yet most of that sample did not act upon this knowledge. This line of argument does not discount the importance of educational initiatives to improve understanding of how the body works and why it should be kept active. Indeed this type of work has a prominent position within the National Curriculum for Physical Education. However, its limitations should be recognised and knowledge should be seen as a starting point for behavioural change rather than an end in itself. It should also be noted that, from a physiological perspective, it does not matter if you are active because of a rational, educated decision or simply because of an almost unconscious habit.

ATTITUDES

Most health professionals who have been involved in health promotion campaigns will have attended a meeting at which it has been suggested that they need to 'change people's attitudes'. Indeed, the Health Education Authority's Active for Life campaign has as one of its specific aims the desire to change attitudes toward physical activity. Implicit within these goals is the belief that by changing attitudes you will ultimately change behaviour. This point was powerfully made by Fishbein and Ajzen (1977) when they wrote, 'attempts to predict behaviour from attitudes are largely based on a general notion of consistency. It is usually considered to be logical or consistent for a person who holds a favourable attitude toward some object to perform favourable behaviours, and not to perform unfavourable behaviours, with respect to the object.'

This quote suggests that those who are active may have very different attitudes to those who are sedentary. A problem occurs when health professionals become confused over the meaning of the term 'attitudes' and the most appropriate way of change them. Before reading further, write down your own definition of the word 'attitude' and compare it with that of the 'experts'.

Hewstone *et al.* (1988) defined an attitude as 'an enduring positive or negative feeling about some object (some person, object or issue)'. If your definition did not match this wording you can take some comfort from Jasper (1978), who wrote that 'although it has been described as one of the key concepts of social psychology or even the most distinctive and indispensable concept in (American) social psychology, no commonly accepted definition of the concept of attitude exists.' It is always important to ask someone what they mean by the term 'attitude' before agreeing to its use in the wording of targets set at the start of a health-promotion campaign. The danger of not agreeing on a working definition of the term is that you may find your project is evaluated using inappropriate criteria.

Arguably the most important attitudinal perspective in relation to exercise adherence is the Theory of Reasoned Action/Planned Behaviour (Fishbein and Ajzen, 1977; Ajzen, 1985). Fishbein's and Ajzen's approach to attitudinal measures is built on the concept of *correspondence*. They argue that measuring attitudes in general terms (e.g. to exercise) will tell us very little about actual behaviour and that we need to look at attitudes that correspond to very specific target behaviours (such as walking to work tomorrow morning). To achieve correspondence we should consider four factors.

1. *Action*: the attitude and the behaviour must be assessed in relation to a specific action, such as riding a bike, rather than a general attitude object, such as physical activity.
2. *Target*: reference should be made to specific target groups, such as cyclists, or to specified significant others, such as partners or motorists.
3. *Context*: reference should be made to the context within which the behaviour takes place; for example, on a designated cycleway as opposed to a main road.
4. *Time*: time should be specified in identifying attitudes; for example, cycling next week or next winter.

From their starting point of correspondence Fishbein and Ajzen argued that behaviour can be predicted by a combination of intention, attitudes, social norms and perceived behavioural control. Their theory is illustrated in Figure 4.1.

Fishbein and Ajzen have also postulated that attitudes and social norms can be broken down into their constituent parts. These indirect measures of attitudes and social norms can be presented in the form of equations:

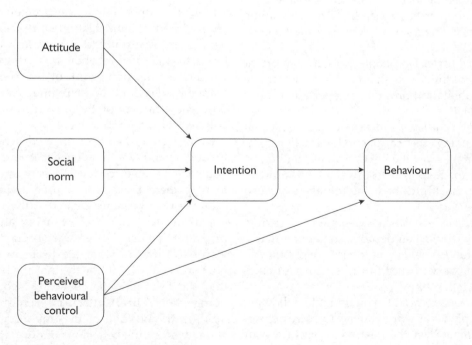

Figure 4.1 The Theory of Planned Behaviour

Attitude = Outcome belief

×Outcome evaluation

and

Social norm = Normative belief

×Motivation to comply

Where: *outcome beliefs* are what people think will happen if they carry out the target behaviour; *outcome evaluations* are how good or bad they think the outcome of the behaviour will be; *normative beliefs* are what people think important others want them to do; and *motivation to comply* is whether they want to do what important others think they should do.

Researchers have attempted to predict exercise behaviour using questions based on the different components of the Theory of Planned Behaviour. The sample questions below correspond in terms of action, target, context and time to a very specific behaviour.

- *Intention question*: Do you intend to attend the cardiac rehabilitation programme over the next six weeks?
- *Attitude question*: Do you think that attending the cardiac rehabilitation programme over the next six weeks would be good or bad?
- *Social norm*: Do people who are important to you think you should attend the cardiac rehabilitation programme over the next six weeks?
- *Outcome belief questions*: Do you think that attending the cardiac rehabilitation programme over the next six weeks will (a) be fun (b) help you lose weight (c) improve your health (d) be tiring (e) take too much time?
- *Outcome evaluation*: Generally speaking, how would you describe something that is (a) fun (b) helps you to lose weight (c) will improve your health (d) is tiring (e) takes too much time?
- *Normative belief*: Do you think the following people want you to attend the cardiac programme over the next six weeks: (a) your GP (b) your family (c) your friends?

- *Motivation to comply*: Generally speaking, how often do you do what the following people tell you to do: (a) your GP (b) your family (c) your friends?
- *Perceived behavioural control*: Are you confident that you will be able to attend the cardiac rehabilitation programme over the next six weeks?

On a questionnaire all of these items would be measured on a five or seven-point Lickert scale with semantic endpoints such as highly likely/highly unlikely. Research using this approach has had some success in explaining variance in exercise behaviour (adherence or drop out). A meta-analysis by Shepherd *et al.* (1988), which combined the results of 87 studies with a total sample size of 11 000 found a correlation between intention and behaviour of 0.53. The correlation between attitude and social norm with intention was 0.66. Godin (1993) reported that 30% of the variance in subjects' intention to be physically active could be explained by the theory and concluded that 'when attitude is measured within a proper theoretical framework, it seems an important determinant of exercise behaviour.' Returning to our example of attitudes to a cardiac rehabilitation programme we can use the framework of the Theory of Planned Behaviour to help understand the different attitudes of the adherer and non-adherer, as shown in Table 4.1.

By using the theory of planned behaviour to understand your patients in more detail you may be able to develop new strategies to help them to stick to a programme. For example, if it becomes clear that the wife of a patient does not want him to attend a programme it may be necessary to contact her to try to find out what the problem is and how you can help. It may be that she believes that the last thing her husband should be doing after a heart attack is exercising. By tackling the attitude of the important other we may affect the behaviour of our patient in a very direct and significant way.

Table 4.1 Hypothetical comparison of an adherer and a non-adherer to a cardiac rehabilitation programme

Theory	Adherer's attitude	Non-adherer's attitude
Behaviour	Attending a six-week cardiac rehabilitation programme	Not attending a six-week cardiac rehabilitation programme
Behavioural intention	I intend to attend the six-week cardiac rehabilitation programme	I do not intend to attend the six-week cardiac rehabilitation programme
Attitude	I think that attending the six-week cardiac programme would be pleasant/rewarding/good	I think that attending the six-week cardiac rehabilitation programme would be unpleasant/unrewarding/bad
Social norm	People who are important to me want me to attend the six-week cardiac rehabilitation programme	People who are important to me either don't care if I attend the programme or do not want me to go
Perceived behavioural control	I am confident that I will be able to stick to the six-week programme	I am not confident that I will be able to stick to the six-week programme so what's the point in starting?

It is clear from the scientific evidence that attitudes have an important role to play in helping us to understand why some people exercise and others do not. They can also be used as a basis for constructing intervention measures. However, as this section has shown, attitudes are a more complex phenomenon than many people imagine and are bound up with both our social environment and our perceptions of control.

CONFIDENCE

If you reflect upon your own behaviour it is not difficult to identify tasks that you avoid because you lack confidence in your ability to complete or succeed at them. At this very moment you might be consulting this book for an essay or project that you have put off until the last minute because you think it is very difficult! Arguably the leading theorist on confidence and behaviour is Bandura, who developed the concept of self-efficacy (Bandura, 1986). Central to his thinking was that confidence is situationally specific. In other words, confidence is not a global construct that we carry into every area of our life but something that is altered by our environment. This can be seen when the high-flying businessman who is extremely confident within the workplace finds himself embarrassed and lacking in confidence during an exercise to music class. Given that we often ask previously sedentary adults to begin an exercise programme, in what for them may be the rather strange environment of the gym or leisure centre, self-efficacy is an important concept for us to understand. Bandura (1986) expressed the essence of self-efficacy when he defined it as 'peoples' judgements of their capacities to organise and execute courses of action required to attain designated types of performances. It is concerned not with the skill one has but with the judgements of what one can do with whatever skills one possesses.'

A number of studies across a wide range of settings, including exercise adherence (Kaplin and Atkins, 1984), have indicated that self-efficacy does predict behaviour. Indeed, a threshold of self-confidence may be needed simply for the patient to walk through the doors of the exercise centre. There are a number of things that health professionals can do to enhance the confidence of their patients to exercise:

1. Ensure that the venue is non-threatening. For example, make sure reception staff are friendly and helpful, that there are pictures of real people exercising to show that shape and size are not a barrier. Attention should also be paid to any music used: if it is too loud or not to most people's taste it can turn people away from the centre.
2. Self-efficacy is likely to be increased if new exercisers can see people like themselves having fun on the programme. This means introducing newcomers to people who have had a good experience on the course. You may also want to experiment with peer-group led sessions. Don't forget that exercise leaders do not always have to be young and slim.
3. Health professionals must give lots of verbal encouragement to people who lack confidence at the start of an exercise programme. This means noticing them doing something right and giving unconditional positive reinforcement during activity sessions.

SUMMARY

In this section a variety of reasons, from genetics to confidence, have been suggested to explain why so few people live an active lifestyle. Other authors may identify a completely different sets of reasons which could be equally well argued for, although we have come a long way since Sallis and Hovell (1990) stated 'overall, it must be concluded that we understand nothing about why some begin exercising'. However, it is clear that no one explanation will unlock the exercise adherence puzzle; we must seek mulitivariable explanations for this complex behavioural process. This may mean that to get 'more people, more active, more often'

health professionals will have to work within interdisciplinary teams incorporating exercise specialists and physical educators.

INTERVENTIONS TO PROMOTE ACTIVE LIVING AND EXERCISE ADHERENCE

As health professionals have become more aware of the benefits of physical activity and the low levels of public participation in health-related exercise, they have begun to pay more attention to interventions aimed at getting 'more people, more active, more often.' This is demonstrated by the publication 'Promoting physical activity: guidance for commissioners, purchasers and providers' (Health Education Authority, 1995), which is a valuable resource for health professionals bidding for resources. In the following section we will present intervention strategies targeted at whole communities and then those designed for use on a one-to-one basis with patients and clients.

COMMUNITY-BASED INTERVENTIONS

For the purpose of this section communities will be defined as groups of people who, through a shared location, set of beliefs or perceived self-identity, have common agreed needs and collective aspirations. Given the many different types of communities within which health professionals may work (from hamlet to World Wide Web) it will be impossible to look at all possible community-based interventions. However, it is hoped that the following settings will find a resonance with the reader.

1. Schools
2. The workplace
3. Sport and leisure centres
4. Voluntary groups and special interest networks
5. Cyberspace communities
6. The nation.

SCHOOLS

Perhaps the most worrying aspect of our increasingly sedentary society is that our children are becoming habitually inactive. Landmark research by Neil Armstrong concludes that 'this series of studies has shown that British children have surprisingly low levels of habitual physical activity and that many children seldom experience the intensity and duration of physical activity associated with health-related outcomes' (Armstrong *et al.*, 1990).

By intervening in school communities we may not only tackle the need established by Armstrong to help our children be active but may also affect their participation levels as adults. Without doubt one of the most important intervention strategies within the school is the National Curriculum for Physical Education. It often comes as a surprise to health professionals that the first general requirements for PE across Key Stages 1–4 (age range 5–16 years) does not include reference to prowess in sport or team games and reads:

'1. To promote physical activity and healthy lifestyles, pupils will be taught:
a) to be physically active
b) to adopt the best possible posture and the appropriate use of the body
c) to engage in activities that develop cardiovascular health, flexibility, muscular strength and endurance
d) the increasing need for personal hygiene in relation to vigorous physical activity.'

Given the statutory obligation upon schools to meet this requirement we should be confident that our children are being given both the experience of and the desire to be physically active. However, the delivery of the National Curriculum within schools has not been without its critics. For example, although this general requirement focuses upon physical activity and health, the areas of activity used to deliver it to children tend to be based on traditional team games and sports. This means that flexibility may be taught through cricket and aerobic fitness through football. Some children may find this approach fun, but others may be put off by a competitive sports environment. However, health professionals should not overlook the opportunity to work with PE teachers in helping to deliver the National Curriculum. Health-promotion staff could work with PE staff to improve the teacher's knowledge of health and in return learn practical skills related to the promotion of physical activity to children.

One of the great unknowns about exercise promotion within the school environment is whether childhood activity patterns are associated with participation or dropout in later life. Although some research (for example the Allied Dunbar National Fitness Survey, 1992) suggests that active children become active adults much of the evidence is inconsistent and weak (Powell and Dysinger, 1987). For example, Bollaret *et al.* (1992) indicated that whilst the Belgian PE curriculum was dominated by competitive sport, when given the choice pupils would opt for individual pursuits, thereby breaking the school–community leisure link. Within the UK Glyptis (1992) has argued that it is too simplistic to argue that adults make choices based solely on the basis of their school PE and goes on to contend that the activity patterns of adults are determined by a much wider context. Even if school PE does have an effect on participation levels in later life we must not assume that this effect is positive. Qualitative research by Crone-Grant and Smith (1998) has shown that some adults hold very negative memories of school PE, which still put them off exercise; for example, one subject said 'my PE teacher was an old dragon who made me go into the pool and I still have a fear of water to this day.'

Before leaving the school it is appropriate to reflect upon the fact that PE classes represent only a small percentage of the child's waking week. If we were to rely solely on these classes to deliver our children's physical activity needs we would find an ever-increasing incidence of hypokinetic disease. For a school to be an effective promoter of physical activity it must consider:

- how children travel to and from home;
- whether the environment around the school is safe for children to walk, ride and play in;
- the active lifestyle options available for children at break, lunch time and after school, and whether they are all based on sport and competition;
- how effectively physical activity is taught across the curriculum;
- the example staff set in terms of their own levels of physical activity;
- how the school can contribute to meeting the needs of the local community to live physically active lifestyles.

The concept of 'The Active School' has been explored by Cale (1997), who argues that schools need to promote active living through their policy, ethos, environment, care and support networks, community links and formal and informal curricula. For such an approach to work PE teachers will need to continue to redefine their roles and will have further need of professional development opportunities in health-related areas.

THE WORKPLACE

Like the school, the workplace is a location in which the health professional has a 'captive audience' and is able to work with large groups of people in one convenient location. Worksite exercise promotion is a global phenomenon, with programmes being developed in Japan, Canada, the USA and Europe. Within the UK we have often looked to American examples of good practice to guide our work. Although this has been a helpful starting point the limitation of importing American health-promoting models should be recognised. For example, American companies pay large health insurance premiums for their staff and therefore have a very different motivation for supporting health-promoting behaviours than

British companies, who operate within the context of the National Health Service. If American companies are motivated by the health insurance dollar, British companies often limit their approach to health to that laid down in Health and Safety legislation. This means that, whilst most companies have stringent rules about the use of dangerous equipment and chemicals, their canteens serve high-fat foods and their shift patterns can be so arranged as to negate the possibility of adequate leisure time.

Given this context, why has the workplace been suggested as good place to promote exercise? Commentators have suggested the following reasons.

1. The historical link between work and exercise. Redmond (1987) points to the 'military legacy', by which he refers to the significant number of people within our society who work or have worked in the armed services and have been exposed to physical training as part of their occupation. Within the civilian sector a number of companies have a long tradition of providing sport and exercise facilities for their staff. This historical legacy still provides opportunities for a health professional to enter the workplace to promote physical activity.
2. Although many occupations have become less labour intensive some roles still require physical fitness. In reviewing the need for occupational fitness, Gettman (1988) points to police officers as one group that need to be fit. A similar argument can be made for fire officers and members of other uniformed services.
3. In the late 1980s and the early 1990s a new health-promotion agenda has developed, in which the workplace is considered an influential environment in which the health professional can work with established groups using structured communication channels.

A number of health promotion programmes – for example 'Good Health Somerset' – emphasised the major benefits that the

Table 4.2 Suggested benefits for corporate fitness programmes

Employer	Employee
Enhanced corporate image and higher company morale	Higher morale
More effective work force	Health gain
Positive effect on productivity, staff turnover and absenteeism	Access to free facilities and advice

employer could achieve by promoting health-related behaviours. The benefits to the employer and employee are summarised in Table 4.2.

Given the perceived benefits of workplace exercise promotion schemes it is not surprising to find that there are a number of different intervention models. These are summarised, along with their strengths and weakness, in Table 4.3.

As this section has shown, the workplace is an attractive environment for the health professional to target adults with a physically active message. Unfortunately the workplace also presents a number of challenges which, whilst well known by the health professionals who work in them, appear to be under-reported within the exercise science literature. Chief amongst these are the low levels of adherence that exercise interventions achieve. Evidence of this problem can be found in the conclusion of Shepherd (1988): 'Despite occasional overly optimistic claims, no more than 20% of eligible workers are usually recruited to a corporate fitness programme, and only half of those who are recruited become long term adherents.' These figures should not surprise us, for the workplace is staffed by the same people who find it hard to exercise in their local leisure centre or build physical activity into their life. Their motivation and adherence to exercise does not change simply because the exercise centre is within the factory rather than on the high street.

The potential economic benefits to the company and the employer should not be overstated: the reported increase in productivity and reduced absenteeism that occur in association with the establishment of an exercise centre might be only *related to* (not *caused by*) the intervention, for one could argue that a management team that is enlightened enough to establish an exercise centre will also be the type that invests in its people and stresses the importance of good communication. In short it may be the management style which leads to both the decision to build an exercise centre and the increase in productivity!

It can be argued that corporate fitness programmes reinforce the responsibility of the individual to look after their own health but distract attention from the need to change the work environment itself. In other words building an exercise centre may be a lot cheaper and easier than changing working patterns and systems to give staff less stress and more opportunities for recreation. Mills (1998) presents a 'radical' critique of workplace health promotion using a structuralistic perspective which leads him to conclude that 'the impact of workplace health promotion on disease-related behaviour has been both overstated and confined to those least in need.' He attributes this lack of success to a failure to tackle key issues in the work place on the concept of rewarding and unrewarding work (job satisfaction). Arguing that those with unrewarding work are more likely to engage in behaviours tending to instant gratification, for example eating sugary and fatty foods. In this type of analysis the role of the health professional is to facilitate institutional and, arguably, political change.

Despite the criticisms detailed above, health professionals should continue to engage companies in their work to promote physical activity. However, more evidence-based practice is needed in the area and the following research agendas should be considered:

- A UK-based research agenda, which develops examples of good practice specific to our cultural setting and corporate structure, is needed.
- There is a need for an interdisciplinary approach combining exercise scientists and health economists to explore both the financial and health benefits of worksite schemes.
- Qualitative work is required to explore the agendas of senior management teams involved in approving or disapproving worksite health-promotion schemes.

Table 4.3 Strengths and weakness of different types of exercise interventions within the workplace

Intervention	Strengths	Weaknesses
In-house exercise facility owned and operated by the company (for example installing a gym within a factory)	1. Helps to overcome the time barrier to exercise 2. Service clearly identified with the company helping to improve the image of management	1. Adherence levels to such initiatives have at times been very low. 2. Costly to set up and run.
Development of a health-promoting company. This would include provision of cycle racks and showers, paying travel mileage for cycling and having a healthy eating canteen	1. Promotes a holistic lifestyle approach which many staff could adopt 2. Ingrains a health policy into all aspects of the company's work	1. Actual action can 'get lost' in well meaning committee meetings and initiatives 2. Calls for long-term senior management support which may not always be forthcoming
Corporate membership to local health clubs, which becomes free at the point of delivery for the company's staff	1. Links the company with specialist providers of exercise services within the community 2. Calls for little commitment from the company's management (except signing an annual cheque!)	1. Experience suggests that only those who are already fit will take up member ships 2. The company may feel that it 'has done its bit' and not develop, for example, a 'healthy eating' policy
Fitness-testing programmes (as used for example by the police and fire brigade)	1. Lays down set standards that staff are asked to meet and which they can compare themselves against 2. Provides a structured opportunity for education and motivation related to exercise and fitness	1. Testing by its nature implies pass and fail. Those who fail may not be motivated to change their behaviour, deciding instead to drop out 2. Fitness testing within a field setting is not always valid and reliable, possibly leading to incorrect results
Visits to the workplace by health-promotion teams to run a lifestyle display with talks and stands	1. Provides an opportunity for staff to focus on health issues and talk to health professionals 2. Builds a bridge and trust between the company and local health professionals	1. The event may raise expectations about exercise opportunities that the company cannot meet 2. May be seen by the management as an easy option

SPORTS AND LEISURE CENTRES

Through the work of local authorities and the Sports Council most urban populations have been provided with either a sports centre or a leisure centre. As we discussed in the introduction, whilst some members of the community feel very much at home in these facilities others can feel out of place because they are 'not the sporty type'. Herein lies the paradox of a habitually sedentary nation within reach of adequate (and even good) facilities. Indeed with the use of National Lottery funding to provide more sports facilitates the number of exercise suites and lifestyle centres is likely to increase. This is not to dispute that more facilities are needed nor that those that exist are not very busy and provide excellent services for many people; rather it is to recognise that sports centres tend to attract people who are already committed to sports and exercise and that these individuals often make many repeat visits, leading to large usage figures for most centres.

The challenge, then, is to encourage those who are sedentary to take the first step and use their local facilities. A number of models can be used.

GP referral schemes

Biddle *et al.* (1993) identified that one form of 'exercise prescription schemes' involved GPs sending patients to structured and supervised exercise programmes in leisure centres. An essential element of this approach is that the GP refers patients he/she thinks will benefit from an exercise intervention. This means that people who would not of their own volition have entered a leisure centre are encouraged to participate by their GP, who is often perceived as a high-status significant other with whom they wish to comply. In a number of schemes this has resulted in leaders finding themselves working with patients with a range of conditions from hypertension to osteoarthritis. This introduction of previously sedentary adults to

a structured and supervised exercise environment is arguably the greatest achievement of GP referral schemes. In short they 'encourage those who do least to do a little bit more'. These programmes are built on good communication and understanding between exercise and health professionals.

Specialist classes and courses

Many leisure centres provide exercise classes that are designed for special populations. Traditionally these have included weight loss classes, 'keep fit for the unfit!' and courses for the over 50s. The major challenge within these schemes is to market them effectively and convince the target audience that the programmes will not be too hard. A number of centres have found innovative ways of doing these – including appropriate timetabling of courses, reducing fees, reinforcement of a group identity and ensuring that exercise leaders are appropriately qualified and trained.

Outreach services

It is pleasing to see that a number of leisure centres have begun to develop outreach services that meet the needs of the wider community. This can take the format of organising exercise classes in the workplace or running community-based charity events. This not only provides more opportunities for people to be active but it may also encourage people to visit the centre.

Health-promoting leisure centres

Whilst leisure centres, by their very nature, have a good track record at promoting physical activity, they sometimes have a less impressive track record in relation to other areas of health promotion. Perhaps you would like to reflect upon your leisure centre's vending machines (chocolate and fizzy drinks?), canteen (chips and sausages?), bar (alcohol and crisps?) and relaxation suite (sunbeds?).

Although not wanting to paint too bleak a picture, particularly given that some leisure centres have tackled these issues admirably, some still have a long way to go.

Sports and leisure centres are undoubtedly a key resource in achieving the goal of 'more people, more active, more often' and many deserve more support and recognition from health professionals. In evidence of this praise, leisure centres actively promote family involvement in sport and exercise. Many provide first-class crèche facilities and run mother and toddler classes. If you're not convinced go down to your local leisure centre on a Sunday morning and look at all the families swimming!

VOLUNTEER COMMUNITY GROUPS AND SPECIAL INTEREST NETWORKS

One of the strengths of British sport is its volunteer workforce who organise, coach and run sports teams and clubs. The Sports Council has done much in recent years to identify and support these groups but their potential remains to be fully exploited by health professionals wishing to promote health-related physical activity. With guidance and perhaps minimum financial support these groups can achieve a great deal in terms of promoting physical activity at a local level.

Recently organisations have developed with a special interest in promoting new activities in a non-competitive way. The case study below illustrates how one such organisation is helping to develop mountain biking for women.

CYBERSPACE COMMUNITIES

It is still too early to say if the claims being made about the impact of the Internet and Cyberspace on how we will live our lives will prove to be true. However, it is a sobering thought that two similarly revolutionary technological developments – the car and the television – have radically altered both the type of social world we live in and the quality and health of our day-to-day lives. Clearly, the Internet and e-mail will continue to transfer information, and it is important to explore ways of exploiting this potential to carry health-promotion messages to sedentary computer users.

Straying nearer to science fiction than exercise science, we may speculate that the future leisure (and even sporting) pursuits of the next generations will be played, not on muddy sports fields but on computer screens and not through physical movement but through virtual reality. This may lead to an even greater number of our children being habitually sedentary. Innovative and positive measures

---

Case Study: 'Women on Wheels'

'Women on Wheels' runs an introductory programme to mountain biking for women. These sessions are run by qualified female coaches and the aim is 'to encourage women of all ages and abilities to just get out on a bike and get active' (Karen Hambly, WOW co-ordinator). The introductory sessions are run over two days with the emphasis being on fun and enjoyment. Whilst most of the course is spent on the bike there is also an introduction to basic mechanics, nutrition and cycling technique. These courses provide an opportunity for women to increase their self-confidence and to ride a mountain bike in a safe and friendly environment.

Acknowledgement: Lucy Darbishire and Karen Hambly.

are needed to prevent those communities bound by information technology from suffering hypokinetic diseases. This means moving away from a 'knee jerk' rejection of all that is new and finding ways in which the new technologies can be put to good use. This may range from programming desktop computers to encourage their users to turn off and take a walk to developing new sports that enable people to interact with their computer through purposeful physical activity.

THE NATION

One way agencies like the Health Education Authority can support health professionals who work with community groups at the local level is through national campaigns. A good example of this type of support is the Active for Life programme. Arguably, the most significant contributions these national campaigns can make is the promotion of a key message. Based on considerable evidence (published in *Moving On*; Health Education Authority, 1995) the Active for Life programme has campaigned on the clear and unambiguous message that people should take 'half an hour's physical activity five times a week'. This was put across in television adverts during peak time viewing shows such as *Coronation Street* and *The Bill*. In addition, a poster campaign and adverts in the popular press ensured that many different target audiences were exposed to the message.

A particularly impressive part of the Active for Life campaign was the briefing days and materials provided to health professionals 'on the ground'. This has ensured that members of the public have been targeted both through the national media and from within their local communities. Surely it is through this combined and reinforcing approach that the public's attitudes and behaviour will change. Another major achievement of the Active for Life campaign has been to put physical activity onto the centre of the health-promotion agenda. Before this initiative there had never

been a national programme to promote physical activity, which may have contributed to the perception of physical activity as a marginal issue dwarfed by the attention that was paid to diet and smoking.

INTERVENTIONS WITH INDIVIDUALS

The section on community-based interventions dealt with how health professionals could work with large groups of people and the locations in which they can find themselves promoting physical activity. However, much of our work is conducted on a one-to-one basis, with a client either in the clinic or at one of the locations described earlier (for example, the workplace). This section will look at the tools available for this one-to-one work, and attempt to evaluate their effectiveness.

1. Fitness testing
2. Exercise counselling and stages of behavioural change
3. Attribution restructuring.

A NOTE ON EVALUATION

As one would expect from a discipline as new as exercise science, information on the effectiveness of a number of intervention strategies is extremely limited. Indeed, at the time of writing the Health Technology Assessment Unit of the NHS is commissioning a major research project investigating the effectiveness of GP referral schemes to exercise courses. When this, and work from other projects, is published we will have a much clearer idea of the best way to promote physical activity. However, at this stage we can make two tentative observations. The first is that most intervention techniques which aim to promote exercise will have a significant (and sometimes dramatic) decay factor – in the weeks just after the interventions the behavioural change recorded will be greater than many months or years later (see Dishman, 1988 for a review of work in this area). The second observation is that health professionals and exercise leaders are using a large number of intervention techniques to promote physical activity to individuals. Leith and Taylor (1992) reviewed 31 studies that had investigated intervention procedures: 22 different techniques had been used and 26 of the studies reported positive results. The types of interventions reported are illustrated in Figure 4.2.

What are we to conclude from the apparent success of so many different intervention strategies? One approach is to try and identify common denominators within the different approaches. With the exception of 'self-monitoring', all bring the client into direct and positive contact with an exercise leader or health professional. It may be that the actual contact time and desire to comply with a significant other is more important than the actual intervention method employed – it may not be what you do, but how you do it!

FITNESS TESTING

It might at first seem a little strange in a section about behavioural change to find an item on fitness testing. However, at the start of many exercise programmes in leisure centres and on GP referral courses clients are inducted to the course via a fitness test. Unfortunately these tests are often justified and designed purely from a physiological perspective with reference to health and safety and the need to find baseline information on which to prescribe the frequency, intensity and duration of the programme. These are important reasons for fitness testing but, to ensure that a proper context is achieved, they should be combined with an understanding of the motivational dimension. In 1988 the Council of Europe (Committee for the Development of Sport) published the European Test of Physical Fitness (EUROFIT, 1988), which it recommended that every child

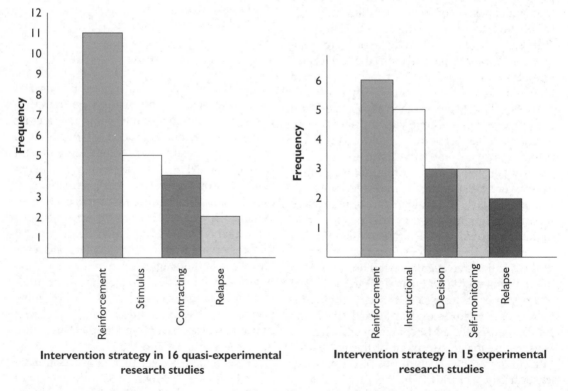

Figure 4.2   Types of interventions identified by Taylor and Leith (1992)

in Europe should undergo on a regular basis. Within this publication it was stated that fitness testing could help children become 'better motivated to maintain or improve his or her fitness'. It is laudable that the EUROFIT project recognised the psychological component of fitness testing but it is inappropriate to suggest that the motivational effect will always be positive. This point can be made quite effectively by reference to an analogue with which many readers will empathise. Remember your worst subject at school; now suppose that your teacher explained that at the start of the new term there was to be a test in that subject. Would you find that motivational? Is it not more likely that the members of the class who were least able at the subject would perceive the test as a threat and even bunk off? If we apply this reasoning to fitness testing do we not identify potential problems for those who perceive themselves as over-fat and unfit? Not only may they be concerned about the prospect of having an exercise leader or a health professional conducting a test which may strike at the very centre of their physical self-esteem (e.g. body composition) but they may worry about the possible discomfort of the test (e.g. an aerobic test).

This critique of fitness testing is not intended to discredit the procedure or recommend that it should not be used. Fitness testing does play an important role in providing some of the background information needed to design safe and effective exercise programmes (see pp. 89 and 99). However, people who run fitness test packages need to reflect closely upon the psychological effect of the test battery. Table 4.4 suggests five steps to better fitness tests.

If fitness testing is conducted for the right reasons by empathic and caring staff it can be both an educational and motivational experience for the client. This is particularly so if a series of tests can be conducted over time to chart progress and to provide a formal appointment at which the exercise leader can talk about adherence and related issues.

EXERCISE COUNSELLING AND STAGES OF BEHAVIOURAL CHANGE

Some exercise programmes begin with a counselling or interview session as well as, or in place of, the more traditional fitness test. The objectives of these sessions are to identify the needs of the client (e.g. to lose weight) and the barriers that they may face (e.g. lack of time) and to suggest strategies to promote adherence (e.g. time management skills). As with any talk-based approach it is important that these sessions have a theoretical basis to give them structure and focus. One approach that has been used is the Stages of Change model (Prochaska and DiClemente, 1984), which suggests that motivation and behaviour can be classified into five stages.

1. *Pre-contemplation:* Individuals at this stage do not intend to change their behaviour and may lack basic knowledge about the health consequences of their actions. Interviews (if the client turns up!) could focus on giving basic knowledge and increasing the client's confidence about their ability to change.
2. *Contemplation*: Individuals at this stage intend to change but have not yet done anything about it. Interviews at this stage would need to build a bridge between positive attitudes and actual behaviour; this may include looking at barriers to exercise.
3. *Preparation*: Individuals at this stage are about to act and may have framed a definite plan of action (that may be why they are having the interview). Interviews at this stage could focus on rewarding the positive steps already taken and setting short-term, realistic and achievable goals to continue the process of change.
4. *Action*: Individuals at this stage have taken the first steps to be active, which defines

Table 4.4 Five steps to better fitness testing

Step	Suggested action	Possible outcome
1. Do not use the term 'fitness test'	Consider terms such as 'lifestyle assessment' or 'health-related fitness profile'	May appear less threatening to sensitive clients and remove connotations of pass and fail
2. Clearly identify and write down the goals of the 'fitness test'	Do not think in terms of measuring fitness unless you are working in a British Association of Sports and Exercise Sciences (BASES) accredited laboratory. Focus on estimating fitness and (perhaps more importantly) educating and motivating the client	Helps you to build a bridge from the 'fitness test' results to new behaviour and a new health-related fitness status
3. Reflect upon your procedure for informing the client about the nature of the 'fitness test'	Ensure that the client under-stands why you want to conduct a 'fitness test' and how they will benefit from the procedure. This can be done by a leaflet which clearly explains that the test is optional and not compulsory	Will ensure that the client under stands what is going to happen to them and gives you the oppor-tunity to correct any misunder-standings. This process may enhance the client's perception of control
4. Ensure that the tests are conducted in a non-threatening manner	Never do a test before explaining exactly what you are going to do. Work hard to create a professional feel without confusing the client with jargon	This action will enhance the client's perception of your professionalism and should lead to a positive experience
5. Review your feedback of results procedure	Avoid comparing the subject's results with national norms that may label them 'poor' or 'average'. Instead, relate the results to the needs of the individual in their everyday life	By appropriate feedback you avoid the problem of 'failing people' or reinforcing the 'I am not the sporty type' barrier

the starter period (which lasts up to six months). Interviews at this stage may need to consider issues related to practical concerns such as muscular stiffness and how to commit to long-term adherence.

5. *Maintenance*: Individuals at this stage have built their new behaviour into their habitual behavioural pattern (at any stage from six months to one year). Interviews at this stage may need to focus on how to manage potential threats that could change normal behavioural patterns (e.g. a new job) and may need to suggest new ways of exercising to promote motivation and stop staleness.

The Stages of Change model is helpful in both identifying the type of support that is needed for the client and in assisting the health professional to set realistic and achiev-able goals for themselves and the client. For example, moving a client's cognitive state from one of pre-contemplation ('what do you mean, I need to exercise?') to preparation ('I have found an exercise class near work!') is a major achievement, which could be over-looked if we evaluated our performance simply in terms of actual behaviour. In other words, the move from pre-contemplation to preparation is a major change in cognitive and motivational orientation but does not involve the client in actually doing any exercise.

As well as being a basis on which to build intervention studies the Stages of Change model has been used extensively in research. Interested readers are directed to Lee (1993), Prochaska *et al.* (1994) and Myers and Roth (1997); these are studies which look at a range of health behaviours, in different populations and make links with other theoretical areas such as attitudes and barriers.

At the time of writing the Stage of Change model and motivational interviewing approaches are very popular, just as fitness testing was in the 1980s. It is interesting to speculate that in the first decade of the new millennium the two approaches may merge to form an induction and ongoing motivational intervention that delivers psychological motivational techniques through a physical medium.

ATTRIBUTION RESTRUCTURING

As we have seen earlier in this chapter, many health professionals are familiar with the need to change attitudes toward physical activity. Fewer may be familiar with the concept of attributions and how they, like attitudes, may alter behaviour. Biddle (1993) defined attributions as 'perceived causes or reasons that people give for an occurrence related to themselves or others.' We are concerned with attributions here because they help us understand how our clients answer the question 'why did I drop out/stick to that exercise course?' The answer may help us to understand future attitudes toward exercise and actual behaviour. We may then be able to use this information to intervene and help the client stick to an active lifestyle.

Attribution Theory has been developed by a line of psychologists – from Heider (1944, 1958) through Kelly (1967) and onto Weiner (1979, 1985), whose work is arguably most important within the present context. Weiner postulated that people explain their behaviour in relation to four attribution elements: ability, task difficulty, effort and luck. Weiner's work suggests that if you ask a patient why they dropped out of your exercise programme their response should be classifiable into one of these four dimensions. Each dimension can be ascribed certain characteristics which relate to its locus of causality (does the person have control over it or is it external?) and its stability (does it change over time?).

- *Ability*: Internal (related to the person) and stable (it might be determined by genetics or a personality trait).
- *Effort*: Internal (you decide how hard you will try) and unstable (sometimes you try hard, sometimes you don't).
- *Task difficulty*: Stable (walking a mile does not get any shorter) and external (outside the person's control).
- *Luck*: Unstable (sometimes you win, sometimes you lose) and external (you have no control over it).

Theoretically we can argue that a person who attributes their adherence to an exercise programme to their ability and effort will be more likely to stick to it in the long term than an individual who attributes their current attendance to task difficulty and luck. In other words it is best to attribute to dimensions that are internal and over which you have control. However, Weiner's work has been criticised for ascribing characteristics to the four dimensions (internal/external and stable/unstable) and assuming that all subjects agree with this classification. For example some people might disagree with the view that 'ability' is internal and stable and argue that ability can be changed even in the short term.

Qualitative work by Smith and Biddle (1991) has shown that adherers and dropouts from a private-sector health club made attributions that could be categorised into each of Weiner's attribution dimensions and which gave an insight into their motivational perspective. A selection of these statements is shown below.

- *Ability*: 'I have been suffering from health problems for the past year, which have restricted my physical activities and will do so for the immediate future.'
- *Effort*: 'I believe I have adopted a sedentary lifestyle basically because I am lazy.'
- *Task difficulty*: 'I have yet to find any exercise which I enjoy. If I did, I would do more. I do particularly enjoy competitive sports but I am a very bad loser, which defeats any stress relief from the activity.'
- *Luck*: 'The amount of time I have spent/will spend on physical activity is directly governed by work and family commitments.'

Quantitative research by Smith and Biddle (1991) has also shown that adherers and non-adherers to an exercise programme have significantly different attributional perspectives (differing most in relation to effort and task difficulty) – so what can be done to restructure unhelpful attributions? A number of suggestions are given in Table 4.5.

As well as restructuring the attributions of their patients, health professionals may also need to restructure the attributions they make to explain the behaviour of others. For example, if a health professional thinks that a person has dropped out of a programme because of 'lack of effort' but the patient attributes their drop out to 'lack of physical ability' it is likely that they will talk at cross-purposes and not agree on the best way forward.

CONCLUDING REFLECTIONS

Despite the large amount of evidence to show that habitual physical activity is related to good health very few people exercise. To take us to a healthier future through physical activity we need to get 'more people, more active, more often'. To do this, health professionals must continue to develop their role and competence in promoting both the uptake and long-term adherence to physical activity. In

Table 4.5   Attributional restructuring

Attributional statement	Comment	Suggested change
Ability: 'I'm just not the right shape to exercise ... I was born with big bones'	This internal and stable attribution implies that the client can take no action which would help them stick to an active lifestyle	Move to 'There are lots of different types of physical activity which cater for lots of different body shapes. What I need to do is find one that suits me'
Effort: 'When I get home from work I feel too lazy to put any effort into exercise'	This is an internal but unstable attribution that implies the client is taking responsibility for their own behaviour. This is a good starting point for action	'I do feel lazy of a night so perhaps that's not the best time for me to exercise. I feel wide awake and motivated in the morning so perhaps I should try and jog in the park before breakfast'
Task difficulty: 'I tried jogging but it was too hard and made my knees hurt so I decided exercise is not for me'	This is an external and stable attribution related to the physical stress of one activity	'Jogging might have been a difficult task for me so perhaps I should try swimming, which is a very different type of exercise'
Luck: 'My boss is very erratic and she keeps altering my workload, which makes establishing an exercise routine very difficult'	This statement implies that the subject's exercise behaviour is controlled by someone else and is outside their control	'My boss may be erratic but I need to be assertive and establish those bits of the day which are special and which can only be used for what I think is important'

light of the important role health professionals will have in developing active communities and individuals the following points may help you to reflect more closely on the individual role you can play.

- Research by Smith (1997) shows that 36% of the variance in the intention of health professionals to promote physical activity is explained by their perceived behavioural control (confidence) and their personal attitudes. As confidence often comes from training these results suggest the importance of exercise science courses for health professionals.
- The same research (Smith, 1997) showed that out of a sample of 83 health professionals involved in promoting physical activity a sizeable minority (32%) were sedentary. Although it may be unscientific to draw conclusions from this simple statistic our clients may be less sympathetic in reaching their own conclusions if we don't practise what we preach.
- In a systematic review of the few randomised controlled trials published Hillsdon and Thorogood (1996) showed that people exercise more if they are regularly followed up and contacted.

Ending on a positive note, if we know that people need regular prompts to stay active can we not harness the new information technologies which threaten so many people with inactive lifestyle, and use them as a means of staying in touch with our clients?

REFERENCES

Allied Dunbar National Fitness Survey (1992). London: Sports Council and Health Education Authority.

Armstrong, N. *et al.* (1990). Patterns of physical activity among 11 to 16 year old British children. *British Medical Journal*, **301**, 203–205

Armstrong, N. and Sparkes, A.C. (1991). *Issues in physical education.* London: Cassel.

Azjen, I. (1985). From intention to actions: A theory of planned behaviour. In *Action Control: From cognitions to behaviour*, Kuhl, J. and Beckmann, J. (eds). Heidelberg: Springer; 11–39.

Bandura, A. (1986). Self-efficacy: Toward a unifying theory of behavioural change. *Psychology Review*, **84**, 191–215.

Biddle, S.J.H. (1993). Attribution research and sport psychology. In *Handbook of research on sports psychology*, Singer, R.N. *et al.* (eds). New York: Macmillan; 437–464.

Biddle, S.J.H. (1996). Editorial: Embracing exercise in 'sport' psychology. *Journal of Sports Science*, **14**, 109–110.

Biddle, S.J.H. and Mutrie, N. (1992). *Psychology of physical activity and exercise.* London: Springer–Verlag.

Biddle, S.J.H., Fox, K. and Edmunds, L. (1993.) *Physical activity promotion in primary care. London:* Health Education Authority.

British Medical Association (1992). *Cycling towards health and safety.* Oxford: Oxford University Press.

Bollaret, L., De Knop, P. and Theeboom, M. (1992). *The leisure relevance of a physical education curriculum.* Paper presented at the Olympic Scientific Congress, Benalmadena, Malaga, Spain.

Cale, L. (1997). Promoting physical activity through active schools. *The British Journal of Physical Education.* Spring.

Crone-Grant, D. and Smith, R.A. (1998). Exercise adherence: A qualitative perspective. *Journal of Sports Science*, **16**(1), 75.

Dishman, R.K. and Gettman, L.R. (1980). Psycho-biological influences of exercise adherence. *Journal of Sport Psychology*, **2**, 295–310.

Dishman, R.K. (1988). *Exercise adherence: Its impact on public health.* Champaign, IL: Human Kinetics.

Dishman, R.K. (ed.) (1995). *Advances in exercise adherence.* Champaign, IL: Human Kinetics.

EUROFIT (1988). *'Eurofit' European test of physical fitness.* Rome: Council of Europe Committee for the Development of Sport.

Finch, H. and Morgan, J. (1985). *Attitudes to cycling.* Research Report RR19. Crowthorne: Transport Research Laboratory.

Fishbein, M. and Ajzen, I. (1977). Attitude–behaviour relations: A theoretical analysis and review of the empirical research. *Psychology Bulletin*, **84** (5), 888–918.

Gettman, L.R. (1988). Occupational-related fitness and exercise adherence. In *Exercise adherence: Its impact on public health*, Dishman, R.K. (ed.). Human Kinetics.

Glyptis, S. (1992). Leisure lifestyles: Present and future. In *Physical activity and health*, Norgan, N.

(ed.). Cambridge: Cambridge University Press; 230–245.

Godin, G. (1993). The theories of reasoned action and planned behaviour. Overview of findings, emerging research problems and usefulness for exercise promotion. *Journal of Applied Sport Psychology*, **5**, 141–157.

Health Education Authority (1995) *Promoting physical activity: Guidance for commissioners, purchasers and providers*. London: Health Education Authority.

Heider, F. (1944). Social perception and phenomenal causality. *Psychology Review*, **51**, 358–374.

Heider, F. (1958). *The psychology of interpersonal relations*. New York: Wiley

Hewstone, M. *et al.* (1988). *Introduction to social psychology*. Oxford: Blackwell.

Hillsdon, M. and Thorogood, M. (1996). A systematic review of physical activity promotion strategies. *British Journal of Sports Medicine.*

Jasper, J.M.F. (1978). The nature and measurement of attitudes. In: *Introduction to social psychology: An analysis of individual reaction and response*, Tajfel, H and Fraser, C. (eds). London: Pelican.

Joshi, M. and Smith, G. (1992). Cyclists under threat: a survey of Oxford cyclists' perception of risk. *Health Education Journal*, **51**, 188–191.

Kaplin, R.M. and Atkins, C.J. (1984). Specific efficacy expectations mediate exercise compliance in patients with COPD. *Health Psychology*, **3** (3), 223–242.

Kelly, H.H. (1967). Attribution theory in social psychology. In *Nebraska symposium on motivation*, Levine, D. (ed.). Lincoln, NB: University of Nebraska.

Killoran, A. *et al.* (1995). Who needs to know what? An investigation of the characteristics of the key target groups for the promotion of physical activity in England. In Killoran, A. et al. (eds) *Moving on: International perspectives on promoting physical activity*. London: Health Education Authority.

Lee, C. (1993). Attitudes, knowledge and stages of change: A survey of exercise patterns in older Australian women. *Health Psychology*, **12** (6), 476–480.

Leith, L.M. and Taylor, A.H. (1992). Behaviour modification and exercise adherence: A literature review. *Journal of Sports Behaviour*, **15** (1), 60–74.

(1997) Medicine and Science in Sports and Exercise. A collection of physical activity questionnaires for health related research. vol. 29. no. 6, June 1997.

Messner, M.A. and Sabo, D.F. (eds) (1990). *Sport,* *men and the gender order: Critical feminist perspectives*. Champaign, IL: Human Kinetics.

Mills, M. (1998). A radical approach to health promotion. *Occupational Health Review*, January/February.

Myers, R.S. and Roth, D.L. (1997). Perceived benefits of and barriers to exercise and stage of change adoption in young adults. *Health Psychology*, **16** (3), 277–283.

Powell, K.E. and Dysinger, W. (1987). Childhood participation in organized school sports and physical education as precursors of adult physical activity. *American Journal of Preventative Medicine*, **3**, 276–281.

Prochaska, J.O. and DiClemente, C.C. (1984). *The transtheoretical approach: Crossing traditional boundaries of therapy*. Pacific Grove, CA: Brooks/Cole.

Prochaska, J.O. and Marcus, B.H. (1994). The transtheoretical model: Applications to exercise. In *Advances in exercise adherence*, Dishman, R.K. (ed.). Champaign, IL: Human Kinetics; 161–180.

Prochaska, J.O. *et al.* (1994). Stages of change and decisional balance for 12 problem behaviours. *Health Psychology*, **13** (1), 39–46.

Redmond, G. (1987). Historical aspects of fitness in the modern world. In: *Physical activity in early and modern populations*, Malina, R.M. and Eckert, H.M. (eds). Champaign, IL: Human Kinetics.

Roberston, N. and Mutrie, N. (1989). Factors in adherence to exercise. *Physical Education Review*, **12**, 138–146.

Sallis, J.F. and Hovell, H.F. (1990). Determinants of exercise behaviour. *Exercise and Sport Reviews*, **18**, 307–330.

Sallis, J.F. (1993). Epidemiology of physical activity and fitness in children and adolescents. *Critical Reviews in Food Science and Nutrition*, **33**, 403–408.

Somerset Health Authority (1992). *The Somerset Lifestyle Survey 1992*. Taunton: Somerset Health Authority.

Shepherd, R.J. (1988) Exercise adherence in corporate settings: Personal traits and program barriers. In *Exercise adherence: its impact on public health*, Dishman, R.K. (ed.). Champaign, IL: Human Kinetics.

Smith, R.A. (1997). Health professional attitudes toward physical activity. *Proceedings of the British Association of Sport and Exercise Annual Conference 1997, York.* Abstract published in *Journal of Sports Sciences*, **16**, 1998.

Smith, R.A. and Biddle, S.J.H. (1991). Psychology and the promotion of physical activity and exercise. In: *Exercise and sport psychology: A European perspective,* Biddle, S.J.H. (ed.). Champaign, IL: Human Kinetics.

Sparkes, A.C. (1989). Health related fitness: An example of innovation without change. *British Journal of Physical Education,* **20** (2), 60–63.

Surgeon General (1997). *Physical Activity and Health.* Washington, DC: US Government.

Weiner, B. (1979). A theory of motivation for classroom experiences. *Journal of Education Psychology,* **71**, 3–25.

Weiner, B. (1985). 'Spontaneous' causal thinking. *Psychology Bulletin,* **97**, 74–84.

Wigmore, S. (1996). Gender and sport: The last 5 years. *Sport Science Review.* **5** (2), 53–71.

THE PRINCIPLES OF EXERCISE PRESCRIPTION

5

THE EFFECTS OF DIFFERENT TYPES OF EXERCISE

Most forms of exercise will involve all the major components of fitness to a greater or lesser extent: muscular strength, joint mobility/flexibility, cardiovascular/aerobic fitness and muscular endurance. The classification of an exercise as being, for example, aerobic or strengthening really refers to its primary effects, which may not always be the sole benefit. For example, a particular exercise may have the primary objective of increasing hip mobility but it may also enhance the strength of the muscles around that joint. Similarly, press-ups are primarily prescribed to enhance arm and shoulder strength, yet they may also enhance the strength/endurance of the abdominal muscles which have to work as fixators throughout the exercise. The situation becomes even more complex when the exercise session is activity based, as in the case of swimming or gardening: such activities will have many effects upon numerous aspects of fitness (joint mobility, strength, endurance and cardiovascular fitness) and involve different parts of the body. A further aspect to be considered is the effect of exercise upon proprioception, kinesthetic awareness and the learning of motor skills; learning to control the lowering of a weight on a multigym or pedalling a cycle ergometer can provide great benefits to those with motor learning difficulties.

It is also important not to forget the psychological implications of exercise participation. Many individuals derive great benefits and much pleasure from the participation in exercise, whether in the context of therapy, social activity or competitive sport.

THE PRINCIPLES OF EXERCISE AND FITNESS TRAINING

When discussing the effects of exercise upon the body and suggesting appropriate exercises, certain principles need to be considered. With some slight modification these principles are appropriate for anyone participating in exercise, ranging from the patient recovering from myocardial infarction or stroke to the elite athlete rehabilitating from a strained muscle. The rigour with which these principles are applied in an exercise programme will depend upon the individual circumstances. For example, when rehabilitating after an injury restoration of physical capacity will be of primary concern in the short term and the optimum physical programme should be devised to do this, even if the client does not find it very enjoyable. However, if the programme has more long-term objectives such as modifying an individual's lifestyle to one which is more active, then the issues of motivation and long-term adherence will be of vital importance. The content of a programme for such a client should be adjusted to include exercise sessions which will maintain their interest, produce some benefit and be enjoyable, rather than insisting upon a monotonous set of exercises which might be slightly better physiologically but which the individual does not enjoy and will give up. The principles of exercise prescription will be discussed under the following headings:

- The training effect
- Overload
- Specificity
- Intensity
- Duration
- Frequency
- Dose-adaptation response
- Recovery
- Progression
- Reversibility
- Motivation and adherence

These principles are applicable in a variety of situations, including applied activities as well as the fitness gym or clinical setting where they may be used by the physiotherapist, nurse and occupational therapist. In the wider context of exercise prescription the physiological aspects must be combined with the psychological issues of motivation and adherence. After all, even the most well designed 'physiological' exercise programme will not be effective if the client is unmotivated and drops out after a few weeks. The points made in Chapters 3 and 4 should be considered when reading this section.

THE TRAINING EFFECT

Appropriate forms of exercise stimulate the body to improve its physical capacity. If an appropriate form of exercise is repeated often enough it will promote long-term adaptations to the exercise: this is called the 'training effect'. The type of adaptations, and hence the training effect induced by the exercise, are very specific to the form of exercise undertaken. For example:

- strengthening exercises will stimulate the muscles and tendons to adapt by becoming stronger;
- aerobic exercises will stimulate improvement in the cardiovascular system by changes in the condition of the heart, blood, blood vessels and even the muscles themselves;

- stretching exercises improve an individual's flexibility and joint mobility.

Training effects may be observed within days or weeks of commencing an exercise programme. The rapidity and extent of the improvement will depend upon a number of factors, including the nature of the exercises being undertaken and the condition of the participant.

OVERLOAD

Overload refers to the principle that, for the physical condition to improve, the body must experience a suitable amount of physical stress. Typically, this stress would be greater than that usually encountered in a more sedentary existence. Overload is required to develop any component of fitness, including flexibility/joint mobility, muscular strength and cardiovascular/aerobic fitness.

To improve an individual's flexibility/joint mobility the muscles and tendons must be stretched and the joint must be moved through a greater range of motion than it would normally encounter in everyday life. This can be achieved by specific exercises, which may be performed with the assistance of another person or external object.

The principle of overload can also be illustrated in the development or maintenance of muscular strength. In order for a muscle to maintain its strength it must be used; if it is not used it will lose strength and may atrophy. This is most clearly illustrated when a limb is immobilised and put in a cast, as occurs in, for example, the case of a broken leg. For a muscle or group of muscles to gain strength they must be exercised more intensively. This can be achieved with the use of exercise machines, free weights or exercises that require the muscles to work against the resistance of the individual's body weight. The exact nature of the exercises needed will depend upon the individual's physical condition. Examples are given in Chapter 8.

For cardiovascular and aerobic fitness, overload is applied by increasing the muscle's demand for oxygen and energy for a prolonged period by sustained rhythmic activities such as walking, swimming, jogging and cycling. The body responds to these activities by making the cardiovascular system work harder – by raising the heart rate, stroke volume, cardiac output and pulmonary ventilation. Repeating this form of activity will induce long-term adaptations in the cardiovascular system and muscles.

SPECIFICITY

The specificity of an exercise or exercise programme relates to a number of exercise factors.

The improvements in physical condition are almost exclusively observed in the parts of the body that are being exercised and hence experiencing overload. For example, arm exercises will improve the strength of the arm muscles but not that of the leg muscles. Similarly, exercising the right side of the body will not significantly improve the condition of the left, although there may be a slight effect due to an improvement in the neurological signals being sent from the central nervous system.

The type of training effects produced by the exercise are specific to that type of exercise. In practical terms this means that in order to develop muscular strength strengthening exercises are needed: loosening and joint mobility exercises will not improve strength. Similarly, cardiovascular fitness will only develop from exercises that overload the cardiovascular system. When planning an exercise programme these factors should be borne in mind. However, it should also be noted that many forms of physical activity use a combination of strength, flexibility and cardiovascular fitness and will therefore physically stress the body in a number of different ways – and may enhance all three aspects of fitness. This is especially true in the case of activity-based exercises such as swimming or remedial gymnastics.

Specificity also refers to the way in which muscles are used. For instance, exercising the biceps through a limited range of motion: by doing biceps curls from a fully extended elbow to one that is flexed at 90° may improve the strength of the biceps through this particular range of motion but may not have such a substantial effect upon their strength through the range of motion from 90° to full elbow flexion. Specificity also refers to the speed with which the muscles are contracted and the sequence in which they are used to produce a particular movement. Hence, to improve a particular movement, the muscles must be used and exercised through the required range at the required speed. However, during the early stages of training and/or rehabilitation it is often advisable to break a movement down into its component parts and target a specific weakness, perhaps via isometric contractions, then slow isotonic contractions, before increasing the speed and introducing any eccentric loading. This has specific implications for therapists rehabilitating individuals with an injury, as the exercise programme must progress gradually from slow controlled movements up to full speed over a period of weeks. Attempting to work the muscles at maximum speed too early in a rehabilitation programme is likely to result in re-injury because the tissues will not be able to withstand the stresses of the movement.

INTENSITY

Intensity refers to the degree of difficulty of the exercise. In terms of strengthening exercises lifting a light object or pushing against a slight resistance would be considered as a low-intensity exercise; lifting a heavy object or pushing against a large resistance would be considered as a high-intensity exercise. The concept of intensity can also be applied to aerobically based exercises. For instance, walking, swimming or cycling at a relatively slow, easy pace would be considered as low intensity whereas running, cycling or swimming fast, where the individual really has to work hard, would be considered as high-intensity exercise.

Exercise intensity may be expressed as an 'absolute' exercise intensity or a relative exercise intensity (REI). An absolute exercise intensity is a defined numerical value – for example, a specific power output of 200 W, or a running speed of 17 km h^{-1}, or a resistance of 60 kg. A 'relative' intensity is proportional (relative) to an individual's current level of fitness: this might be 60% of an individual's VO$_{2max}$, 80% of the maximum weight they can lift, or 75% of their maximum power. The use of relative exercise intensity in many exercise prescription contexts helps to ensure that individuals experience the desired level of physiological stress (and hence exercise benefits). For example, two people doing a set of 12 arm-strengthening exercises at 60% of maximum should experience similar levels of fatigue and a similar training effect, regardless of the actual weight they are moving. Contrast this with the situation whereby both were asked to lift 40 kg. One might find this very easy and gain no benefit, the other might find it too heavy to lift and also gain no benefit. Similarly, a running speed of 12 km h^{-1} may be very easy for an elite athlete (who would rate it as a low intensity), whilst an unfit individual would find it very fast and rate it as a very high intensity. If, however, they were both told to run at a speed corresponding to 70% of their aerobic capacity the fitter runner might run at 14 km h^{-1} and the less fit one at 7 km h^{-1} – but they would gain similar benefits from the activity. This emphasises the point that it is important for any form of exercise to be pitched at an appropriate intensity for the individual concerned because the same exercise may be too easy for some and too difficult for others. In summary, any exercise programme needs to be 'personalised' or 'individualised' to ensure that it is appropriate.

It is also common to express intensity in terms of 'multiples of the individual's basal metabolic rate' (METS). An exercise/activity which increases a person's metabolic rate by 3 would be described as an intensity of 3 METS and an exercise which resulted in a sevenfold increase in metabolic rate, 7 METS. Very fit individuals may be able to work at up to 10 METS, whereas the maximum for less fit individuals may be around 3–6 METS.

DURATION, REPETITIONS AND SETS

The duration of an exercise refers to how long it lasts. The duration of aerobically based exercises tend to be recorded in terms of time or distance. The duration of an exercise is often linked to its intensity, since high-intensity exercises cannot be maintained for as long as low-intensity exercises. A simple example would be that of cycling – an individual may be able to sprint (high intensity) for only a few seconds before becoming fatigued and having to slow down but if they were to pedal more slowly (low intensity) they would be able to continue the exercise for far longer.

When performing stretching exercises an individual may be advised to hold the stretched position for 15 seconds.

In some forms of exercise repetitions are more applicable than duration; for example, when performing strengthening exercises it may be appropriate to recommend that an exercise is repeated 20 times rather than suggesting that it should be continued for a duration of, say, 30 seconds. Both duration and repetitions can be used to determine the length of time spent on the exercise, but in practical terms it is often easier to count repetitions. This could also be true of an activity such as swimming, when specifying the number of lengths may be the most practical way of prescribing a duration (provided that the length of the pool is known).

Some forms of exercise, especially strengthening exercises, need to be of a fairly high intensity if they are to be effective. This means that the duration of the exercise will be relatively short, i.e. only relatively few repetitions will be achieved before fatigue ensues and the participant needs to rest. Since a single short bout of a particular exercise is unlikely to convey any substantial benefits the bout will need to be repeated. This is achieved by incorporating 'sets' into an exercise session. The participant will complete a number of specified repetitions of one exercise (one set), rest and then repeat the exercise. For example, if someone was to step up and down on a step 30 times, rest, repeat the exercise, rest and then repeat the exercise again this would be described as 'three sets of 30 repetitions'. Strengthening, mobility and stamina exercise sessions can all be organised in this manner to optimise their effectiveness.

FREQUENCY

The frequency refers to how often an individual performs an exercise session; for example, three times a week or twice a day. The frequency of an exercise session will depend upon numerous factors, including the content of the session, the condition of the individual and the other demands of his or her lifestyle.

DOSE–ADAPTATION RESPONSE

The dose–adaptation response is the relationship between the amount of exercise/physical activity performed and the responses/adaptations of the individual to that exercise. For most physiological adaptations a larger dose of exercise will evoke a greater response/adaptation; for example, more aerobic exercise will induce greater improvements in aerobic fitness. However, this relationship may not be simple, and it is also possible that different health factors could have a different dose–adaptation response relationship. For example, lipid profiles, blood pressure and fibrinolytic factors may not adapt equally to the same dose of exercise. The link between

activity and coronary health is not linear but curvilinear, greatest improvements in health being attained when changing from doing no activity to doing some. Further increases in activity produce additional benefits but of lesser magnitude: at very high levels of activity little or no additional coronary health benefits are observed beyond those attained from more moderate exercise regimens. Therefore for some factors there may be a 'ceiling' to the dose–response relationship. Conversely, for other factors a threshold level of activity may be required before any responses/adaptations are observed. This threshold could be the total amount of exercise, or the amount above a certain intensity, or the amount above a particular intensity after a certain duration. It is also possible to overdose on exercise, additional exercise beyond a defined limit having adverse rather than beneficial effects.

Initially much of our understanding of the dose–adaptation response, and consequently our prescription for healthy exercise, was based upon observations of athletic individuals training for athletic performance. During the last 20 years our appreciation and understanding of the subtle differences between training for sport and physical activity for health has developed but many questions still remain unanswered. For further details see the reviews by Haskell (1994) and Shephard (1997). However, many of the questions raised in Shephard's review remain to be resolved.

RECOVERY

Recovery can refer to rest periods taken within an exercise session, and/or to the rest interval between exercise sessions: both are important. In exercise sessions that include sets of relatively high-intensity exercise the recovery periods are required to allow the body to remove waste products from the muscles and restore itself to a condition that will enable it to repeat the exercise. The exact nature and duration of the recovery period will depend upon the nature of the exercise session and the condition of the participant. Recovery within an exercise session may be passive or active. A 'passive' recovery will take the form of a complete rest. An 'active' recovery may take the form of a period of relatively low-intensity exercise that is sufficiently easy to enable the body to recover or a different exercise. For example, during a strength training session participants may exercise their upper body and allow those muscles to recover while they exercise their leg muscles, after which they may again exercise their upper body. This form of recovery maximises the amount of time spent exercising within a session.

Recovery between exercise sessions is also important. As a general rule, the more intensive the exercise the longer the recovery period required. Relatively low-intensity exercise can be repeated daily; high-intensity exercise can put a large amount of stress upon the body, and up to 48 hours may be required to recover. Repeating the exercise session before the body has fully recovered is likely to result in the rapid onset of fatigue and may therefore reduce the effectiveness of the session. Repeatedly exercising without adequate recovery can lead to over-fatigue, which will reduce rather than increase the body's physical capacity, and may lead to overuse injuries.

PROGRESSION

When the body is subjected to an appropriate physical overload it will respond by adapting to the physical demands placed upon it. If the exercise is of an appropriate type, intensity, duration and frequency, distinct physical improvements will occur. These improvements increase the individual's ability to cope with the same type of exercise. The exercise will thus become easier and, as a result, will begin to have less of an 'overload' effect. This is fine if the desired level of activity and fitness has been reached but if improvement is to continue the exercise sessions will need to be altered so that they once again place an appropriate amount of overload upon the individual. This is referred

to as *progression*. Progression, or a 'progressive overload', can be achieved through a number of alterations to an exercise programme. In practice, it can be implemented by manipulating one or more variables in the exercise programme: by altering the intensity (walking faster or lifting heavier weights) or the duration (by lengthening the time spent exercising and/or the number of repetitions and sets included within the session). Further means of applying progression include increasing the frequency of the exercise, reducing the recovery time, adding extra exercises or swapping the exercises for more difficult versions (this would have the added advantage of providing variety in the programme). In summary, progression may be achieved by altering one or a combination of factors, with the exact means of progression depending upon the individual circumstances. Examples of progression are given in each of the chapters that describe the different forms of exercise.

In all situations it is important for progression to be gradual. If progression is too rapid the new level of overload will be too demanding. Too much overload will reduce the benefits of the exercise and in some cases may even be detrimental, as frequently happens when an individual tries to do too much too soon. For example, an individual can strain a muscle when trying to lift a weight that is too heavy, or may develop an overuse injury by exercising for too long. Overuse injuries can also occur if the frequency of sessions is increased to the extent that the body does not have enough time to recover between bouts. However, on a positive note, by applying a steady gradual progressive overload that is within the capabilities of the participant and basing any further adjustments on perceptions of physical strain or undue fatigue such occurrences will be prevented.

REVERSIBILITY

Reversibility refers to the fact that if a body part or system (such as a muscle or the cardiovascular system) is not used, or if the amount of work it performs is substantially reduced for a period of days or weeks, then its physical capacity will decline. In simple terms this means that if someone stops exercising for a prolonged period his or her physical capacity will be diminished. In the case of strengthening exercises, if an individual stops exercising the muscles will become weaker. Similar effects can also be observed with the flexibility and stamina aspects of fitness.

The rate of reversibility will depend upon the individual and his or her physical condition. However, since a noticeable reversal in physical condition will not manifest itself for days, or even weeks, the relatively short period required for full recovery from an exercise session (perhaps a few days) will not cause a person's physical capacity to decline. Health also has an element of reversibility; individuals who had an active lifestyle 10 or more years ago but have since become sedentary exhibit health risks similar to those of people who were not as active in their youth.

MOTIVATION AND ADHERENCE

The exercise practitioner must always be aware that exercise prescription cannot be based solely on physiological factors. Prescription of optimal activities, intensities and durations will be completely ineffective unless the individual decides to undertake the exercise session. Participants will only benefit from exercise if they are sufficiently motivated to adhere to the regimen of prescribed activities. Therefore the practitioner must take these considerations into account when designing a programme and presenting it to their patient. Details of these issues are discussed more fully in Chapter 4.

WHAT IS HEALTH-RELATED FITNESS?

According to Bouchard and Shephard (1994), 'Health related fitness refers to those components of fitness which relate to health status.'

Table 5.1 Components of fitness that relate to health status (Bouchard and Shephard, 1994)

Morphological components:
  Body mass for height
  Body composition
  Subcutaneous fat distribution
  Abdominal visceral fat
  Bone density
  Flexibility
Muscular components:
  Power
  Strength
  Endurance
Motor components:
  Agility
  Balance
  Co-ordination
  Speed of movement
Cardiorespiratory components:
  Sub-maximal exercise capacity
  Maximal aerobic power
  Heart functions
  Lung functions
  Blood pressure
Metabolic components:
  Glucose tolerance
  Insulin sensitivity
  Lipid and lipoprotein metabolism
  Substrate oxidation characteristics

In their consideration of the topic they list a number of components (Table 5.1).

Therefore when planning an exercise programme the range of potential objectives and goals, along with diversity of responses and adaptations, must be remembered. Different individuals will require different programmes to achieve different goals and may respond/ adapt in different ways and to a different extent. Knowing the details of their current physiological condition and state of health may help to predict the potential adaptations, but until further research sheds greater light on the topic very precise prescriptions remain elusive. Therefore the skill and knowledge of the exercise adviser is essential in their ability to respond to their client's needs and individual circumstances.

PLANNING AND INDIVIDUALISING AN EXERCISE PROGRAMME

The aims of an exercise programme can be complex: it may be undertaken to improve, to maintain or to minimise the deterioration of an individual's condition. Similarly an exercise programme may be implemented with the intention of conveying various psychological and/or sociological benefits. Regardless of the kind of exercise programme being embarked upon or the reasons for prescribing it, it should be designed with specific short-term and long-term goals. Short-term goals are usually set over a period of 6–8 weeks and provide the participant with something to aim for. They also give the programme a point of focus rather than letting it remain a series of exercise sessions with no apparent direction. Setting out the exercise sessions for the next few weeks in a written format helps to clarify the programme for both the participant and their adviser and can have the added psychological benefits of demonstrating the direction and progression of the programme to the participant.

It is often useful to commence an exercise programme by assessing the participant's current physical condition. Depending upon the goals of the programme this assessment could include measuring their mobility at different joints, assessing the response of their heart and cardiovascular system to exercise and assessing the strength of particular muscles. It could also involve more detailed assessments, including those of a medical nature if the situation warrants, such as the measurement of haematological and cardiac factors. Assessments that are undertaken in an objective and quantitative manner may provide very valuable information which can be used immediately to design the initial programme and referred to later to provide a means of monitoring the effectiveness of the programme and modify it when necessary.

The overall effect should be to produce a programme which includes exercise of an appropriate type with suitable levels of intensity, duration, frequency and overload and which will therefore be far more effective than a random series of exercise sessions that lack appropriate specificity and progression. A more detailed coverage of the uses and benefits of physiological assessments is presented in Chapter 6.

In the short term, most exercise programmes should be planned for a period of about 6–8 weeks since this is the duration over which some distinct improvements can be expected. However, within this time span the programme should be dynamic and subject to any changes he or she feels necessary. Changes may be necessary if the individual finds the exercise programme too easy or a complication (such as a minor illness) may require the programme to be interrupted and then modified to make it easier in the weeks immediately following the illness. Modifications may also be precipitated by factors such as the participant's personal likes or dislike and motivation.

To maximise the benefits, an exercise programme must be specific to the individual's condition, needs, likes, dislikes and goals. For example, an exercise programme for a 55-year-old man who is rehabilitating after a heart attack will be different from that of a 22-year-old woman who is recovering from a broken leg. Personal likes and dislikes affect motivation and are especially important when the individual may be asked to undertake parts of a programme unsupervised. If someone dislikes the prescribed programme they are less likely to adhere to it. This is important if the exercise adviser is seeking to produce a lifestyle change in their client. In some cases it is, of course, not always possible to give someone a programme that is 'enjoyable' but possible options and alternatives can be discussed with the participant. The ease of access to exercise facilities, such as a gym or swimming pool, will also have some bearing upon the precise content of a programme.

WARMING UP AND COOLING DOWN

Warming up and cooling down are very important aspects of any exercise session and should never be neglected. Warming up is the preparatory phase at the beginning of an exercise session. It generally involves a few minutes of low-intensity exercise that prepares the body for the more strenuous aspects of the session. It has an important role in reducing the risk of injury. The cooling down phase involves a short period of low-intensity exercise at the end of the exercise session which gradually returns the body to its 'resting state'. It is believed to reduce the chances of muscular soreness occurring the day after an exercise session and also reduces the risk of fainting or collapsing at the end of a strenuous exercise session.

WARMING UP

All exercise sessions should commence with a warm-up period. In some cases this may take the form of a distinct series of preparatory exercises; in other sessions it will simply involve performing the activity at a relatively low intensity before gradually increasing the intensity to the desired level. A warm-up period is important for the following reasons.

- Cold muscles, tendons and connective tissues do not stretch very easily. Stretching without a warm-up is therefore unlikely to be beneficial. Warming up also relaxes the muscles, which allows them to be stretched more effectively. It is also believed that cold muscles and tendons are more prone to tear as they are less elastic.
- In the case of aerobic-type exercises, a warm-up prepares the cardiovascular system and muscles for the activity. A warm-up gradually increases the heart rate. If a participant attempts to perform strenuous activity without an adequate warm-up cardiac arrhythmias (irregular activity of the heart) can occur, even in those without heart disease.

- A warm-up diverts the blood to the exercising muscles. The blood vessels leading to the working muscles dilate (enlarge) whilst those leading to the parts of the body not involved in the exercise, such as those leading to the gut, constrict. In this way the blood is diverted towards 'priority' areas such as the muscles that require an increased supply of oxygen during exercise.
- Attempting to exercise strenuously without a warm-up may result in the muscles having to work without an adequate supply of oxygen, forcing them to use anaerobic processes to supplement ATP production. As a consequence, lactic acid accumulates and the muscles may become fatigued at an exercise intensity that they would be quite capable of sustaining had they been adequately warmed up.
- A warm-up increases the temperature of the body. This speeds up many of the processes associated with exercise metabolism: the rate of nerve impulse transmission, the rate of oxygen delivery to the muscles and the speed of the reactions associated with ATP production. Therefore, a warm-up may be said to optimise the condition of the body, preparing it for the strenuous physical activity to follow.
- In the case of strengthening exercises a warm-up prepares the muscles for the physical demands of the exercise by increasing their temperature. This increases the rate of ATP production and reduces the risk of muscles being damaged by over-stretching when cold.

In general terms the warm-up prepares the body for the exercise that follows. It optimises the participant's physical condition, enabling them to cope more easily with the demands of the activity. It also enables them to obtain the most benefit from the exercise session. The warm-up can also be used to re-familiarise the participant with the content of the session, especially if it includes specific movements that will be used in the main part of the session.

A typical warm-up will involve some gentle 'loosening' exercises, followed by a few minutes of low-intensity aerobic activity, and then a series of preparatory stretching exercises. It may last for 5–10 minutes, depending upon the intensity of the session that follows. During the warm-up the participant usually wears additional clothing to ensure that their overall body and muscle temperature is sufficiently elevated. The loosening exercises at the start of the warm-up can include activities such as 'heel raises' and 'shoulder circling' (see Chapter 9). These are gentle activities which begin to prepare the body for exercise and are especially important if the participant has been inactive for a while, as would be the case if he or she had just got out of a car or had been sitting at a desk for some time.

The aerobic component of a warm-up may involve a low-intensity activity such as cycling on an exercise cycle, walking around the room or some modified exercise for those unable to walk. This increases the heart rate, stroke volume and ventilation; it also diverts a greater proportion of the blood (cardiac output) to the exercising muscles and raises their overall temperature, increasing the supply of oxygen to the muscles and preparing the heart for more strenuous activity.

Stretching exercises (the final phase of a warm-up) ensure that the muscles and tendons are prepared for the exercise to come. An important reason for stretching is to prevent overstretching the muscles and tendons during the session. This aspect of the warm-up will also prepare the joints for physical activity, preventing or minimising any joint problems.

In some cases the final stage of the warm-up will include performing part of the exercise session at a low intensity. For example, if the session involves the use of weights a person may do a few repetitions of very light weights as part of the final warm-up or, if the session involves cycling on an exercise cycle, the person may spend the first few minutes pedalling against a very light resistance.

COOLING DOWN

The cool-down is a short period at the end of an exercise session during which time the metabolic activity of the body is gradually reduced almost to its resting level. Therefore the cool-down often involves a period of low-intensity aerobic exercise, followed by a few gentle stretching exercises. This has a number of effects:

- The gentle aerobic activity helps to get rid of any metabolic waste products that may have accumulated during the exercise session. Various research studies have demonstrated that gentle active recovery is better in achieving this than simply stopping the exercise (a passive recovery). The benefits of an active recovery are believed to be related to the muscles continuing to receive oxygenated blood, which will also assist the removal of metabolic waste products.

- The cool-down assists the general functioning of the cardiovascular system. During exercise the blood is pumped more rapidly around the body by the increased action of the heart. Blood from working muscles is assisted in its return to the heart (venous return) by the active contraction of the working skeletal muscles. If a person stops exercising suddenly the heart continues to beat fast, sending blood around the body but, because the exercise has ceased, the blood is no longer assisted in its return to the heart. This is thought to be one of the reasons why people who stop suddenly sometimes feet faint immediately after the exercise. During a cool-down the heart rate is gradually lowered to its resting level and the venous return continues to be assisted by the actively contracting muscles, thereby preventing this problem.

A few minutes after the end of a cool-down the participant's heart rate is unlikely to be completely at its resting level but should be within about 30 beats of what it was before the exercise session started. This will, of course, be influenced by the overall physical condition of the individual and any medication that he or she may be taking. It can also be influenced by the content of the session, more demanding sessions requiring a more prolonged cool-down.

The cool-down period also provides the opportunity for additional stretching exercises, which are especially desirable if they were not included as part of the main session. The inclusion of stretching exercises within the cool-down period not only helps to gradually lower the activity level of the body at the end of the session but it may also prevent stiffness the following day. The cool-down is also likely to be performed when the body is warm, making the muscles responsive to a good stretching routine.

SAFETY CONSIDERATIONS FOR EXERCISE SESSIONS

The overall health, well-being and safety of the participant(s) are paramount in all exercise sessions. A number of factors are important:

- warming up and cooling down;
- use of appropriate clothing and footwear;
- correct exercise technique;
- appropriate progression;
- safety of the equipment and the exercise environment;
- food and drink.

WARMING UP AND COOLING DOWN

The importance of a warm-up and cool-down have already been discussed extensively. In summary, a lack of warm-up may result in premature fatigue, may increase the risk of ruptures and strains and will increase the risk of overuse injuries such as tendonitis. The benefits of a cool-down include gradually returning a number of metabolic and physiological processes to their resting state, reducing the risk of post-exercise dizziness or fainting and reducing the risk of post-exercise soreness.

APPROPRIATE CLOTHING AND FOOTWEAR

In any exercise situation appropriate clothing must be worn. Approximately 71% of the energy used by the body during exercise is released as heat. This is why it is usual to commence a session wearing a number of layers of clothing, some of which may be removed after the warm-up and at appropriate intervals during the session as the participant feels necessary.

In general terms clothing needs to permit movement and facilitate the regulation of body temperature. In a cold environment and/or at the beginning of an exercise session it needs to provide adequate warmth. In a warm environment and/or when the body is generating excess heat the clothing must permit heat loss via the evaporation of sweat and the convection of cool air over exposed skin. In very hot conditions, light clothing can also reduce radiative heat gain from the environment. Whilst exercising for health there is no merit in trying to perspire excessively; this can result in severe dehydration and the associated weight loss is water not fat. This water must be replenished if the body is to remain healthy – therefore the use of plastic sweat suits and similar items is not recommended. Athletes who sometimes wear excess clothing in an attempt to acclimatise for a competition in a hot humid climate must also ensure that they drink copiously; even the most elite are vulnerable to the adverse effects of dehydration.

Clothing must also be appropriate for the activity. Excessively loose garments can become caught in exercise machines or multi-gyms. Some activities will have specific clothing requirements or recommendations, such as safety helmets for cycling or protective glasses for squash.

Appropriate footwear is very important in weight-bearing activities. Wearing inappropriate shoes (or, worse, not wearing shoes at all) can place excessive stresses upon the muscles, bones and joints: adequate cushioning is most desirable. Comfort and protection are the key factors. Even indoors, shoes will protect the feet from grit, abrasions and infection, to which they may otherwise be susceptible. In some activities the wearing of specifically designed footwear will help the individual to cope with the particular stresses of the activity. For example, if taking up jogging then a proper pair of running shoes will provide the greatest protection, especially if they are chosen to suit the individual's running style. This is because particular problems are associated with certain running gaits, such as excessive pronation or supination.

CORRECT EXERCISE TECHNIQUE

Much concern has been expressed over safety during certain forms of exercise. This stems from the knowledge that if certain exercises are performed incorrectly minor injuries can result. This concern covers all forms of exercise, including those used to develop flexibility, strength and muscular endurance. For this reason it is important that the participant always follows the correct technique for all the exercises included in their programme. Demonstrating the exercise is often more informative than describing it, since the participant may visualise an exercise differently to their exercise adviser. This could result in them performing an inappropriate and potentially unsafe exercise when unsupervised. Supervision is especially important during the initial stages of the programme when the participant may be unsure of the exercises prescribed. Inappropriate technique can result in strained muscles and back pain and will be less effective in developing the participant's

physical conditions. These factors are discussed further in Chapters 7–9.

APPROPRIATE PROGRESSION

In any exercise programme it is important that the participant progresses steadily. Improvement in an individual's physical condition provides positive motivation, which may cause him or her to wish to progress more rapidly than is advisable. It should be remembered that any form of exercise, however beneficial, places certain physical stresses upon the body. The body needs time to adapt to these stresses and if progression is too rapid overuse injuries may result. For example, in strength training the force produced by the muscles is conveyed to the bones via the tendons. It is generally believed that the tendons take longer than the muscles to adapt to the stresses of strength training. If the participant progresses at the speed which is dictated by the increased strength in their muscles they may exceed the capability of their tendons. This could overstress the tendons, resulting in injuries such as tendonitis or (in extreme cases) rupture. It is therefore up to the adviser to design an exercise programme which is progressive, and which the participant sees as being progressive, yet does not progress too rapidly. Gradual progression should include the duration, intensity and frequency of the exercise.

SAFETY OF THE EQUIPMENT AND THE EXERCISE ENVIRONMENT

Safety of the equipment involves a multitude of factors, most of which will be highlighted by the manufacturer. It will include the requirements for regular servicing, oiling of moving parts, ensuring that weights are securely fixed by collars and that the participants cannot hurt themselves on moving parts. Other safety factors include the use of mats for floor exercises such as sit-ups and the use of the correct keys (not makeshift alternatives) when using multigym equipment.

A further concern is the safety of the environment itself. Users may bump into poorly arranged apparatus and hurt themselves. It is also important that apparatus is not left lying around the exercise room in dangerous positions for someone to trip over. Such safety considerations should be strictly applied – and they become even more important if the room is crowded.

FOOD AND DRINK

As a general rule it is not advisable to eat within one hour of exercising or to exercise within three hours of a substantial meal. This is because of the discomfort caused by a full stomach and the possibility of recently ingested food causing nausea. It can also place additional strain upon the body to ask it to cope with the demands of digestion and food assimilation as well as those of the exercise; in the case of swimming there are serious additional risks.

However, liquids should be readily available and taken at liberty during an exercise session since it is undesirable for the participant to become dehydrated. Dehydration will cause unnecessary fatigue, discomfort and lack of concentration and will therefore reduce the effectiveness of the session. Whether the adviser permits liquids into the exercise area or recommends that they are consumed elsewhere will depend upon the circumstances, but for safety reasons glass should not be brought into an exercise area.

GETTING STARTED

Knowing how and where to begin an exercise programme can be the most difficult stage for the novice exercise adviser. Therefore, some basic guidelines and suggestions are presented here. It should be remembered that physical fitness is very specific. Even if the participant is fairly fit they will not necessarily be able to cope easily with all forms of exercise. If an individual wishes to try something new, they should begin at a relatively easy level and progress gradually. For example, cycling puts slightly different stresses on the body than running and someone who cycles regularly may not be completely fit for jogging. This aspect of specificity is important and too many unfamiliar stresses should not be placed upon the bones, joints and muscles: even the fittest can overexert themselves when trying something new and experience a few unwanted aches and strains the following day. Therefore, if an exercise is unfamiliar it is better to start at relatively easy level than to attempt to do too much too soon. The exercise adviser should also be aware that if a participant is overweight then activities such as jogging may put too much stress on the joints. For these individuals alternative, non-weight-bearing activities such as swimming and cycling are often preferable.

Points that the exercise adviser should consider when designing an exercise programme:

1. Try to choose exercises that the participant will enjoy and will stick with.
2. Choose exercises that will easily fit in with the participant's daily routine.
3. Gradually increase the amount of exercise.
4. Do not exceed the participant's capabilities.
5. Vary the exercise routine to prevent boredom.
6. Try to ensure that the exercises are done frequently and regularly.
7. Make exercise part of a daily or weekly routine.
8. If necessary include strength and suppleness exercises as well as aerobic exercises in the programme.
9. Remember that if the participant is serious about his or her physical condition and health, the commitment to exercise should be for life and not just a few weeks.
10. Record and monitor the details of the exercise sessions. This will help to reveal

progression and assist with the production of the following phase of the exercise schedule.

MEDICAL CLEARANCE BEFORE STARTING AN AEROBIC EXERCISE PROGRAMME

Many authorities recommend a complete medical check-up before beginning an exercise programme. This is particularly prudent if the individual has not exercised for some considerable time. A check-up can include a basic questionnaire, assessment of blood pressure, analysis of body composition, resting electrocardiogram, analysis of blood cholesterol and even an exercise stress test (where the activity of the heart is monitored during strenuous exercise). Such medical evaluations may be performed at various venues and may be conducted in several stages, with only those people deemed to be of a high risk going on for the more extensive form of assessment. In practice, these assessments tend to be precautionary only: most individuals are cleared to exercise. For exercise specialists working in a medical environment it is likely that most of the individuals they work with will have been referred by their medical consultant. If this is not the case, it may be necessary to clear the patient with their medical consultant and find out whether any specific factors need to be considered when devising an exercise programme.

In all cases the pre-exercise questionnaires serve a useful function. If the client is found to possess several potential risk factors the exercise adviser should seek further medical advice before proceeding with the programme.

WHEN NOT TO EXERCISE

It is widely established that appropriate exercise can convey numerous benefits to many people. However, there are a few occasions when it is inadvisable to exercise. It is unwise for anyone to exercise whilst suffering from a basic viral infection such as influenza. Many individuals erroneously believe that a hard exercise session will enable them to 'sweat it out' and accelerate their recovery but medical evidence would suggest that if a person infected with a virus attempts to exercise the virus can cause a greater amount of inflammation, and even permanent damage to body tissues. Of greatest concern in this context is the possibility of the virus affecting the heart and causing pericarditis, which can cause permanent damage. It has also been shown that the incidence of cardiac arrhythmia is increased in those exercising with a virus even if they have no apparent cardiac disorders and are otherwise healthy. A further cause for concern are the post-viral fatigue syndromes, including myalgic encephalopathy (ME). The exact cause of these disorders remains unclear, although evidence suggests that individuals are more susceptible if they are physically fatigued and/or under mental stress. It is therefore inadvisable to exercise when suffering from a viral infection.

A further factor to consider when recommending that someone should not exercise is the presence of specific injuries. Although exercise, if undertaken at the correct time, can provide a useful form of rehabilitation, exercises performed at the wrong time may aggravate an injury. The timing of the inclusion of certain exercises into a programme is thus important. For instance, if the participant is suffering from tendonitis then it may be advisable to stop or minimise any form of exercise that places stress upon that particular tendon until the condition improves sufficiently to permit exercise without pain or subsequent soreness. A typical example would be in a jogger suffering from tendonitis of the Achilles tendon: an alternative form of exercise, such as swimming, should be pursued until the inflammation is sufficiently reduced and return to exercise should be gradual, involving strengthening exercises and walking before attempting to jog. Failing to do this is likely to cause recurrence of the injury, because the tissue will not have developed the resilience required to withstand the rigours of jogging.

Basic muscle injuries such as simple partial ruptures tend to respond well to exercise after an initial rest of approximately 48 hours. Gentle exercise at this time appears to enhance the healing process, but should not be commenced earlier as it can aggravate the injury by damaging the weak tissues. Once exercise has been introduced into a rehabilitation programme the intensity, duration and frequency should be increased very gradually in accordance with the limitations imposed by the injury. Exceeding these limitations is likely to aggravate the injury and therefore emphasis should be placed on working within the individual's capabilities and not at their limit. In the case of all injuries, resumption of exercise should be undertaken with caution and progression should be gradual.

In practical terms the question may not simply be whether to exercise or not but whether a particular form of exercise is appropriate for a particular individual at that particular time. For example, circumstances may suggest that a person should stop one form of exercise and take up an alternative. This could occur at any stage of an exercise programme and may also involve a change in the intensity of the exercise. It should also be remembered that what is beneficial to one individual may not be beneficial to another, once again emphasising the importance of personalising exercise programmes. There are certain individuals who have specific conditions that will make their participation in certain forms of exercise inadvisable. For instance, a blind person who has no other disabilities will be capable of exercising as hard as an individual with sight (indeed, many blind individuals actively train and compete in sports such as athletics) but an individual rehabilitating after a coronary heart attack will require a very different level of exercise intensity.

EXERCISE AND MEDICATION

Certain forms of medication may preclude an individual from exercising. It is therefore important that the exercise adviser is aware of any drugs that the participant is taking and of any implications that they may have. This information should be gained directly from the participant's medical practitioner or an appropriately qualified specialist.

Beta-blockers are drugs that reduce the heart rate. When a person taking beta-blockers exercises, the normal increase in heart rate is suppressed, resulting in an artificially low pulse and any prescription of exercise intensity based upon heart rate must be modified in such patients. It will be inappropriate to expect a person taking beta-blockers to exercise within the usual heart rate training zones (p. 13). It is more appropriate for such people to exercise to a perceived exertion – for example, at an intensity which makes them 'slightly breathless', but no harder. A more quantitative assessment of an individual's perceived exertion, such as the 'Borg scale', may be used (see p. 104).

In certain contexts exercise enhances the effectiveness of medication. For example, a number of studies have shown that exercise aids the reduction of moderately high blood pressure and reduces the amount of medication required by the individuals involved. This is not uncommon: exercise has been shown to increase the body's sensitivity to insulin, reducing the amount required by insulin-dependent diabetics.

PSYCHOLOGICAL PRINCIPLES OF EXERCISE PRESCRIPTION

Perhaps the most fundamental tenet of exercise prescription is that we must prescribe for adherence. As indicated in Chapter 4, most people will either not start an exercise programme or will drop out very soon after they have started unless they are well motivated. We must design routines which people will enjoy and which will enhance rather than detract from motivation. To achieve this, health professionals should apply the following principles:

- promote intrinsic motivation;
- link intensity to perceived and preferred exertion;
- set goals.

PROMOTE INTRINSIC MOTIVATION

An individual is intrinsically motivated when they take part in an activity for its own sake and the pleasure and internal satisfaction they feel from doing so. This can be contrasted to an individual who is extrinsically motivated and who takes part in an activity for rewards such as money, trophies or external approval from significant others. As intrinsic motivation is not dependent on these external reinforcers (which may not always be present) it is more likely to promote long-term adherence. Intrinsic motivation can be fostered by carefully matching the individual with the activity. This matching is more likely if a proper needs analysis has been conducted and if a range of possible activities is available from which the individual can choose.

LINK INTENSITY TO PERCEIVED AND PREFERRED EXERTION

Exercise intensity is not just a physiological factor: different intensities result in different levels of perceived exertion. Borg (1982) has developed a scale to measure perceived exertion (Figure 5.1).

The Borg scale can be used by health professionals to estimate exercise intensity in place of, or in conjunction with, other measures such as heart rate telemetry. It can also be used to promote a dialogue with the client on their *preferred* level of exertion. For example, one client may like and enjoy working at level 15 (hard) whilst another may find this level demotivating. These preferences should not be

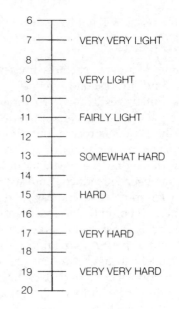

Figure 5.1   The Borg scale of perceived exertion

overlooked when prescribing an exercise or activity programme, for to do so may reduce intrinsic motivation and the probability of long-term adherence. As yet unpublished work by Buckton indicates that health professionals may also need to be aware of *observed* exertion. This refers to the intensity at which the exercise leader *thinks* the client is working, based on subjective observation in the gymnasium. Any discrepancy between actual and observed exertion may lead to inappropriate and unhelpful attributions and comments. For example, if the client has a high perceived exertion but the exercise leader thinks 'this client is not working hard enough' it is unlikely that preferred exertion will be achieved.

SET GOALS

Many health professionals will be aware of the importance of goal setting in promoting behavioural change. However, difficulties arise when a goal-setting regimen is imposed upon an individual who is not the goal-setting type or when the following issues are not addressed.

1. Goals should emerge from the client, not be imposed upon them by the health professional. They should meet the client's needs and take into account the client's level of motivation.
2. Although goals should be recommended and formalised they should not be 'cast in concrete'. Goals should be regularly revisited and changed in light of progress, regression and changed circumstances.
3. Goals should emphasise the process rather than the outcome. For example, they should relate to the frequency, intensity and duration of physical activity required rather then to the amount of weight to be lost. Promote the behaviour and the health outcome will take care of itself!
4. Goals should be realistic and achievable. Put simply, they should be easy to achieve – goals that are not lead to feelings of guilt and reduced perceived behavioural control. How many of us give up trying because we have failed to meet a set of goals so many times?
5. It is often suggested that goals should be set for the short, medium and long term. Whilst we do not wish to contradict the many writers and researchers who have proposed this format, we recommend that health professionals adopt a sense of realism when attempting to set long-term goals. In our experience it is difficult to set long-term goals which, at the point of recording, do not appear 'unrealistic and unachievable'. Since we all live in the present, short-term goals, which affect our behaviour in the 'here and now', seem the most important. This being the case it may be most effective to set a series of short-term goals over an extended period.
6. Consideration should be given to whether goals should be shared with important others or kept between the client and the health professional. Although in many cases sharing will facilitate a supporting and understanding environment it may also lead to 'Mickey taking' and jealousy. To avoid these problems the health professional should discuss with the client both their motivation to comply with important others and the attitudes they hold.
7. Goals should be reviewed. Notice that we have refrained from saying that 'goals should be evaluated': evaluation implies pass or fail, success or failure approaches which are hardly likely to promote continued effort. Rather, goals should be reviewed and restructured to promote continued commitment to behavioural change.

CONCLUSION

By putting the principles of this chapter into practice health professionals will be able to meet the exercise needs of a wide range of clients and community groups. An important principle of exercise prescription is that *health professionals should continue to update their knowledge base and reflect upon their professional practice related to exercise prescription*. The Chinese curse 'may you live in interesting times' certainly applies to the research agenda and debate currently surrounding the science of exercise prescription. Although we are confident that the principles outlined in this chapter will apply for many years their emphasis and application will undoubtedly continue to evolve.

REFERENCES

Bouchard, C. and Shephard, R.J. (1994). Physical activity, fitness, and health: The model and key concepts. In *Physical Activity, Fitness and Health. International Proceedings and Consensus Statement*, Bouchard, C., Shephard, R.J. and Stephens, T. (eds). Champaign, IL: Human Kinetics.

Borg, G.A. (1982). Psychophysical basis of perceived exertion. *Medicine and Science in Sports and Exercise*, **14**, 377.

Haskell, W.L. (1994). Health consequences of physical activity: understanding and challenges regarding dose-response. *Medicine and Science in Sports and Exercise*, **26** (6), 649–660.

Shephard, R.J. (1997) What is the optimal type of physical activity to enhance health? *British Journal of Sports Medicine*, **31**, 277–284.

PHYSIOLOGICAL AND PSYCHOLOGICAL ASSESSMENTS

6

REASONS FOR CONDUCTING A PHYSIOLOGICAL ASSESSMENT

Assessing a client's motivation, goals and physical condition before commencing an exercise programme can help to ensure that the prescribed exercise regimen is most appropriate and effective. The formality and depth of assessment can range from an informal chat to a full clinical evaluation, depending upon circumstances.

A physiological assessment can provide valuable information about the physical condition of the client, and may be conducted for a number of reasons.

1. It provides information on the client's current physical condition that may be used to devise suitable exercise loads and personalise an exercise programme. Later assessments may then be used to modify the programme.
2. It provides initial data against which later assessments can be measured. This enables the adviser to see whether the programme is suitable and effective. It also provides positive feedback and motivation for the participant.
3. An assessment can provide information about the client's current physical condition relative to others and national norms. Such comparisons may be appropriate when assessing certain characteristics of health but for other factors it is often better to emphasise the comparison between an individual's initial and current results.

4. A comprehensive assessment that includes clinical tests can detect problems associated with the client's health, such as hypertension or atherosclerosis. The subject may then be cleared for exercise, or their exercise programme modified according to any identified problems.
5. The assessment session can provide an opportunity for assessor and client to discuss aspects of exercise, health, and (where appropriate) the reasons for incorporating exercise into the lifestyle.
6. An assessment can be used as a short-term goal, giving the participant an objective to aim for and providing a focus within the programme.

The exact content of the physiological assessment will depend upon the condition of the participant and the aims of the exercise programme. It must be appropriate for their physical capacity; exhaustive tests are clearly unsuitable for many individuals, but may be appropriate for others. The assessment must also be relevant to the person's needs; monitoring strength may be appropriate as an ongoing process, but improvements in strength cannot be expected if strengthening exercises are not included within the programme.

MULTISTAGE ASSESSMENT BEFORE DEVELOPING AN EXERCISE PROGRAMME

Before commencement of any exercise programme it is usually advisable for the participant to undergo some form of assessment and/or medical check-up, although the extent and nature of the assessment will vary considerably depending upon age, medical history and current level of activity. The exercise adviser may require their client to complete one or all of the following stages:

- *Stage 1:* pre-exercise questionnaire on medical history and current exercise participation.
- *Stage 2:* health-related assessment of factors such as blood cholesterol, lipoproteins and blood lipid profile, body composition, lung function and blood pressure.
- *Stage 3:* further medical screening if there are contraindications to exercise.
- *Stage 4:* physical fitness assessments, which could include measurements of strength, flexibility and aerobic capacity.

STAGE 1

This basic lifestyle questionnaire should be used to gain information about the client's current levels of physical activity, medical disorders and any medication that they are currently taking, smoking habits, stress, family history of CHD, diet and age. The questionnaire should provide the exercise adviser with information on the participant, risk factors which they exhibit, and preliminary information about the participant's capabilities and expectations. Such a questionnaire can also be used to discover the forms of exercise the participant might enjoy.

STAGE 2

The initial questionnaire may be followed by evaluation of blood pressure (if this information is not already available) by a suitably qualified individual. If it should reveal hypertension, additional care should be taken when the individual undertakes certain forms of exercise. If the exercise adviser is not medically trained and is presented with a client with blood pressure values of around 165/95 (systolic/diastolic), he or she should not conduct any further exercise tests on that individual until appropriate assurances have been obtained from the participant's medical specialist. High blood pressure will not normally preclude all forms of exercise but some (especially isometric work) will be inadvisable, and the intensity of the prescribed activities will need specific consideration. For example, in the initial assessment the assessor may simply evaluate the individual's aerobic fitness using very light exercise intensities, which would be substantially less than those used for a person with normal blood pressure.

Other tests which could be included at this stage are measurements of blood cholesterol, lipoproteins and blood lipids and body composition. The results of these tests will generate a 'profile of risk' on the client. For details on the assessment of body composition see Eston and Reilly (1996).

STAGE 3

If the client reveals a significant profile of risk, the exercise adviser may wish to attain assurances of their suitability to exercise before proceeding further. A letter from their medical practitioner may be sufficient, but in a few cases a more extensive medical exercise stress test with an electrocardiogram (ECG) may be needed. Such a test should be conducted by a specialist who can then liaise with the exercise adviser over the condition of the participant and the content of the exercise programme.

One reason for performing an exercise stress test is that many individuals with CHD will exhibit a normal resting ECG; the ECG becomes abnormal only whilst exercising at relatively high intensities. However, even this test will not detect all CHD sufferers (25% of CHD sufferers will still exhibit a normal ECG whilst exercising). For the 75% of sufferers that are detected, appropriate precautions can be taken with their exercise programmes. If an abnormal ECG is detected further tests may be required, after which the individual may or may not be cleared to exercise. The information obtained from such tests can also be used by the specialist to determine a suitable level of exercise intensity.

Some authorities suggest that in an ideal situation everyone should undergo a regular, extensive physiological assessment which includes an ECG stress test – especially those over 40 years of age. However, such procedures are expensive, time consuming, the facilities are not always available and (as previously indicated) may not detect all those with a heart problem. Extensive assessment procedures may put off some individuals from embarking on a programme. Therefore a balance needs to be obtained between the most extensive form of assessment available and what is practically feasible.

STAGE 4

A basic physical assessment of aspects of physical capacity can include a submaximal assessment of the individual's aerobic capacity and/or joint mobility measures and/or measurements of strength. The results of these tests can then be used directly in prescribing the exercise loads to be incorporated into the exercise programme.

REPEATED PHYSIOLOGICAL ASSESSMENTS AND MONITORING

Once a participant has spent some weeks on an exercise programme it may be useful to reassess his or her physical fitness. Repeat assessments can be conducted every 6–12 weeks if desired and can be useful in a number of ways.

- They can act as a short-term or intermediate goal for the participant.
- They provide information about whether the exercise programme has been effective.
- The data from such assessments can be used to modify the exercise programme and to provide positive feedback for the participant.

With most assessment procedures a key aspect of the evaluation is the comparison between the current and previous scores, thereby monitoring any progress. Relating scores to standardised norms may be helpful for some factors but it is often inappropriate because of the highly individual nature and circumstances of the participant with whom the exercise adviser is working. However, if working in a specialised area, the adviser may

Pre-Study Medical Screening Questionnaire *strictly confidential*

> **OFFICIAL USE ONLY:**
> **Subject Number**

Please complete *all* pages of this form and answer each question by circling either YES or NO.

1. Are you currently, or have you recently had a cold, flu or other respiratory chest infection?   **YES / NO**
   If yes, please give approximate date when started ....

2. Are you recovering from an **illness and/or operation?**   **YES / NO**
   If yes, please give details of the illness and/or operation with approximate dates
   ....
   ....

3. Are you **pregnant, or have you had a baby in the last 12 months?**   **YES / NO**
   If yes, please give the date when the baby is due or when the baby was born
   ....

4. Do you consider yourself to be overweight?   **YES / NO**
   If yes, by approximately how much? ....

5. How many units of alcohol do you consume each week? ....

6. Do you smoke?   **YES / NO**
   If yes, how many cigarettes do you smoke each week? ....

7. Are you worried that any of the assessments may affect your health?   **YES / NO**
   If yes, in what way? ....
   ....

8. Do you consider your health to be **Poor / Fair / Good / Excellent?**
   (Please circle where applicable).

9. Do you have chest problems such as asthma or bronchitis?   **YES / NO**
   If yes, do you take any medication?
   If yes, please give details ....   **YES / NO**
   ....

10. Has a doctor ever said you have heart trouble?   **YES / NO**

11. Have you ever had angina pectoris or sharp pain or heavy pressure in your chest as a result of
    exercise, walking or other physical activity, such as climbing a flight of stairs?   **YES / NO**

12. Do you experience sharp pain or extreme tightness in your chest when you are hit by a cold blast
    of air?   **YES / NO**

13. Have you ever experienced palpatations or rapid heart beat?   **YES / NO**
    If yes, please give the approximate date ....

14. Have you ever had a real or suspected **heart attack/coronary occlusion/myocardial
    infarction/coronary insufficiency/thrombosis?** (Please circle one or more if applicable.)   **YES / NO**
    If yes to any of these, please give dates ....

15. Has more than one blood relative (parent, brother or sister, first cousin) had a heart attack or
    coronary artery disease before the age of 60?   **YES / NO**
    If yes, please state which member of your family ....

Figure 6.1   Example of a pre-assessment questionnaire

16. Have you ever had rheumatic fever? **YES / NO**
    If yes, please give approximate date ....

17. Do you have **diabetes/high blood pressure/sugar in your urine**? **YES / NO**
    (Please circle where applicable).

18. Do you have high **blood pressure/hypertension**? **YES / NO**
    (Please circle where applicable).

19. Does any of your family have high **blood pressure/hypertension**? **YES / NO**
    If yes, please state which member of your family ....

20. Have you ever taken medication to lower your blood pressure? **YES / NO**
    If yes, please state what medication and approximate dates ....
    ....

21. Have you ever taken digitalis, quinine or any other drug for your heart? **YES / NO**
    If yes, please give type of medication and approximate date when this was
    ....

22. Have you ever taken nitroglycerine or any other tablet for chest pain – tablets that you take by
    placing under the tongue? **YES / NO**
    If yes, please give type of medication and approximate date when this was
    ....

23. Have you ever had a resting or stress electrocardiogram that was not normal? **YES / NO**
    If yes, please give approximate date when this was ....
    ....

24. Have you ever **taken any medication** / **been on a special diet** to lower your blood
    cholesterol? **YES / NO**
    If yes, please give type of diet and or medication and approximate date when this was
    ....
    ....

25. Do you have any other physical condition that is not covered by the above questions? **YES / NO**
    If yes, please state ....
    ....

OFFICIAL USE ONLY
Comments
....
....
....
....

Figure 6.1 continued

accumulate a quantity of data which could enable specialised norms or standards to be produced for use in his or her own setting. For certain health factors such as lipid profiles a longer duration (12–18 weeks) may be required before reassessment.

CHARACTERISTICS OF ASSESSMENT PROTOCOLS

The assessment process is usually multistage, with only those individuals revealing a high number of risk factors in the basic assessment being recommended for more comprehensive tests. Tests of aerobic fitness, joint mobility and strength are likely to be conducted by the exercise adviser but specialised assessments, such as the measurement of exercise ECGs, should be undertaken by appropriate experts. Other types of fitness test, such as measurement of $\dot{V}O_{2max}$ through maximal exhaustive exercise and the lactate threshold (T_{LAC}; see p. 123) are more specific to sports performers and are not normally appropriate in a health-related context. However, even though not all exercise advisers are likely to conduct these tests they may well encounter individuals who have undergone them. Since many of the test protocols used in a health-related setting are submaximal modifications of the maximal tests, the physiological basis and responses to maximal tests are briefly described in this chapter to help explain the rationale and interpretation of the sub-maximal versions.

SELECTING AN ASSESSMENT TEST: VALIDITY, RELIABILITY AND ACCURACY

For an assessment to produce meaningful information it needs to be valid and reliable. Collecting inaccurate data not only wastes time but can also undermine the assessor's credibility and demotivate the participant. Before devising their own set of tests an exercise adviser is strongly recommended to investigate whether established tests that have been checked for their validity and reliability are already in existence. If used correctly these will ensure the validity of the assessor's data and prevent any problems arising when attempting to design a new test. Established tests should have clear instructions on how to implement the test, standardise the procedures and interpret the data. Validation of a new test and determining its reliability are lengthy processes which are likely to require more time and resources than typically available to most exercise advisers unless such research is a component part of their activities. Examples of texts that provide this information are included in the list of references for this chapter.

Test validity refers to whether it measures what is intended. For example, if the aim of the test is to assess the strength of a particular group of muscles does it achieve this?

Reliability refers to how repeatable the measurements are – how similar the data would be if the test was repeated on the same individual under the same conditions. Some small variation is inevitable due to measurement error, differences in individual technique and the limits to which equipment can be calibrated. Knowing the repeatability of measurements will enable an assessor to determine whether any measured differences are genuine or within the likely test variation. For example, when monitoring an individual it is not possible to say whether an improvement of 5 kg in their muscular strength is likely to be real or not unless the test reliability has been determined to be significantly less than 5 kg. If this were the case then any difference of this magnitude or greater would be a genuine difference in muscular strength.

An important aspect of ensuring test reliability is precise calibration of all equipment. The assessor should not assume the values given by a piece of equipment are correct unless it has been calibrated recently. It is vitally important to check the resistance of cycle ergometers, treadmill speeds, calliper and dynamometer pressures. Additional variations in test results can be caused by slight differences in the measurement techniques of the different assessors (inter-assessor reliability). Therefore the standardisation of technique between assessors is also vital if more than one adviser is working with a set of clients.

THE ASSESSMENT OF FLEXIBILITY AND JOINT MOBILITY

The objective assessment and monitoring of a person's flexibility may fulfil many functions. It can reveal lack of mobility at specific joints and hence indicate those which need special attention. An initial assessment can also provide an objective measure of the amount of mobility at specific joints. These measurements can then be compared with subsequent measurements, thereby enabling any changes in joint mobility to be objectively monitored. They can also be used to provide positive feedback to the participant as well as informing the exercise adviser of the effectiveness of the exercise programme.

It is essential that the methods of measurement and the conditions under which the measurements are taken are standardised. For example, the assessor may choose to measure the participant's mobility after he or she has completed an exercise session and conse-

quently is already warm. If so, all comparative measurements should be taken following a similar session since the participant is likely to be more flexible after a session than before it. Ideally, the same time of day should be also used for each assessment since most people are far less flexible first thing in the morning. The room in which the assessment takes place should be comfortably warm; the person is likely to be less flexible if he or she is cold. Whether the individual is relaxed or tense is also likely to be a factor. A few preparatory stretches are advisable before all assessment sessions since this could have a substantial effect upon the results.

MEASUREMENTS OF JOINT MOBILITY/ FLEXIBILITY

Individuals vary in their level of joint mobility/flexibility due to certain inherited factors. This applies to both their current level and their potential to improve. Therefore, although norms may be applied in the assessment of joint movement the key issue is the comparison between that person's current and previous scores. Careful measurement is important and a comprehensive set of records should be kept for each individual. The use of appropriate movement terminology will aid in the precise description of the test and clear communication of the results (see Chapter 11).

Using a goniometer

The instrument commonly used to measure joint mobility is the clinical goniometer, which can be used to assess movement at virtually any joint. The instrument is placed on the body part to be moved, the dial is set to zero, the limb is moved (either actively or passively depending upon the aspects of mobility being measured) and the assessor records the degree of movement. There are several variations on the goniometer but all are basically simple to use and an assessor can become proficient in their use with relatively little practice. More sophisticated versions tend to produce greater reliability and validity. The assessor's technique must also be reliable and repeatable, otherwise the results lose their value.

When measuring joint angles and limb movements it is essential to isolate the joint being assessed. For example, if assessing hip abduction it is vital that the pelvis remains fixed and is not tilted; failure to prevent lateral flexion of the spine and associated pelvic tilting may result in an artificially high score. Similarly, because the hamstring muscles cross both the hip and knee joints a much greater degree of hip flexion will be recorded if the knee is flexed than if it remains extended. Standardisation of technique is thus essential – as is the accurate positioning of the measuring device. An illustration of the use of a goniometer is given in Figure 6.2.

Alternative methods for assessing flexibility involve standardised tests such as the sit and reach test or back hyperextension test. These are less applicable in the clinical setting because they tend to measure movements over a range of joints and are therefore less specific in the readings they produce. For details of flexibility assessments refer to Eston and Reilly (1996).

ASSESSMENT OF JOINT FLEXIBILITY/
MOBILITY IN A CLINICAL SETTING

The range of motion available at certain joints is often of great relevance clinically, and goniometers are usually used to assess this. Often, comparing the ranges available in the same joint on either side of the body helps to detect an abnormality. Goniometric measure-

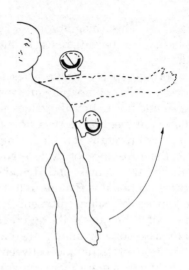

Figure 6.2 Use of a goniometer to measure shoulder abduction

ment may be used to monitor stiffness at a joint, but will not in itself reveal the cause of stiffness. Recording of both active and passive ranges will distinguish the range that can be achieved by the activity of the muscle working upon the joint (active) from the range available if the joint is moved by some external source (passive), as when the movement is helped by a clinician. Such differences are often useful in helping the clinician to diagnose a problem, and repeated measurements will show decline or improvement over time.

ASSESSMENT OF MUSCULAR STRENGTH

Muscular strength is defined by the amount of force generated by a muscle or group of muscles. The International System (SI) unit of force used in strength testing is the newton (N), and is the unit most likely to be used on a dynamometer (1 N is the amount of force required to accelerate 1 kg by 1 m s^{-2}). However, when using multigyms or other weight-training equipment, it is common for the resistance to be quantified in pounds or kilograms. This makes comparison between equipment difficult and in many cases impossible due to the effects of different lever systems and ranges of movement produced. To give an indication of the force required in a straight lift with free weights, since the force acting on the weight is gravity (which causes an acceleration of $9.8\,\mathrm{m\,s^{-2}}$), lifting 1 kg is equivalent to 9.8 N and 1 lb to 4.45 N.

When conducting strength tests the assessor should be aware that occasionally what is actually being assessed is *power*. Power is the 'rate of doing work' and therefore is determined by the force of the muscular contraction and the speed of the movement. The unit of power is the watt (W). When movement is involved the term strength is sometimes applied somewhat loosely. However, whilst such distinctions are important in a scientific context and the exercise professional must be aware of them, in a practical context the term 'strength assessment' is often used loosely to avoid complicating the issue from the client's perspective.

As with other fitness components, the assessment of muscular strength may be used to identify relative strengths and weakness, determine exercise loads and monitor the effectiveness of a training or rehabilitation regimen. An appropriate level of strength is important for everyone, not just those involved in strength-related sports. For example, an appropriate level of strength can reduce the likelihood of potentially injurious falls in elderly people, reduce the incidence of back complaints, and (by encouraging the correct balance of strength in different muscles groups) can reduce the risk of both chronic and acute injuries. Therefore assessment of strength and interpretation of the results are important skills which an exercise professional can use to good effect.

When constructing a battery of strength assessments the exercise professional must consider the aims of the assessment and the test's specificity. In doing so it is important to consider factors such as which muscle groups are involved, how they are used, the range of movement and the speed of movement. Specificity is important: if an inappropriate test is used it will fail to assess the intended factors and will therefore lack validity. In practical terms this means that test results will be misleading. Furthermore, because strength gains tend to be specific to the range and speed of movement used in training, if the selected test assesses a different movement it may not detect improvements and could have a negative and discouraging effect.

When evaluating muscular strength and endurance a number of assessment methods are available:

- subjective resistance tests;
- dynamometers for assessing maximal isometric strength;
- tests of maximal dynamic strength using free weights machines or body resistance;
- muscular endurance tests using free weights machines or body resistance;
- isokinetic machines;
- electromyography.

The appropriateness of each method will depend upon the individual, their condition and the aspect of muscular strength that the exercise adviser wishes to evaluate. An initial assessment incorporating one or more of these methods may assist with the design of a programme by providing an indication of the participant's capabilities and potential. Repeated assessments can then be used to monitor the participant's progress and the effectiveness of the exercise programme.

It is also evident that when assessing muscular strength the exercise professional is working with a continuum from maximal strength, assessed via a single maximal contraction to muscular endurance, which is the capacity of the individual to repeat or maintain a contraction of a specified force. It may be that, even for a specific action, measures of both maximal strength and muscular endurance are required to assess whether either (or both) are limiting the individual's ability to function. Therefore a battery of tests must be devised, allowing sufficient recovery time between each to prevent the effects of fatigue adversely affecting the results. The test equipment used may be determined by availability but if a choice is available the assessor should balance the advantages of the additional safety inherent in using exercise machines against the potential for machines to not place as great a demand on the muscles involved in controlling and/or stabilising a movement. This could be an important limiting factor in determining the individual's functional strength. Exercise machines may therefore have less validity in terms of assessing functional movements than free weights.

Isokinetic machines can provide very detailed information about muscular strength/power in an isolated joint movement, including quantifying the force produced at various stages of a movement and at different speeds. This can be very useful in the comparison of opposing muscle groups and identification of muscular imbalances. More recently developed isokinetic machines can assess eccentric as well as concentric muscle action, thereby providing more detailed information about the condition of the muscles.

PRETEST CONSIDERATIONS

To produce valid and reliable results specificity is important. As previously indicated, this requires consideration of the position of body parts and joint angles and (in the case of dynamic actions) the type, range and speed of movement. All equipment must be calibrated correctly and the testing environment should be appropriate. Changes in temperature and time of day can have significant effects upon the results. The physical status of the participant is likewise important; for example, whether they are fresh or fatigued from previous exertion. A pretest warm up may be advocated before many tests to facilitate optimal performance. Further differences may be caused by the psychological state of the participant, whether they are confident or tentative in their surroundings and of the test procedures.

Regardless of the method of assessment, some familiarisation is necessary. If time permits the test protocol should be repeated until a consistent set of reproducible results is attained. Failure to incorporate a period of familiarisation will reduce the reliability of the test and may result in an incorrect evaluation.

During the test the level of feedback and encouragement can have a significant effect. The assessor must establish a consistent protocol in these aspects – for example the level of verbal encouragement and/or whether the results displayed by the equipment are visible to the participant during the test – as they can provide additional motivation.

SUBJECTIVE RESISTANCE TESTS

In these tests the exercise adviser will ask the participant to perform a movement, such as knee extension or elbow flexion. They will then resist this movement using their hands in the same way that resistance is applied during accommodating resistance exercises. Whilst this form of assessment will not produce a quantitative measure of strength it can indicate the participant's general strength for that movement and any obvious weakness. In the case of a rehabilitation programme, comparing the strength of opposing limbs is often informative.

A commonly used system of assessing strength clinically is the British Medical Research Council grading scale (Table 6.1). This is a subjective scale which gives a gross indication of the strength available within a muscle or muscle group. It is often used in conjunction with other tests to diagnose a patient's problem, although an indication of muscle weakness revealed by this test will not uncover the cause of weakness. This scale is used clinically to indicate abnormalities in muscle function. The best available score (5)

Table 6.1 The British Medical Research Council grading scale

Grade	Level	Description
5	Normal	Motion through full range against gravity and maximum applied force
4	Good	Motion through full range against gravity and less than maximum applied force
3	Fair	Motion through full range against gravity and hold
2	Poor	Motion through full range with gravity eliminated
1	Trace	Palpable contraction but no movement
0	Zero	No palpable contraction

indicates normal muscle function, and this is often decided upon by comparing with the opposite side, as long as the condition does not affect both sides. This scale is often used as a crude indicator of change.

DYNAMOMETERS FOR ASSESSING MAXIMAL ISOMETRIC STRENGTH

Dynamometers require the participant to squeeze, pull or push; the dynamometer registers their maximal isometric strength in a quantitative manner. Dynamometers are commonly used to measure grip strength, back strength and leg strength. Owing to the maximal nature of the required contraction care should be taken when using the back and leg dynamometers: overexertion can cause strained muscles, and this risk makes this form of assessment inadvisable for some individuals. Another consideration with all forms of isometric exercise is its effect in increasing blood pressure. Therefore isometric work and isometric testing of individuals with high blood pressure and related cardiovascular problems may be inadvisable.

Isokinetic machines set at a velocity of 0 can also be used for isometric testing, with the added advantage that specific joint angles can be assessed. Comparing the force produced at different angles can reveal weakness through specific ranges of movement that can then be targeted in a training programme.

TESTS OF MAXIMAL DYNAMIC STRENGTH

Any exercise that uses free weights or a multigym can be used to assess maximal isotonic strength. Indeed, a body-resistance exercise such as a press-up can also be utilised as a gross indicator of functional strength. For maximal strength the assessment requires the participant to complete one lift or movement with a set resistance or weight. If he or she is successful then the weight or resistance is increased. The new load is then attempted and the process repeated until the participant is unable to complete the lift or movement. The heaviest weight or resistance lifted successfully is recorded as the participant's maximum (one repetition maximum – 1RM) for that particular exercise. The maximal exertion required for these tests makes it unsuitable for many individuals and conveys a risk of injury. When using body resistance exercises increasingly difficult variations of a movement may be attempted to determine physical ability.

If the test is being used to determine suitable 'training' loads rather than to produce a value for maximal strength it can be modified – rather than attempting to lift a maximum, the assessment may proceed with the participant attempting three repetitions of each weight until difficulty is encountered. The perception of a resistance as being difficult should inform the exercise adviser of the participant's capabilities and enable him or her to prescribe suitable resistances in the programme. Since the participant is likely to be required to complete 12–15 repetitions per set within the programme, the prescribed weight will be slightly below that attained in the assessment when only three repetitions were required – this is usually in the region of 60–80% of their maximum.

For examples the exercise adviser should refer to any exercise included within the chapter on strengthening exercises, but (as previously highlighted) validity, reliability and standardisation of technique are important.

A suggested protocol for the assessment of maximal strength (1RM) should include a light warm-up with loosening exercises followed by 5–8 repetitions of the movement using a light-to-moderate resistance. The resistance is then increased and the participant attempts one repetition at this resistance. If successful they rest for 3–5 minutes, and then attempt one repetition of a greater resistance. This process is repeated until the participant is unable to perform the movement successfully. The greatest resistance they were able to lift successfully is then taken to be the 1RM. In this process the assessor should increase the resistance at a rate which reaches the participant's actual maximum after 3–5 increases by appropriate questioning after each successful attempt. In practice, when assessing a 1RM for the first time the final successful lift may be slightly below the true maximum because of the amount of increase in resistance between the final successful attempt and the unsuccessful attempt. The assessor should be aware of this fact and/or repeat the assessment within a couple of days and design the test so that the participant attempts resistances between their provisional 1RM and the resistance that was above their capacity.

In other contexts the assessor may wish to assess an individual's strength by determining the amount they can lift three times without a pause. This is referred to as their three repetition maximum (3RM) and is a good indicator of maximal strength – but the final weight at which the individual is successful will inevitably be lower than that for a 1RM. Likewise, 5RM and 10RM may be used as indicators of muscle strength; whilst the values achieved for all of these will be slightly lower than that in the 1RM they have the advantage of using slightly less weight,

which can reduce the risk of injury. The basic protocol for determining 3RM, 5RM and 10RM is essentially the same for the 1RM. However, the greater the number of repetitions used the less informative the assessment is in terms of the individual's maximum strength. The practitioner must decide on the appropriate number of repetitions for what they are assessing: if purely maximum muscle strength then it will almost certainly be the 1RM, but if they are looking for a combination of muscular strength and muscular endurance a 10RM may be more appropriate.

TESTS OF MUSCULAR ENDURANCE

These are essentially fatigue tests and usually involve the participant completing a number of repetitions of an exercise in a specified time or to exhaustion. Alternatively, the participant is required to maintain a force of muscular contraction for a set duration.

In the former case, the rate at which the exercise is undertaken may be dictated by a specified rhythm, as in the standardised National Coaching Foundation Abdominal Conditioning Test. This is an incremental protocol in which the rate of performing the exercise is increased every minute until the participant is unable to perform any more. In alternative tests the participant will attempt to complete as many repetitions of an exercise as possible within a set time limit – for example as many sit-ups as possible in a minute or press-ups in 30 seconds. The selected duration of the test will depend upon the individual: 20–30 seconds is appropriate for many individuals whilst a minute may be used for those who are very fit. A set time limit or specified rhythm is used in preference to simply asking the participant to do as many as possible, because the rate of performance significantly influences the number achieved. For example, performing sit-ups quickly can be more tiring than performing them slowly, where the participant has the opportunity to pause between each one.

With this form of assessment and monitoring the exercise adviser is evaluating a combination of strength and endurance. The exercises that are incorporated into the exercise programme should be used, as this will indicate suitable numbers of repetitions to be included within the programme. It will also ensure the specificity of re-testing when monitoring progress. When administering these tests standardisation of the exercise is essential: failure to do so may make the results meaningless. For example, when doing a sit-up test the position of the hands will affect the level of difficulty, as will the rhythm and whether the participant has their feet anchored or free; the angle of shoulder and elbow flexion will affect press-ups or dips and must be standardised. One way of achieving this is to position an object at the end range of the movement and ensure that the participant touches it each time. For press-ups this could be a small block at a set height which their chest must touch; in dips the test administrator could position their clenched fist at the height to which the participant's shoulder must be lowered to make their upper arm parallel with the floor. Whatever the standardisation, it should be recorded for use at a later date. Further standardisation will be necessary if more than one assessor is involved in the testing; inter-tester reliability can be quite poor, with each person tending to interpret the instructions differently.

For the measurement of sustained muscular contraction computerised strain gauges and load cells are becoming more readily available. With these devices the participant is asked to maintain a force of contraction for a designated duration or to maintain a force of contraction above a set level for as long as possible. A common protocol for this would be to ask them to maintain 75% of their 1RM and provide feedback on the amount of force which they are applying. If the force of contraction falls below this level they must restore it immediately to above the threshold level. The test is terminated once the force of contraction falls below the required level for the third time. The time elapsed since the start of the test is recorded as the muscular endurance score.

Use of isokinetic machines for assessment of muscular strength and power

Isokinetic machines record the force of a contraction at a specified speed through a predetermined range of movement. Owing to the length–tension relationship of muscles, the maximum amount of force produced during a movement will vary at different points in the range of motion (ROM). This means that, in addition to assessing maximum force, isokinetic machines can assess the force applied at each point in the ROM, thereby detecting joint angles at which the force produced may be particularly weak. Force measurements are recorded by the machine's computer software, with the information being displayed in tabular and graphical form.

The more advanced isokinetic machines allow assessment of both eccentric and concentric muscle action. A key feature of isokinetic devices is that they enable maximum force to be applied throughout the entire range of movement, whereas other forms of testing that use general exercise machines and free weights permit the application of maximal force at only one point in the movement (the weakest), with only submaximal force being required to produce the movement through the remainder of the ROM. This has further implications when isokinetics are used for strengthening exercises; a training effect can be attained throughout the full ROM, unlike the use of free weights where the maximum resistance applied is determined by the amount of force that can be produced at the weakest part of the movement, thereby limiting the training effect at other points in the ROM.

The large number of variables and performance measures generated from an isokinetic test make evaluation of the data complex. Researchers and practitioners are still in the process of developing our current understanding of the implications and applications of these test results. Interpretation of the data generated by isokinetic machines is a specialist area requiring some expertise, and specific diagnosis can be subject to debate.

In isokinetic testing the participant will be required to repeat a movement a specified number of times at a speed dictated by the machine. With some variations due to make and model type, most machines can work at speeds ranging from 0 to 450° s^{-1} for concentric contractions and up to 180° s^{-1} for eccentric movements. Most of the machines available are designed with attachments that enable all major joint movements to be assessed. A number of isokinetic devices have been designed for specialist movements, such as isokinetic swim benches, although these are primarily training devices rather than assessment tools.

During an assessment the participant is required to exert as much force as possible against the resistance and the force applied is measured and recorded by the machine. This produces a large amount of detailed information concerning the strength of the muscles and any weaknesses during particular phases of a movement. The data can also be used to identify muscular imbalances, a commonly used example being the comparison of the strength ratio between the hamstrings and quadriceps; this is typically about 0.6 (60%) but alters with the angular velocity.

When conducting isokinetic tests it is important to isolate the movement and the joint involved. To do this the participant is strapped to the device to prevent other body movements contributing to the registered force. As with other forms of strength testing, an appropriate rest (typically 1–3 minutes) is required between sets of repetitions.

When conducting an assessment the rate of movement is defined as the angular limb velocity, using the units of degrees per second (° s^{-1}) (SI units radians per second; rad s^{-1}).

The selection of an appropriate angular velocity is important as the amount of force produced tends to be greater at slower velocities. Therefore an angular velocity appropriate to functional movement should be chosen. When possible, a number of different speeds may be used to attain a fuller profile of muscle strength. For example, three tests (at about 60, 120 and 180° s^{-1}) could be used to assess hamstring strength. The force applied by the participant in an isokinetic test will usually be expressed as 'torque', which is a combination of the force applied and the distance moved. The units of torque are newton metres (N m).

An isokinetic test will generate various measures of strength including data on peak torque, torque at a specific joint angle, the total work performed, time to peak torque, mean torque throughout for the entire movement and fatigue indexes. Each of these can be produced at different angular velocities and with different muscle groups. This therefore produces a profile of performance measures which must be interpreted appropriately. Further information on the use of isokinetics can be attained from texts such as that by Chan *et al.* (1996).

As previously indicated, isokinetic machines can also be used to assess isometric strength if the velocity of movement is set to zero. The process of comparing isometric strength at different joint angles may help to identify weakness at specific ranges of movement which can then be focused upon in the resultant exercise prescription.

ELECTROMYOGRAPHY

When a muscle contracts in response to a nerve impulse it produces a measurable amount of electrical activity, the study of which, electromyography, is used in the assessment of muscle function. Within clinical settings it can help to identify neuromuscular disorders where muscles respond inappropriately to the nerve impulses they receive. To measure the electrical activity of a muscle, electrodes are placed on the surface of the skin: if more specific sites of activity are being investigated, fine-wire electrodes can be inserted into the muscle. Surface electrodes detect the sum of the electrical activity (action potentials) occurring within their range of measurement. Electrodes should be positioned parallel to the orientation of the muscle fibres and set a distance apart that will maximise the assessment of electromyographic activity from the designated muscle, without collecting unwanted signals from other muscles within its vicinity.

The electrical activity produced from an electromyogram (EMG) can be matched with the force of muscle contraction and movement patterns to detect whether a muscle is contributing appropriately to a movement or whether there is a dysfunction.

The electrical activity within a muscle is influenced by the recruitment of the motor units and the frequency of action potentials. When undertaking electromyography key points to consider are the placement of the electrodes, the preparation of the skin, and the interface with the electrodes. Other factors that can affect the results include interference from other electrical sources, such as cables, and other muscular activity. Therefore extraneous sources of electrical signals must be minimised to reduce the amount of unwanted 'noise' in the recorded signals. This may be achieved by 'shielding' the equipment from sources of electrical signals and ensuring that as far as possible the muscles that are not being assessed remain relaxed throughout the data collection.

The raw electrical activity recorded in an EMG includes both positive and negative action potentials. To facilitate the analysis of the data it is usual for the negative action potentials to be converted to positive values. This is referred to as 'rectifying' the signal. The data may be further processed or smoothed to account for the recorded peaks and troughs in the signal. Data collected from an EMG include the amplitude of the activity

in microvolts (μV) and the duration of the signal in seconds. Integrating these two gives the total amount of activity in microvolt seconds (μV s). Other forms of data manipulation include the calculation of the root mean square (RMS) of the electrical activity. The RMS has been shown to correlate with the amount of force generated by a muscle; it can thus provide information about whether the strength of contraction is appropriate for the electrical activity produced. For example, a 'weak' individual will display a higher RMS for a given force of contraction than a stronger person (Shephard, 1987). Similarly, the RMS increases as an individual becomes fatigued during a sustained contraction, and it can therefore be used as a fatigue test.

In a clinical setting the speed of nerve impulse transmission can be used to detect neurological disorders. Using specialist equipment the signals produced by the muscle can be used to generate biofeedback in the form of sound, light or other visual displays. This gives the participant information about the strength of muscle activity. Biofeedback has particular applications in rehabilitation and training programmes. For further information on electromyographic analysis and the application of biofeedback see Prentice (1994); additional texts with sections on EMG include those by Hamill and Knutzen (1995) and Hall (1995).

ASSESSMENT OF AEROBIC FITNESS

The aerobic capacity of an individual is largely determined by their ability to utilise oxygen. The reasons for its consideration in a health-related exercise programme are, firstly, the contribution of aerobic fitness to an individual's capacity to undertake everyday activities and, secondly, the general link between fitness, activity and aspects of health. The exact relationship between these factors is inevitably complex but the evidence suggests that regular involvement in aerobic exercise promotes aerobic fitness, improves an individual's physical capacity and reduces the risk of certain diseases.

An individual's capacity to use oxygen (VO_{2max}) can be measured using sophisticated laboratory apparatus, but to do so requires the participant to exercise to exhaustion. Such tests are therefore not likely to be suitable for the vast majority of individuals that the exercise adviser will encounter. Maximal tests are usually employed only in the contexts of 'sport science', when evaluating the fitness of competitive sports performers or in specific exercise-related areas of research. However, submaximal predictions of VO_{2max} are quite commonly used in a health-related exercise setting. Submaximal tests require the participant to exercise at much lower exercise intensities. These tests are primarily based upon the findings that the 'fitter' an individual is the lower will be that individual's heart rate during a specified bout of exercise. The observed lower heart rates of the 'aerobically fit' are related to the increased stroke volume of their heart and the improved efficiency of their cardiovascular system, both of which are enhanced by regular exercise.

Therefore the protocol for maximal tests will be outlined only briefly before describing the submaximal variations that have been developed from them. Comments about conducting assessments for individuals with a substantially reduced physical capacity such as those who are postoperative, rehabilitating from illness, recovering from injury or suffering from certain chronic conditions, are given in a later section. Generally, submaximal tests rely upon the collection of heart rate measurements at known submaximal intensities and extrapolating the information to predict the subject's maximal performance characteristics without requiring them to exercise at maximal levels. In some of the more sophisticated forms of submaximal testing the heart rate data is supplemented by the collection of oxygen use measurements (VO_2) during submaximal exercise. However, since these tests incorporate an element of prediction the data

obtained from them must be viewed in the knowledge that some element of predictive error will be present in the results. This does not invalidate them, provided that they are used in the correct context. When interpreting the results the exercise adviser may wish simply to state what has been measured – i.e. heart rates at specific workloads – and only cautiously use them to predict VO_{2max}. Indeed, when monitoring fitness a reduced heart rate at the specified workload may be considered as an adequate indicator of an improvement in fitness rather than introducing the potential error of comparing two predicted VO_{2max} values. However, a further note of caution must be made concerning the use of submaximal tests for the assessment of the fit sports performer: the validation of many submaximal tests has generally used moderately active and/or sedentary individuals. These tests are therefore often unsuitable for those with a very high aerobic fitness, particularly if the results are used to estimate VO_{2max}, as the participant's actual VO_{2max} may not fall within the range of the test. So, for the very fit sports performer the more strenuous, sport-specific assessments should be employed as these will give more valid and informative data.

The relevance and applicability of each type of test will depend upon the participants being assessed and the reasons for assessing them. Simple non-quantitative assessments may involve a basic evaluation of an individual's capacity to perform prolonged forms of exercise such as walking. A more quantitative assessment could attempt to evaluate how far a person could walk in 10 minutes or how long it takes that person to walk a mile. These examples would require a reasonable level of fitness and therefore the exercise adviser will need to devise variations that use times or distances appropriate for the individual being assessed. Substantially shorter tests should be used for the less fit, with whom it may also be important to ensure that there is no element of competition in order to prevent over-exertion. For active individuals who are already physically fit, involved in strenuous sport and familiar with maximal exertion, more strenuous variations are available: examples include a number of 'shuttle running' tests, or simply recording how quickly a person can run 1.5 miles. These tests are maximal and will be appropriate only for those who are already physically fit and motivated. They are not appropriate for use in assessing the health-related fitness of less active and non-sporting subjects.

LABORATORY MEASUREMENT OF VO_{2MAX} USING MAXIMAL PROTOCOLS FOR THE SPORTS COMPETITOR

The VO_{2max} is a measure of the maximum amount of oxygen that a person can utilise. It is usually measured in litres of oxygen per minute ($l\,min^{-1}$). Assessment of VO_{2max} requires sophisticated apparatus to measure oxygen consumption, carbon dioxide production and a number of other factors. It is therefore usually conducted in a laboratory setting using an ergometer appropriate to the participant's sport (treadmill, cycle ergometer, rowing or canoeing ergometer). During the assessment the participant is required to exercise at an intensity that produces exhaustion, during which time the individual's oxygen consumption is measured. In general, there is a good correlation between an individual's VO_{2max} and his or her capacity to perform endurance exercise. In basic terms this means that the higher a person's VO_{2max}, the fitter that person is for aerobically based sport. Thus, VO_{2max} is an important component of sports fitness.

However, the correlation between VO_{2max} and performance is not perfect and other factors will contribute towards a person's aerobic fitness. One of these factors is the intensity of exercise that can be performed without accumulation of large amounts of lactic acid. Since the accumulation of lactic acid is a major cause of fatigue, the greater the intensity of exercise that can be performed without this occurring is clearly important. For example, if two runners A and B have the same VO_{2max}, but one can run faster before their level of lactic acid rises rapidly (lactate threshold or T_{LAC}) then that runner should be able to run faster than the other in endurance events. In practical terms, if runner A has a T_{LAC} at a speed of $18\,km\,h^{-1}$ while B has a T_{LAC} at $19\,km\,h^{-1}$ and if both were to run at $18.5\,km\,h^{-1}$ A would exceed their T_{LAC} and hence would become fatigued while B would remain below their T_{LAC} and would be able to maintain the pace. The T_{LAC} is important in many endurance sports including running, cycling, canoeing, rowing and swimming.

The measurement of VO_{2max} generally involves use of an incremental protocol during which the subject commences exercise at a modest intensity but is then required to exercise at progressively higher intensities as the test proceeds. During the test the subject's oxygen use, heart rate and other physiological variables are measured. As the exercise intensity increases so will their VO_2, heart rate, ventilation and perceived exertion. The highest recorded VO_2 value is generally referred to as the VO_{2max}, although to be designated as a VO_{2max} it must fulfil certain criteria: a plateau in oxygen utilisation despite an increase in workload, a heart rate within 10 beats min^{-1} of their age-predicted maximum (220 minus age), a perceived exertion of 19 or 20 on the Borg scale (see p. 104), a respir-atory exchange ratio (carbon dioxide produced/oxygen consumed) in excess of 1.1 and a blood lactate concentration in excess of $8\,mmol\,l^{-1}$. If these criteria are not fulfilled then the highest oxygen use should be designated as the subject's peak VO_2. Typical values for VO_{2max} are shown in Table 6.2.

For active adults the observed decline in VO_{2max} with age is approximately 4–8% per decade after the age of 30. For inactive adults the decline is greater and may be in the region of 8–12% per decade.

Table 6.2 $\dot{V}O_{2max}$ values. Exact values will vary depending upon the sport, activity and position played within the sport.

Group (aged 25–35 years)	$\dot{V}O_{2max}$ (ml kg^{-1} min^{-1})	
	Men	Women
Elite endurance athletes	70–80	60–70
Highly trained team games players	55–65	48–60
Active young adults	44–52	38–46
Average for young adults	40–45	34–39

MEASUREMENT OF BLOOD LACTATE

The amount of lactate in the blood indicates the amount of physical stress being experienced by the subject. Low levels (<2 mmol l^{-1}) generally indicate that the participant is coping with the exercise and finding it relatively easy. During an incremental test the subject will reach a stage when blood lactate levels start to rise quite rapidly. At this point the individual will begin to perceive the exercise as difficult and will not be able to sustain exercise intensities above this level for very long: this level is generally referred to as an individual's lactate threshold (T_{LAC}). The higher the workload at which this occurs the fitter the individual is deemed to be. The interpretation of lactate data can be quite complex and the costs involved generally mean that it is reserved for assessing sportsmen and women, or for exercise research.

The following features may be seen with an increase in fitness.

1. At the final maximal workload:
   - The attainment of a higher final workload or the ability to sustain the same final workload for a longer duration.
   - A higher maximal oxygen uptake ($\dot{V}O_{2max}$ or peak $\dot{V}O_2$).
2. At each submaximal workload:
   - A lower heart rate at each workload. This is a useful indicator when monitoring one individual, but (due to individual variations) it may not be as good when comparing different individuals, especially those of a similar level of fitness.
   - A lower blood lactate concentration at each workload.
   - A lower perceived exertion at each workload.

For those involved in sport rather than a health-oriented exercise programme, a number of sport-specific exercise tests are available, ranging from the relatively simple

Table 6.3 Responses of fit and unfit individuals to exercise

Speed (km h^{-1})	Heart rate (beats min^{-1})	RPE*	$\dot{V}O_2$ (l min^{-1})	Blood lactate (mmol l^{-1})
Aerobically fit individual:				
9	106	7	1.30	0.68
11	117	8	1.83	0.86
13	129	9	2.27	0.89
15	140	11	2.66	0.97
17	154	12	3.20	1.45
19	167	15	3.76	3.17
21	181	17	4.34	6.52
Aerobically less fit individual:				
9	125	9	1.35	0.89
11	148	13	1.93	2.47
13	162	16	2.31	4.67
15	183	19	2.72	6.81

*Ratings of perceived exertion (Borg, 1982)

multistage shuttle test (commonly employed to assess the fitness of team games players) to specific assessments using treadmills, cycle, rowing, canoe and other specialised ergometry. These tests should be confined to those familiar with maximal exertion and should generally be conducted by a sports scientist or, in some cases, a suitably experienced coach.

Recent research suggests that a number of illnesses can significantly reduce the $\dot{V}O_{2max}$ and T_{LAC} of competitive sportspeople and therefore the measurement of these parameters may be relevant in monitoring participants for illness as well as evaluating the effectiveness of their training.

TREADMILL TESTS FOR THE ESTIMATION OF AEROBIC FITNESS

Whilst the laboratory measurement of $\dot{V}O_{2max}$ using sophisticated gas analysis equipment is the most accurate means of assessing aerobic capacity, there are treadmill protocols that enable an estimation of $\dot{V}O_{2max}$. One of the most frequently used is the 'Bruce' protocol. This is an incremental maximum test which, if combined with ECG monitoring, can be used as a diagnostic protocol for CHD. The test protocol commences at a low intensity and increases in speed and gradient every three minutes. The basis of the test is that fitness will be reflected in the individual's ability to reach the higher workloads. An individual with a high $\dot{V}O_{2max}$ will attain a high workload before the test is terminated whereas a less fit individual, with a lower $\dot{V}O_{2max}$ will not reach the higher workloads and the test will be terminated sooner (Bruce *et al.*, 1973). Hence the basis of the test is not dissimilar to that of the 20 m multistage shuttle run test.

The original 'Balke' protocol (Balke and Ware, 1959) was a treadmill walking test, completed at a constant speed of 3.3 mph. During the test the treadmill gradient is increased by 1% every minute until the subject's heart rate reached 180 beats min^{-1}. A number of 'modified Balke protocols' have been developed, which include working to volitional exhaustion, variations in the size of gradient increase and variations in the stage duration. For each of these protocols an equation is then used to estimate the subject's $\dot{V}O_2$ from the final gradient attained. A further variation on this theme is the graded treadmill walking test (GTWT; see below).

GRADED TREADMILL WALKING TEST FOR THE ESTIMATION OF AEROBIC CAPACITY

A GTWT works on a principle similar to that of a submaximal multistage cycle ergometer test. During these tests it is usual to also have the facility for assessing $\dot{V}O_2$ and heart rates. Oxygen use at each submaximal workload can then be plotted against the individual's heart rate at each workload and from this the line of best fit can be extrapolated to their age-predicted maximal heart rate. This can then be used to predict the peak oxygen uptake (peak $\dot{V}O_2$) at the age-predicted maximal heart rate.

A common protocol for a walking test is to use a consistent speed (e.g. 5 km h^{-1}) or one predetermined for the subject. The subject walks at this speed for 4 minutes whilst their heart rate and $\dot{V}O_2$ are recorded. The exercise intensity is then increased by raising the gradient of the treadmill by 2.5% and the subject asked to walk for a further 4 minutes. This is repeated for a total of four stages. For older individuals (above 50 years) it is common to commence the test with the treadmill gradient set at 0%, thereby finishing the fourth stage at 7.5%; for younger individuals the test may commence at 2.5% and finish at 10%. All the required pretest procedures should be employed and the subject allowed to terminate the test at any stage.

SUBMAXIMAL ESTIMATION OF AEROBIC FITNESS FROM HEART RATES

Given the acknowledged risks of strenuous exercise for relatively unfit and older less active individuals, most fitness assessments used in a health context tend to be submaximal rather than maximal. Assessment tests that follow submaximal protocols tend to rely upon the measurement of the heart rate during exercise and/or the measurement of post-exercise recovery heart rates. If the body is given a specified and standardised amount of exercise to do then individuals with a 'fitter' cardiovascular system will be able to perform the exercise with a lower heart rate and, as a consequence, will have lower heart rates immediately after the exercise. For example, if an individual initially performed a standardised test with an exercise heart rate of 150 beats min^{-1}, after a six-week exercise programme designed to improve aerobic fitness that individual should be able to perform the same test with a lower heart rate.

The simplest and most commonly used forms of submaximal testing are the 'step tests'. Submaximal cycle ergometer tests are based upon similar lines but permit variation in the intensity of the exercise. However, if the participant is taking any form of medication, such as beta-blockers (which influence the heart rate), then the exercise heart rate is no longer an appropriate measurement of aerobic fitness and alternatives will be necessary.

The simplest submaximal tests measure heart rate during and/or after a single workload, usually lasting about 5 minutes. These are, arguably, the tests most prone to estimation error. However, they can still be used to detect substantial changes in fitness via comparisons in heart rate. The more involved tests will be multistage, using several submaximal workloads. Some will measure heart rate whilst the more sophisticated will also measure submaximal oxygen utilisation ($\dot{V}O_2$). This information can then be used to predict the individual's fitness, with some tests extrapolating the data to predict the individual's oxygen uptake at their predicted maximum heart rate.

SUBMAXIMAL SINGLE-STAGE HEART RATE RESPONSE TESTS: STEP TESTS

There are a large number of variations on the basic step test. However, they are all based upon the same physiological principles. One of the most widely used is the Harvard Step Test, developed by Brouha *et al.* (1943); most other tests are variations.

The stepping cycle usually involves starting with both feet on the floor facing the bench or step. The participant places one foot on the step, then the other, then lowers one foot to the ground, then the other, and this is repeated in a continuous manner. The test thus involves a repeated four-stage cycle of 'up, up, down, down'. This cycle is performed at a predetermined speed on a bench or step of a specified height. A speed of 25 cycles per minute is appropriate for most individuals in the general population; however, a slower stepping rate (20 cycles per minute) may be more suitable for people whose levels of aerobic fitness may be 'below average'. During the assessment a metronome or prerecorded tape can be used to set the speed, and it is usual to set it to coincide with each phase of the cycle: for a stepping speed of 25 cycles a minute the metronome should be set to 100, for a stepping speed of 20 steps per minute the metronome should be set to 80.

The height of the bench may also be varied in accordance with the physical condition of the individuals being assessed. Step heights of 30–45 cm are fairly standard and will be appropriate in most situations. In reality the exercise adviser is likely to use whatever is available, but if monitoring fitness over a period of time it is important to maintain the same step height and stepping rate so that the results are comparable. It is also important that the participant maintains a consistent stepping technique; this will include extending the knees when on the bench. Alternating the 'leading leg' a number of times during the test is also desirable as it tends to fatigue more rapidly than the other.

The duration of step tests vary from 3 to 5 minutes, although in some variations it is not necessary to complete the full duration of the test as long as the actual time taken is recorded. The participant will stop exercising upon completion of the specified duration, when he or she has had enough, or when the exercise adviser feels that the exercise should stop. Following cessation of the exercise a number of post-exercise heart rates should be recorded (the participant's heart rates should also be recorded during the exercise to provide continuous feedback on how well they are coping with the exercise). With the advent of short-wave telemetry heart-rate monitors this has become relatively easy. The heart rate should be recorded immediately the exercise has ceased; however, if not using a heart rate monitor, the time taken to locate the pulse is likely to mean that it will actually be taken 20–30 seconds after cessation of the exercise.

When palpating the heart rate by hand the pulse should be monitored for 15–30 s. This figure is used to calculate the heart rate in beats min^{-1}. Additional post-exercise heart rates may then be taken at minute intervals to record the rate of recovery. The fitter the individual, the lower their heart rate will be during exercise, the lower it will be after exercise and the sooner it will return to its pre-exercise level.

Repeating the test a number of weeks later will produce a comparable set of results that can be used to evaluate any substantial changes in the fitness of the participant, with lower heart rates indicating an improvement in aerobic fitness.

Exercise heart rate

If the facilities are available, the 'exercise heart rate' should be recorded. This will increase during the exercise and level off some minutes into the test. This exercise heart rate can be used in addition to the post-exercise heart rates to evaluate the participant's fitness. The exercise heart rate is often more informative than the recovery heart rate as it indicates the amount of 'physical stress' the body is experiencing during the exercise. A lower exercise heart rate indicates a greater capacity to cope with the exercise. Significantly lower heart rates should also be associated with a general feeling that the exercise is easier, and will provide further subjective indication of an improvement in aerobic fitness.

Fitness index

If the participant does not complete the specified duration of the exercise the exercise adviser can record the length of time for which the exercise was sustained, and this may then be used as an initial evaluation of their fitness. Alternatively, the duration of exercise and the recovery heart rates may be used to produce a 'fitness index', which will increase as the participant is able to exercise for longer and/or their recovery heart rates are reduced. An example of such an equation is given below (Brouha *et al.*, 1943) and, as with other aspects of the testing procedures, the exercise adviser may like to devise norms for participants in accordance with their own circumstances and the individuals with whom they work.

Fitness index
$$= \frac{\text{Duration of exercise in seconds} \times 100}{\text{Sum of the three recovery pulse rates}}$$

For example, an exercise adviser may devise a 5-minute step test using a gymnasium bench and a stepping rate of 25 steps per minute. Before the test the subject's heart rate should be measured for later comparison. Upon completion of the 5 minutes the participant's heart rate may be measured 30 seconds after the exercise and then at 1 minute intervals for the following 3 minutes to give four post-exercise heart rates.

So, if the participant exercised for the specified 5 minutes (300 s) and the post-exercise heart rates were 152 beats min^{-1} after 30 s, 140 after 1 min 30 s, and 123 2 min 30 s after the exercise, their fitness index would be calculated from Brouha's formula as follows:

$$FI = \frac{300 \times 100}{(152 + 140 + 123)}$$

$$= \frac{30000}{415}$$

$$= 72.3.$$

In subsequent tests any decrease in the post-exercise heart rates would be manifested in an increased fitness index, which would indicate an increase in aerobic fitness. If in an initial test the participant was unable to exercise for the full 5 minutes but was able to continue exercising for longer in subsequent tests, this would result in a larger value on the top line of the equation and therefore a higher fitness index.

Fitness ratings based upon the original Harvard Step Test (Brouha *et al.*, 1943) are shown in Table 6.4.

The example presented above is intended to provide some form of general guidance on how an individual's aerobic fitness may be quantified. It is not intended to represent a rigid testing procedure that is applicable for all individuals: indeed, exercise advisers should modify this assessment procedure, adopting their own form of assessment and calculation of a fitness index appropriate to the individuals with whom they are working. However, when doing so they must be aware of the need to evaluate the validity and reliability of their test protocol. Other validated step test protocols include the Queens College

Table 6.4 Fitness ratings for the Harvard Step Test

Fitness index	Rating
>90	Excellent
80–89	Good
65–79	High average
55–64	Low average
<55	Poor

Step Test (McArdle *et al.*, 1972) and the multistage Siconolfi Step Test (Siconolfi *et al.*, 1985).

The Queens College Step test uses a 41 cm step, a cadence of 88 beats min^{-1} (22 complete stepping cycles a minute) and lasts for 3 minutes. A recovery pulse is recorded for 15 seconds between 5 and 20 seconds post exercise and converted to beats min^{-1}.

The $\dot{V}O_{2max}$ is estimated from the equation

$$\dot{V}O_{2max} = 65.81 - (0.847 \times \text{recovery heart rate})$$

As with many of the other submaximal tests, this is unsuitable for estimating the $\dot{V}O_{2max}$ of the very fit as their actual $\dot{V}O_{2max}$ values exceed the range for which the test was designed.

SUBMAXIMAL MULTISTAGE HEART RATE RESPONSE TESTS: SUBMAXIMAL CYCLE ERGOMETER TESTS

Multistage tests have a number of advantages over single stage protocols. Within the protocol of a multistage cycle ergometer assessment it is possible to increase the intensity of the exercise gradually by altering the resistance of the ergometer. This means that a test can commence at a very easy level and gradually increase in intensity until it reaches a level which is appropriate for the individual. This has a distinct advantage over the single-stage tests, which have a fixed exercise intensity that may be too strenuous to assess some individuals effectively and yet not be sufficiently strenuous for others. The data collected during cycle ergometer tests can be used to produce an objective evaluation of an individual's fitness and, where appropriate, to calculate suitable exercise loads that can be used in the client's prescribed exercise programme.

When using a cycle ergometer the recommended speed of pedalling (cadence) is 50–60 pedal revolutions per minute (rpm). Specifying a pedalling rate is more practical than suggesting specific speeds since for some ergometers a pedalling rate of 50 rpm will correspond to a speed of approximately 18 km h^{-1}

whilst for other ergometers it may correspond to only 12 km h^{-1}. Pedal rates faster than 60 rpm are too rapid and require an anaerobic contribution to the exercise, thereby causing the rapid onset of fatigue. Conversely, pedalling rates of less than 50 rpm are often considered too leisurely. A rate of 50–60 rpm is generally considered optimal for comfort, convenience and for producing a suitable intensity of exercise. However, the exercise adviser may wish to modify the rate slightly to fit the participant and ergometer.

During a cycle ergometer fitness assessment and/or during an exercise programme it is usual to maintain a constant pedal speed (cadence) throughout the exercise. The intensity of the exercise is altered by adjusting the amount of resistance applied to the pedals of the cycle whilst keeping the rate of pedalling constant. With most ergometers the resistance is increased by increasing the tightness of a 'resistance belt' around the rim of the flywheel. Others are electronically braked or use 'wind resistance'. The intensity of the exercise performed by the participant therefore depends upon the speed of pedalling and the amount of resistance offered by the ergometer.

Different exercise cycles display their scale of resistance in different ways: in the simplest examples it may be in the form of an arbitrary scale from 1 to 10 where the units of resistance are not specified; in others the resistance or power output is displayed in kilograms or watts. It is preferable to describe the power output in terms of watts because the watt is the internationally recognised unit in this field of exercise physiology, which will make any dialogue on the topic easier and more meaningful. Accurate calibration of the ergometer is also important to enable meaningful comparisons.

Example protocol

The following example protocol for a submaximal cycle ergometer test is presented to illustrate the general design of such tests. The exercise adviser may modify this protocol in accordance with their own requirements.

1. Check the medical history of the participant and ascertain if he or she is taking any medication. This may be important: beta-blockers will keep the heart rate low (making it an inappropriate measure of exercise intensity).
2. Take the subject's pulse to check its regularity.
3. If appropriate, measure the blood pressure to ensure that the participant is not suffering from hypertension. These preliminary procedures may have been completed by nursing or medical staff before the individual embarks upon the exercise programme.
4. Ensure that the participant is seated comfortably on the ergometer. When seated the knees should be slightly flexed at the bottom of the downstroke. This is the optimum position for pedalling and will ensure that the participant works the knee joint through a full and optimal range of motion without overstretching.
5. Describe the test procedure. The assessor should inform the participant of the exercise protocol and emphasise that the test is not maximal.
6. The exercise adviser should make it clear that the participant can stop the test at any time, especially if he or she feels dizzy, uncomfortable or distressed. The aim is to work moderately hard but not to exhaustion. The test is likely to make the participant slightly warm and breathless but should not cause any distress or discomfort.
7. The test should commence with the participant pedalling at the desired speed against a light resistance. A power output of 25–50 W (or 0.5–1.0 kg) is recommended. Even if the participant is fairly fit the initial workload should be light as it will serve as a warm-up. Commencing

8. The participant should pedal for 2 minutes at the initial workload whilst the assessor monitors their heart rate using an electrocardiogram or pulse meter throughout the tests (alternatively, the pulse could be taken at the end of the 2 minute warm-up). The participant should not stop pedalling while their pulse is being monitored. Some test protocols may use stage durations of up to 4 minutes. The key aspect is to provide sufficient duration for the heart rate to level off at a steady rate.

9. If at the end of 2 minutes the heart rate is still relatively low and the participant is feeling comfortable and is able to continue, the workload may be increased. It is usual to increase the workload by small increments to enable the body to adjust gradually to the increased exercise intensity. Increases of 25–50 W (0.5–1 kg) are recommended. The precise increase will depend upon the fitness of the subject and how easy they find the exercise. Whilst the resistance is being increased the participant should continue to pedal, and thus will pedal continuously throughout the assessment without a break.

10. Stage 9 is repeated until the participant feels that he or she is making enough effort, until the heart rate reaches the top end of the training zone, or until the assessor feels that the assessment should be concluded. During the assessment the participant may get slightly breathless but should still be able to answer questions and should not experience any discomfort or pain. The subject is also likely to become warm, and should remove any excess clothing before or during the assessment to prevent overheating.

11. Following the completion of the final workload the subject should cool down by pedalling steadily for at least a minute against a very easy resistance. This will allow the heart rate to gradually lower until it returns to just above the pre-exercise level.

12. Upon completion of the test the assessor should have a number of heart rate measurements which were taken whilst the participant pedalled against a known resistance. These can then be used in the evaluation of fitness and may also be used to determine future exercise loads on the ergometer if that is to form part of the exercise programme.

13. The data collected during the assessment may be tabulated and/or compared with previous results. Lower heart rates at the specified workloads indicate an improvement in aerobic fitness. By plotting it onto a graph the data may be used to calculate a measure of aerobic fitness called the physical working capacity (PWC) (Wahlund, 1948). The graph can also be used to determine appropriate exercise loads. Astrand and Ryhming (1954) developed a nomogram for the estimation of $\dot{V}O_{2max}$ from heart rate data collected during cycle ergometer tests.

Use of PWC values

The PWC value and exercise loads are calculated by plotting a graph of heart rate against workload and drawing a 'line of best fit' through the points on the graph (Figure 6.3). At the point where this line crosses the horizontal line corresponding to the desired heart rate a vertical line is drawn down to the x axis. The point at which this line crosses the x axis gives the workload required to elevate that person's heart rate to the specified level. For example, a PWC_{170} is the exercise intensity required to elevate a person's heart rate up to 170 beats min^{-1}. The PWC value selected for any individual will depend upon his or her age and condition. As a general guideline, the PWC value

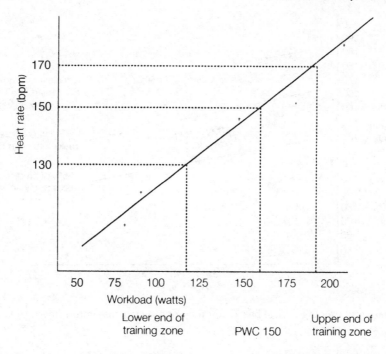

Figure 6.3 The data obtained from a PWC test may be used to determine appropriate training loads

should be towards the upper end of the subject's training zone (see Figure 6.4). For a 20-year-old person PWC_{170} may be appropriate, whereas for someone of 50 PWC_{140} may be more applicable.

These graphs and PWC values may be used to monitor fitness in the following way. An improvement in aerobic capacity will correspondingly lower heart the rate at each exercise intensity, giving a 'line of best fit' below the previous one and also probably with a shallower gradient. This will therefore produce a higher PWC value since a greater workload will be required to elevate the individual's heart rate up to the same level. This means that the fitter the individual, the higher the PWC value will be.

Suitable training loads can be determined using the graph obtained from a PWC test. Firstly, the participant's heart-rate training zone is calculated in accordance with their age (see Figure 6.4). Horizontal lines are then drawn from the points on the y axis to corre-

spond to the lower and upper ends of the heart-rate training zone. Where these lines cross the 'line of best fit' vertical lines are drawn down to the x axis. The points at which these lines cross the x axis are the suggested minimum and maximum exercise loads. Any exercise intensity between these values will elevate the heart rate into the training zone. In the example illustrated in Figure 6.3, if the lower end of the participant's training zone was 130 beats min^{-1}, a horizontal line drawn from 130 until it crosses the 'line of best fit' and then directly down might cross the workload axis (corresponding to the minimum exercise intensity that the participant should work at if aerobic benefits are to be gained from the exercise) at 120 W. The maximum exercise intensity can be calculated by using the heart rate at the upper end of the training zone (e.g. 185 W). Any exercise intensity between these two extremes (in this example 120 and 185 W) is likely to be suitable for the development of the individual's aerobic fitness.

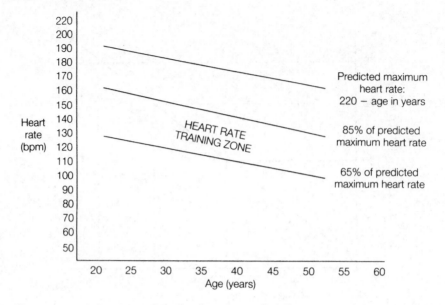

Figure 6.4   Heart rate training zones, based upon age-predicted maximum heart rates (220 minus age in years)

Where repeated assessments indicate an improvement in fitness the appropriate training exercise loads will increase as the participant's capacity to cope with the exercise increases.

The example described in this section is for a basic cycle ergometer. However, similar tests use arm ergometers, rowing machines or even motorised treadmills. By using the same basic principles the exercise adviser can devise appropriate methods for assessing and monitoring the fitness of the individuals with whom they are working.

FIELD TESTS FOR THE ASSESSMENT OF AEROBIC FITNESS

Assessments of aerobic fitness can also be conducted in 'field' settings, such as gyms or halls. These assessments include the multi-stage shuttle running test which is commonly employed with sports teams. Similar, but less strenuous, tests are based on walking; these are likely to be more suitable for most non-sporting individuals. However, 'field' tests are also subject to the considerations of

validity, reliability and specificity. Factors which may influence the results (such as preparation of the subject, the test area, floor surface, clothing worn and, in the case of tests conducted outside, the weather) must all be accounted for. Failing to consider these influences can result in unreliable data, which prevents effective and meaningful monitoring of the participant's fitness.

As with other forms of testing the state of mind of the participant will be important. In field tests which measure the distance covered or number of shuttles completed, the participant's motivation, confidence and familiarity with the activity can all affect the results. In the case of familiarity, if possible the test should be repeated within a few days to detect whether the result was a true physiological assessment. Ideally testing should be repeated at frequent intervals until no further improvements are observed, to provide a true baseline measurement. However, this frequency of testing is usually unrealistic (and indeed participating in the test may have a training effect upon the less fit participants).

Multistage shuttle run

The 20 m multistage shuttle run is a popular field test, commonly used to assess sports teams. It is maximal and exhaustive, and therefore should not be used with very unfit individuals, for whom walking tests are more suitable.

This test requires participants to run between two markers positioned 20 m apart at a pace dictated by a prerecorded tape. The test commences at a relatively slow speed, but pace increases every minute. The participants continue to run between the markers until they are unable to keep up with the dictated speed. At this point they withdraw from the test and the level they have reached is recorded. This test can also be used to estimate $\dot{V}O_{2max}$, although many assessors prefer simply to use the level and number of shuttles completed as the measure of fitness. The rationale for the test is based upon research showing a strong correlation between $\dot{V}O_{2max}$ and the level attained on the test, participants with higher $\dot{V}O_{2max}$ values attaining a higher level.

Maximal effort is important for this test and when assessing groups an element of competition is often involved. When implementing the test the assessor must be aware of the influence of the environment. The test is essentially devised for use indoors with firm flooring, although it may be performed outside, provided that the weather conditions are not adverse. If the ground is soft the results will be adversely affected. The cassette and instructions for this validated test are available from the National Coaching Foundation (Leeds, UK).

Shuttle walking test

The shuttle walking test is based on the same principles as the shuttle running test. However, it requires a less vigorous level of activity and is therefore more suitable for less active individuals.

Run test (12 minute, 15 minute or 1.5 mile)

A number of running tests have been developed to assess aerobic fitness. The strenuous nature of these make them only suited for healthy, young or very fit individuals who run on a regular basis. The effects of pace judgement and specificity will also favour individuals who are familiar with distance running. As with other forms of field testing, weather and underfoot conditions can influence the results. However, despite these reservations, distance runs and timed runs are employed extensively to assess aerobic fitness. Primarily this is due to their relative ease of administration, minimal equipment requirements, relevance to many sporting activities and the facility to assess quite large numbers of subjects at the same time. Consequently they are commonly used to assess sports teams and groups of children. Since these are maximum tests an appropriate warm-up is important to optimise performance and reduce the risk of injury. The results of these tests can be used to estimate the participant's $\dot{V}O_{2max}$; alternatively the assessor may choose simply to use the performance data (distance covered in the designated time or time taken to complete the designated distance) as the fitness measure.

In the 12 and 15 minute runs the participants are required to cover as much distance as possible in the allotted time. They should be conducted on an athletics track or similar surface. The 15-minute run was developed by Balke (1963), who produced an equation to estimate $\dot{V}O_{2max}$ from the distance covered. The 12-minute run, advocated by Cooper (1968a,b), is based upon the same principles, with the results also being used to estimate an individual's $\dot{V}O_{2max}$.

Run tests of 1 and 1.5 miles provide a slight variation on this theme. In these tests the participants are required to cover the designated distance as quickly as possible and the fitness rating is based upon the time taken to complete the distance. Once again a $\dot{V}O_{2max}$

can be estimated from the results (Hazeldine, 1985, based on Cooper, 1968a).

Walking tests

These tests require the participant to walk a prescribed distance as quickly as possible (Kline *et al.*, 1987). The $\dot{V}O_{2max}$ is then estimated from the time taken to complete the distance, combined with the subject's body weight, age and gender. As with other performance tests the assessor may chose to simply use the time taken to complete the distance as the fitness measure. For the Kline 1-mile walking test an estimation of $\dot{V}O_{2max}$ is derived from the following equation:

$$\dot{V}O_{2max} = 132.85 - (0.1694 \times \text{body weight}) - (0.39 \times \text{age}) - (0.0543 \times \text{elapsed time}) - (0.16 \times \text{heart rate}) + (6.32 \times \text{gender})$$

Where body weight is measured in kg, age in years, elapsed time in seconds and heart rate in beats min^{-1}. Gender is given the value 0 (female) or 1 (male).

ASSESSMENTS FOR INDIVIDUALS WITH A SUBSTANTIALLY REDUCED PHYSICAL CAPACITY

Physical capacity may be seriously reduced in a number of circumstances (following surgery, recovery from illness, during rehabilitation from injury, certain chronic conditions). Rehabilitation concerns those with acute conditions (e.g. acute infections such as Guillain–Barré syndrome, or immediately postoperatively) as well as those with chronic conditions. In both cases, rehabilitation involves the use of exercise in the broadest sense, and the assessment techniques used will vary considerably. Exercise programmes are now employed widely in the rehabilitation of people with chronic disease. The importance and application of some assessment techniques for these patients will be considered in this section.

Patients with chronic conditions are entered into a rehabilitation programme involving exercise because their physical status is compromised in some way. This may be due to coronary artery disease, chronic obstructive pulmonary disease (COPD), asthma, chronic renal failure, diabetes or low back pain, to name a few of the patient groups for whom exercise may be an appropriate intervention. For these patient populations it is often more appropriate to take a functional approach to rehabilitation, in which the main focus is upon helping to promote return to normal function and so improve their ability to cope with the activities of everyday life. This may include such simple tasks as climbing steps or walking about the house and therefore assessment and goal-setting must be relevant to these levels of functioning. This is in clear contrast to the fitness assessment and goals of the healthy population, dealing with levels of fitness that are uncompromised by disease.

Measures used for assessment within rehabilitation must be sensitive to changes likely to occur within the specific patient population. Practically, measures commonly used are those of physical performance and health related quality of life.

Clinically, exercise testing is often performed as part of the thorough patient examination and recommended before entry to a rehabilitation programme involving exercise. Other specifics of assessment will depend upon the individual patient and their condition, and are beyond the scope of this chapter. Exercise tests are often used to evaluate a patient's level of disability and their ability to perform day to day activities. Information obtained from such testing will help to determine whether exercise is an appropriate intervention for that individual. Indications of a patient's limitations to exercise, whether cardiovascular, respiratory or peripheral, will also help to determine which type of exercise programme is most likely to be effective. Repeated testing will help to monitor a patient's disorder, as well as showing the outcomes of interventions used.

Both maximal and submaximal exercise tolerance tests have their place in rehabilitation, and are useful in the evaluation of functional capacity when applied appropriately. An end point gained through maximal testing of some patient populations is often referred to as a symptom-limited or peak maximum because exercise may be limited by factors other than the fatigue normally experienced with exercise in a healthy individual. For example, one of several factors likely to limit exercise in patients with respiratory disorders is the inability of their lungs to meet the exercise demands. Similarly, pain may be the limiting factor for those with low back pain. Since the physiological responses to exercise of various patients are different from those in healthy people, care must be taken in prescribing exercise from the information obtained from an exercise test, since this too will differ. For example, the linear relationship between work rate and heart rate seen in healthy individuals is not always present in patients with COPD, making it difficult to prescribe exercise from a submaximal test (Singh, 1997).

In practice, prescription of activity or exercise for very disabled patients must consider such exercise-related symptoms as dyspnoea (shortness of breath), fatigue or anxiety (Jones *et al.*, 1987). Because of the difference in the physiological responses to exercise in some patient groups it is often useful to collect additional data during exercise testing; this may be used later to modify an exercise programme and evaluate progress. Particularly useful are the ratings of perceived exertion (RPE) (Borg, 1982; see Figure 5.1) and the dyspnoea scale (American College of Sports Medicine, 1991; Figure 6.5). The RPE scale is well known and is valuable in helping patients understand appropriate levels of intensities for both exercise and everyday activities. The dyspnoea scale is similar in its application. These tools may be used alone or in combination with other parameters for exercise prescription. They are also useful in evaluating change,

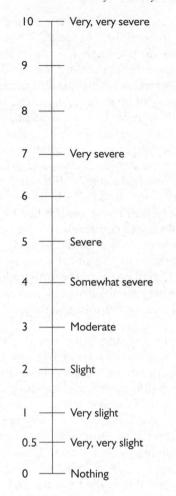

Figure 6.5 The dyspnoea scale (American College of Sports Medicine, 1991).

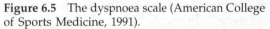

particularly for severely disabled patients in whom improvement is often subjective and difficult to relate to commonly recorded objective measurements. It has been suggested that the measurement of symptomatic changes in this semi-objective manner through the use of rating scales is worthwhile (Jones *et al.*, 1987).

The decision on which exercise test protocol is appropriate will depend upon many factors including age, cardiovascular symptoms, medication, past and present levels of activity and exercise, and psychological status (Pollock *et al.*, 1984). In cardiac patients, the graded exercise test is routinely performed in the belief that it may help to identify those at risk of a future cardiac event. It is also widely considered as the 'gold standard' for the development of exercise prescription and determining the intensity of monitoring in cardiac rehabilitation programmes (Berra and Rudd, 1993).

Research has established guidelines for safe exercise testing in certain patient populations including those with cardiac and pulmonary diseases (Hodgkin, 1987; Miller and Morley, 1987; Berra and Rudd, 1993). These tests are modifications of those used in healthy populations since exercise levels will be comparatively very low. Because of the compromised physical status of patients affected by chronic disease, it may be more appropriate for those who are very disabled to perform tests at a constant level rather than use the graded protocols.

Laboratory testing is not widely available, nor is it considered essential in assessing all patient populations, such as those with little or no risk for cardiovascular disease. Consequently, field exercise tests are often used as an alternative assessment of disability. The simplest and most commonly used tests are 3, 6 or 12 minute walking tests. These are self-paced tests, the patient being required to walk as far as possible in the time allowed. During the test the patient may stop to take a rest if necessary, although the clock continues to run. At the end of the test, final distance walked, heart rate, RPE and level of dyspnoea are recorded. These tests are effective in assessing functional capacity and exercise tolerance and in monitoring progress (McGavin *et al.*, 1976; Lipkin *et al.*, 1986). Clearly these tests may be prone to the influence of motivation and encouragement and it has been recommended that the test is repeated one to three times to obtain an accurate baseline (Belman, 1986).

A recently developed shuttle walking test has proved both reliable and valid for several patient populations including those with COPD (Singh *et al.*, 1992) and low back pain

(Bland and Altman, 1986). This is similar to the shuttle running test used in healthy populations. It is a maximal (symptom-limited) test which requires the patient to walk 10-m shuttles paced by a cassette recording. The pace is increased every minute and the patient continues until he or she can no longer keep up with the pace. Heart rate, dyspnoea and RPE may be recorded. Again, as with all similar tests, patient effort is a factor which may affect the reliability of results. However, there is limited research upon the relationship of all field exercise test results to symptom-limited maximums in patients, and therefore their validity in assessing exercise tolerance must be questioned (Singh, 1997).

Within the functional approach to rehabilitation, it is now well recognised that meaningful measures of health-related quality of life should be used to evaluate interventions within healthcare (Bowling, 1992). Such measures are increasingly used to evaluate the impact of disease upon patients' lives and to determine the effects of rehabilitation. It has already been suggested that patient improvement through rehabilitation may not be detected by standard physiological measurements. In some irreversible or progressive disorders, it may be unreasonable to expect changes in exercise test results. These measurements do not account for the now well accepted psychosocial benefits that may be gained through exercise. In evaluating the outcomes of an exercise intervention, it is therefore important to determine whether it may contribute to a life worth living in social and psychological, as well as physical terms. A wider perspective of functioning is needed, which includes many factors of a patient's life such as function in daily life, productivity, performance, social interaction, emotional stability and life satisfaction. This is a developing area of research, and the ideal tool to evaluate quality of life has yet to be established. There are, however, a number of general and disease-specific questionnaires (e.g. the Sickness Impact Profile (Deyo *et al.*, 1982), the Nottingham Health Profile (Hunt *et al.*, 1986), the Arthritis Impact Measurement Scale (Meenan *et al.*, 1980)) which are applied to evaluate the effects of rehabilitation programmes. However, with such a large number of questionnaires available, it is important to ensure that the tool selected is most appropriate to the patient population.

ELECTROCARDIOGRAM EXERCISE TESTING

While an electrocardiogram (ECG) is an obvious tool in the diagnosis of cardiac conditions in individuals reporting specific symptoms, an exercise ECG can reveal potential problems in asymptomatic people for whom health problems are imminent. Such procedures can therefore help to promote appropriate lifestyle changes and ensure correct exercise prescription in these individuals. In particular, monitoring of the electrical activity of the heart using an electrocardiogram (ECG) can help to reveal cardiac abnormalities, including silent myocardial ischaemia (inadequate supply of blood to areas of the myocardium that does not cause noticeable symptoms during everyday activities). Exercise is commonly incorporated into such assessments because certain ECG abnormalities are not evident at rest but tend to be revealed when the heart has to work relatively hard. However, none of the current procedures can detect all cardiac abnormalities and/or all individuals who may be at risk from strenuous exercise. Those who administer the tests are aware that a small proportion of false negatives do occur and that, whilst a normal ECG usually indicates a healthy heart, it is not an absolute guarantee. False negatives appear to be less common if the test proceeds up to exercise intensities in excess of 85% of maximum. Conversely, exercise ECG tests can produce false positives, which suggest that an individual may have a problem with exercise that they do not in fact have. Shephard (1981, 1994) suggests that up to 66% of individuals with an abnormal ECG may suffer from no serious cardiac problems over the following 5–10 years. Therefore great care must be taken by the professional when interpreting the results of such tests and in making recommendations.

ECG exercise tests generally follow a protocol of small increments in work or a continuous ramp (where the exercise intensity increases in a continuous manner). The treadmill or cycle ergometer are the generally preferred modes of exercise. The basic principle behind an exercise ECG test is that as the exercise intensity increases, so do the demands made upon the heart. This includes an increase in the oxygen used by the myocardium, which, in affected individuals, can alter the ECG. Standard systems for the assessment of ECG use 12 leads placed at specific points, although there is some debate about which combination of locations provides the most informative ECG.

The interpretation of ECGs is a complex practice and should be performed by a specialist cardiologist. The normal ECG (Figure 6.6) consists of a series of waves and points which are associated with the polarisation and depolarisation of the myocardium during the cardiac cycle. These are labelled P, Q, R, S and T. The P phase represents the electrical activity which causes the contraction of the atria, and the subsequent more pronounced Q-R-S complex is associated with the electrical activity that causes the contraction of the ventricles. The final T wave is caused by repolarisation of the ventricles. Abnormalities in the tissues which conduct this electrical activity will result in alterations to the recorded ECG.

When interpreting an ECG the specialist will consider a number of aspects: these include the heart rate and its regularity as well as the

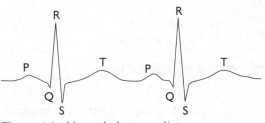

Figure 6.6 Normal electrocardiogram

position and shape of each wave recorded on the ECG. A normal ECG will show consistency in the regularity of the beats (this is measured between consecutive R-R peaks). Significant variations in the time between each beat (as shown by fluctuations in the R-R distance) indicates dysrhythmia (irregular rhythm) or arrhythmia (no rhythm). The shape of each wave, its height on the trace, its duration, the time between each phase and whether each wave is followed by the correct next wave will all indicate whether the electrical activity of the heart is normal. The specialist can attribute abnormalities in these characteristics to specific cardiac problems and thereby diagnose particular conditions.

One of the most common indicators of cardiac abnormalities are changes in the T wave and suppression of the ST segment of the ECG. These tend to indicate myocardial infarction and myocardial ischaemia (inadequate blood supply to a region of the cardiac muscle), which occurs when the amount of oxygen required by the heart to perform exceeds that which is available. This is commonly due to the presence of atheroma which constricts the coronary arteries, thereby restricting the flow of blood and supply of oxygen to the myocardium. If an infarction occurs an area of the myocardium will have been damaged. Cardiac arrhythmia (irregularity of heart beat) is also a common indicator of atheroma, although both can generate false positives. Research suggests that the risk of a future myocardial infarction is 2–6 times greater in individuals with a depressed ST segment than in individuals with a normal ECG. For further details on the interpretation of ECGs see Schaman, 1991.

PSYCHOLOGICAL ASSESSMENTS OF EXERCISE MOTIVATION

REASONS FOR CONDUCTING PSYCHOLOGICAL ASSESSMENTS

At the start of a supervised exercise programme it would be helpful to identify people who are at most risk from dropping out. This would enable allocation of staff time and other resources to these potential non-adherers rather than to people who are well motivated and feel confident that they can stick to the programme. Similarly it would be helpful, when promoting free-living physical activity, if health professionals could identify communities or groups most likely to live sedentary lifestyles because this would allow resources to be targeted at those with the greatest need. Unfortunately exercise psychology is some way from being able to provide either a questionnaire or interview format that can measure motivation or predict non-adherence with the same degree of accuracy as our colleagues in exercise physiology can measure aerobic fitness or flexibility. However, it is possible to offer some suggestions as to how psychological assessments may be able to help health professionals promote physical activity.

QUESTIONNAIRES, INTERVIEWS OR FOCUS GROUPS?

Psychological assessments can be conducted using three basic formats: questionnaires, interviews or focus groups. Each has strengths and weakness and go into and out of fashion with researchers.

Questionnaires

Questionnaires can be used with large groups of people in short periods of time and the data collected can be analysed statistically either by hand or by computer. However, questionnaires which purport to measure motivation are only as good as the items from which they are constructed and at the moment exercise psychology has not clearly identified the variables that discriminate adherers from non-adherers. Questionnaires can also be tedious to fill in and are open to socially acceptable answers – would you want to respond to a question in a way that shows you as lazy and unmotivated? When designing a questionnaire to assess motivation toward exercise or physical activity the following points should be considered.

- Subjects should be told how the information from the question will be used and the benefits that they will receive from it. It should also be made clear that it is not compulsory to complete the questionnaire and that any information given will be treated in the strictest confidence.
- The questionnaire should be kept as short as possible, should include clear instructions on how it should be completed and should use clear and precise language.
- The designers of the questionnaire should know exactly how the data will be analysed and used.
- The questions asked on a questionnaire should be specific to the type of physical activity being provided and the environment in which it will take place.

Interviews

Assessing the motivation of the client to exercise using an interview format offers an opportunity to identify both personality and situationally specific determinants of exercise adherence. Unlike a questionnaire, an interview is a two-way process in which you can interact with your client and change the direction of the questions to uncover more information. However, interviews are relatively time-consuming and can not be used with large numbers of people. Although it is important to allow interviews to develop and themes to emerge it is important to enter into them knowing the questions you would like to ask and having a structure to guide the conversation in the required direction. Patton (1980) suggested that during qualitative inquiry (which includes both interviews and focus groups) the researcher should ask questions related to:

- experience and behaviour;
- opinions and values;
- feelings;
- knowledge;
- sensory perceptions; and
- background and demography.

Although many health professionals who conduct interviews to assess their clients' needs and motivation toward exercise simply internalise the information it is good practice to write up the main points of the interview for future reference.

Focus groups

Over the last decade focus groups have become very popular both with political parties and with marketing companies. They are in effect group interviews which are facilitated by the health professional. As the name suggests, these sessions focus on a specific issue and using prompts, such as those suggested by Patton (1980), allow the group to express both collective and individual opinions. The focus group is lead by a facilitator who keeps the group on the key issue, allows everyone to have their say and records the themes that emerge on flip charts or a blackboard. One of the advantages of focus groups is that the participants can react to and add to the comments of the other group members.

A compromise?

The ideal psychological assessment may be achieved through the use of questionnaire and interview techniques. For example if 100 people have just enrolled on a new exercise course each could be given an exercise motivation questionnaire. If it were possible to identify, for example, 25 subjects who appeared to be at risk from drop-out based on the questionnaire data it may be possible to interview this group to select a group of ten for extra motivation and encouragement. However, although this approach sounds helpful its success is limited by our relative lack of understanding of the determinants of exercise adherence.

WHAT QUESTIONS SHOULD YOU ASK TO IDENTIFY THOSE AT MOST RISK FROM DROP OUT?

Whilst there is a wide range of questions we could ask our clients to assess their motivation to exercise questions should be selected on two criteria:

1. Is the question based on a sound theoretical perspective (e.g. the Theory of Planned Behaviour; Ajzen, 1989) or the results of scientific studies published in refereed journals (see, for example, Kimiecik,1993)?
2. Does the answer to the question help the health professional put in place an intervention that can increase the likelihood of adherence? Just as the exercise physiologist uses the information from a fitness test to prescribe an exercise programme so the exercise psychologist can use the results from a questionnaire or interview to design a strategy to increase motivation and promote exercise behaviour.

To apply these two criteria and develop questions that identify people who are likely to drop out of exercise programmes readers may find it helpful to cross reference the material presented in Chapter 4 (pp. 63–85) with the following.

Current level of physical activity

Assessment format: usually by questionnaire or structured interview. Example format: see the special supplement to *Medicine and Science in Sport and Exercise*, **29**, June 1997, for a collection of physical activity questionnaires for health-related fitness research.

It may sound obvious (and indeed a little unhelpful) to start by saying that those who currently exercise are more likely to be active in the future than those who are currently sedentary. However, by using a measure of physical activity it is possible to rank-order a group of new clients in terms of their current exercise patterns. On the whole we can argue that those in the top 25% need less attention and support than those in the bottom 25%. Unstructured observation shows that exercise leaders at work tend to spend more time with the fitter and more active members of their group than the unfit and more sedentary. This may be because they relate more to people who already share their commitment to exercise or because they find working with those who do least more challenging and stressful.

Previous exercise experience

Assessment format: usually by interview or focus group. Example: see Crone-Grant and Smith (1997).

Just as an individual's current physical activity levels may tell us something about their future exercise patterns so knowledge of their previous experience, including their recollection of school PE, can help to identify those who need more support. Positive experiences of playing sport or living an active life over an extended period of time may indicate that the client has personal experience of the benefits of exercise and may also demonstrate that they have knowledge of how to 'stick with it'. Negative memories of school PE and lack of experience of adhering to an active lifestyle may indicate the need for additional support (Crone-Grant and Smith, 1997). Interviews are probably the most effective way of uncovering these past experiences although on larger programmes focus groups, if appropriately structured, may be useful.

Attitude toward exercise adherence

Assessment format: questionnaire. Example: See Godin (1993).

Attitudes are best measured using a theoretical structure such as that provided by the Theory of Planned Behaviour (see p. 69). People with a poor attitude toward exercise adherence and negative beliefs about possible benefits are less likely to adhere than more

EXERCISE PSYCHOLOGY ASSESSMENT INTERVIEW

Instructions to Interviewers
1. Find a private space to conduct the interview.
2. Explain to the patient that the interview is confidential and the results will only be used to identify those people who need extra help to stick to their exercise programme.
3. If necessary use prompts to encourage the patient to talk, **BUT** beware of influencing their response.
4. Record the key points from the interview in the space provided.
5. Engage in 'active listening' and speak less than the patient!

Patient's name: *Maureen Shepherd* **Sex:** *Female* **Age:** *52* **Referring condition:** *Obesity*

Questions and prompts for patient	Transcription of key points (example responses given in the text)
1. How much exercise did you do as a schoolchild and in your early adulthood? Prompt = PE / Sport / Hobbies Hi risk = Previous history of low activity levels	*I did not like sport at school I was always last in the XC runs and hated my PE teacher! My main hobby when I was younger was reading*
2. How much exercise are you doing now? Prompt = Think about the last seven days Hi risk = No evidence of active living (e.g. walking to work) or active hobbies	*Since I passed my driving test six years ago I don't even walk to the local shops which are only at the end of the street. Most evenings I spend watching the TV with my husband*
3. Are there any problems or barriers that would stop you doing more exercise which you think you could not overcome? Theory = Confidence and attribution theory Hi risk = patient identifies stable and unchangeable problems	*I am worried about my knees which hurt even when I come downstairs at home and am worried about how they will feel when you have me running up and down*
4. Are you looking forward to the programme? Do you think it is going to be fun, rewarding and beneficial or just the opposite? Theory = Attitudes Hi risk = Patient makes consistently negative statements	*I'm very grateful that I have been given the opportunity to come on this exercise programme but I have to be honest and say I don't think I am going to enjoy it. I have tried to lose weight so many times before I can't believe anything could work*
5. How do your partner and friends feel about you coming onto the programme? Theory = Social norm Hi risk = Non-supportive significant others	*My husband is very worried that it might be too much for me and do more harm than good. He said that a lot of these exercise leaders aren't properly qualified*

Instructions to interviewers
Based on the interview, what is your professional judgment of the risk of this subject dropping out of the programme? high / medium / low.

Figure 6.7   Assessment interview questionnaire

positive individuals. Those who are identified as having poor attitudes will require interventions designed to expose them to positive experiences in an exercise environment and will need the health benefits explained to them in a language that they understand using examples that they can relate to.

Confidence toward exercise

Usual format: questionnaire.

Whilst there are many definitions of confidence, and many different tools to measure it, most exercise psychologists would agree that it is an important determinant of exercise adherence. If the health professional can successfully

---

EXERCISE PSYCHOLOGY ASSESSMENT QUESTIONNAIRE

How to complete this questionnaire

1. *The questionnaire is designed to help us identify if you need extra help to stick to your exercise programme. To help us to help you it is important that you answer the questions honestly. All results are confidential.*
2. *To respond to the questions either write your answer or put the number which represents your answer in the space provided.*
3. *If you have any questions please ask the member of staff who gave you this questionnaire.*

Patient's name: *Maureen Shepherd* **Sex:** *Female* **Age:** *52* **Referring condition:** *Obesity*

On a scale of 1 to 10 please answer the following questions:

1. How likely are you to attend all of the exercise sessions over the next ten weeks at the hospital? (1 = very unlikely, 5 = probably, 10 = very likely)	3
2. How active were you at school and in early adulthood? (1 = very inactive, 5 = average, 10 = very active)	3
3. How confident are you that you can overcome barriers which may stop you attending the exercise programme? For example, not having enough time or being too tired. (1 = definitely not, 5 = average, 10 = very confident)	2
4. Do you think that the exercise programme is going to be fun and enjoyable? (1 = definitely not, 5 = it will be OK, 10 = it will be fun)	1
5. Do you think that the exercise programme will help improve your health and be beneficial? (1 = definitely not, 5 = it may, 10 = it will definitely help)	2
6. How supportive do you think your partner, family and friends will be in helping you to attend the exercise programme? (1 = they will not support, 5 = they will be OK, 10 = they will be helpful)	3
(For staff use) total =	14

WHAT HAPPENS NEXT?

A member of staff will add up the total of the answers that you have given. If it is less than 20 they may conduct a short follow-up interview and a decision will be then made as to how we can help you stick to the exercise programme.

Figure 6.8 Drop-out questionnaire

identify people with low levels of self-confidence in an exercise environment they should be able to provide additional support to promote adherence. This may involve spending more time explaining the nature of the exercise programme, introducing the person to others who were nervous to begin with but who are growing in confidence and ensuring that the exercise prescription is at an appropriate level.

EXAMPLES OF A QUESTIONNAIRE AND INTERVIEW FORMAT

Based on the material in the preceding sections it is possible to provide readers with an example of a questionnaire and interview format designed to identify patients who will need extra support to adhere to a new exercise programme. However, these are provided for illustrative purposes only. They should not be used without adaptation to meet the particular needs of individual patients and to correspond with both the goals of your programme and the environment in which it takes place. In these illustrations only one item has been used to explore such complex determinants of exercise adherence as confidence and social norm. Obviously in real assessment instruments it would be necessary to explore these areas in more detail. Both the interview (Figure 6.7) and the questionnaire (Figure 6.8) have been completed by a hypothetical patient called Maureen Shepherd and readers are encouraged to consider how this patient would have responded to the different styles of data collection. Perhaps, more importantly, readers are also encouraged to reflect on how they would use this information to provide the patient with support and assistance.

THE FUTURE OF TARGET INTERVENTIONS IN EXERCISE PSYCHOLOGY

As we find out more about the determinants of exercise adherence we will become more able to match the motivational profile of the client to the appropriate type of physical activity and support them in a more targeted and structured way. However, it is unlikely that this process will become as exact a science as, for example, the prescription of target heart rates from the results of an aerobic fitness test. This is due to the diversity of human nature, which is reflected in the many individual differences we see in personalities and motivation to engage in health-promoting behaviours.

REFERENCES

American College of Sports Medicine (1991). *Guidelines for Exercise Prescription* (4th ed.). Philadelphia: Lea & Feibiger.

Ajzen, I. (1989). *Attitudes, Personality and Behaviour*. Milton Keynes: Open University Press.

Astrand, P.O. and Ryhming, I. (1954). A nomogram for calculation of aerobic capacity (physical fitness) from pulse rate during submaximal work. *Journal of Applied Physiology*, 7, 218–221.

Balke, B. (1963). A simple field test for the assessment of physical fitness. *Civil Aeromedical Research Institute Report*, 63 (6), 1–8.

Balke, B. and Ware, R. (1959). An experimental study of Air Force personnel. *U.S. Armed Forces Medical Journal*, 10, 675–688.

Belman, M.J. (1986) Exercise in Chronic Obstructive Pulmonary Disease. *Clinics in Chest Medicine*, 7, 585–595.

Berra, K. and Rudd, C.L. (1993). High risk and special populations. In *Developing and Managing Cardiac Rehabilitation Programs*, Hall, L.K. (ed.). Pittsburgh: Human Kinetic.

Bland, J.M. and Altman, D.G. (1986). Statistical methods for assessing agreement between two methods of clinical measurement. *Lancet*, 1, 307–310.

Borg, G.V. (1982). Psychophysical basis of perceived exertion. *Medicine and Science in Sport and Exercise*, 14, 377–387.

Bowling, A. (1992). *Measuring Health: A Review of Quality of Life Measuring Scales*. Milton Keynes: Open University Press.

Bruce, R.A., Kusumi, F. and Hosmer, D. (1973). Maximal oxygen intake and nomographic assessment of functional aerobic impairment in cardiovascular disease. *American Heart Journal*, 85, 545–562.

Brouha, L., Graybiel, A. and Heath, C.W. (1943). The step test: A simple method of measuring physical fitness for hard muscular work in adult man. *Revue Canadienne de Biologie*, 2, 86–92.

Chan, K., Maffulli, N., Korkia, P. and Li, R.C.T. (1996). *Principles and Practice of Isokinetics in Sports Medicine and Rehabilitation*. Hong Kong: Williams and Wilkins.

Cooper, K.H. (1968a). A means of assessing maximal oxygen intake. *Journal of the American Medical Association*, **203**, 201–204.

Cooper, K.H. (1968b). *Aerobics*. New York: Evans.

Crone-Grant, D. and Smith, R.A. (1997). Exercise adherence: A qualitative perspective. *Proceedings of the British Association of Sport and Exercise Science Annual Conference 1997, York*. Abstract published in *Journal of Sports Sciences*, **16**(1), 1998.

Daniels, L. and Worthingham, C. (1986). *Muscle Testing*. Philadelphia: W.B. Saunders.

Deyo, R.A., Inui, T.S., Leininger, J. and Overman, S. (1982). Physical and psychological functions in arthritis: Clinical use of a self-administered instrument. *Archives of Internal Medicine*, **142**, 879–82.

Eston, R. and Reilly, T. (eds) (1996). *Kinanthropometry and Exercise Physiology Laboratory Manual*. London: E & FN Spon.

Godin, G. (1993). The theories of reasoned action and planned behaviour: Overview of findings, emerging research problem and usefulness for exercise promotion. *Journal of Applied Sport Psychology*, **5**, 141–157.

Hall, S.J. (1995). *Basic Biomechanics*. London: Mosby.

Hamill, J. and Knutzen, K.M. (1995). *Biomechanical Basis of Human Movement*. Media, PA: Williams and Wilkins.

Hazeldine, R. (1985). *Fitness for Sport*. Marlborough: Crowood Press.

Hodgkin, J.E. (1987). Exercise testing and training. In *Chronic Obstructive Pulmonary Disease Current Concepts*, Hodgkin, J.E. and Petty, T.L. (eds). Philadelphia: Saunders.

Hunt, S,M., McEwan, J. and McKenna, S.P. (1986). *Measuring Health Status*. London: Croom Helm.

Jones, N.L., Berman, L.B., Bartkiewicz, P.D. and Oldridge, N.B. (1987). Chronic obstructive respiratory disorders. In *Exercise Testing and Exercise Prescription for Special Cases*, Skinner, J.S. (ed.). Philadelphia: Lea & Feibiger.

Kimiecik, J. (1993). Predicting vigorous physical activity of corporate employees: Comparing theories of reasoned action and planned behaviour. *Journal of Sports and Exercise Psychology*, **14**, 192–206.

Kline, G.M., Pocari, J.P., Hintermeister, R., Freedson, P.S., Ward, A., McCarron, R.F., Ross, J. and Rippe, J.M. (1987). Estimation of VO_{2max} from a one-mile track walk, gender, age and body weight. *Medicine and Science in Sports and Exercise*, **19**, 253–259.

Lipkin, D.P., Scriven, A.J., Crake, T. and Poole-Wilson, P.A. (1986) Six minute walking test for assessing exercise capacity in chronic heart failure. *British Medical Journal*, **292**, 653–656.

McArdle, W.D., Katch, F.I., Pechar, G.S., Jacobson, L. and Ruck, S. (1972). Reliability and interrelationships between maximal oxygen intake, physical work capacity and step-test scores in college women. *Medicine and Science in Sports and Exercise*, **4**, 182–186.

McGavin, C.R., Gupta, S.P. and McHardy, G.J. (1976). Twelve minute walk test for assessing disability in chronic bronchitis. *British Medical Journal*, **1**, 822–823.

Meenan, R.F., Gertman, P.M. and Mason, J.H. (1980). Measuring health status in arthritis: The Arthritis Impact Measurement Scales. *Arthritis and Rheumatism*, **23**, 146–52.

Miller, H.S. and Morley, D.L. (1987). Low functional capacity. In *Exercise Testing and Exercise Prescription for Special Cases*, Skinner, J.S. (ed.). Philadelphia: Lea & Feibiger.

Patton, M.Q. (1980). *Qualitative Evaluation Methods*. Beverley Hills, CA: Sage.

Pollock, M.L., Wilmore, J.H. and Fox, S.M. (1984). Medical screening and evaluation procedures. In *Exercise in Health and Disease*, Pollock, M.L., Wilmore, J.H. and Fox, S.M. (eds). Philadelphia: Saunders.

Prentice, W.E. (1994). *Therapeutic Modalities in Sports Medicine*. London: Mosby.

Schaman, J.P. (1991). Basic electrocardiographic analysis. In *Resource Manual for Guidelines for Exercise Prescription* (2nd ed.). Philadelphia: Lea & Feibiger.

Shephard, R.J. (1981). *Ischaemic heart disease and exercise*. London: Croom Helm.

Shephard, R.J. (1987). *Exercise Physiology*. Philadelphia: B.C. Decker.

Shephard, R.J. (1994). *Aerobic Fitness and Health*. Champaign, IL: Human Kinetics.

Siconolfi, S.F., Garber, C.E., Laster, T.M. and Carleton, R.A. (1985). A simple valid step test for estimating maximal oxygen uptake in epidemiologic studies. *American Journal of Epidemiology*, **121**, 382–390.

Singh S.J., Morgan, M.D.L., Scott, S., Walters, D. and Hardman, A.E. (1992). The development of the shuttle walking test of disability in patients with chronic airways obstruction. *Thorax*, **47**, 1019–24.

Singh, S.J. (1997). Patient selection and assessment for pulmonary rehabilitation. In *Practical Pulmonary Rehabilitation*, Morgan, M. and Singh, S. (eds). London: Chapman & Hall.

Wahlund, H. (1948). Determination of the physical working capacity. *Acta Medica Scandinavica*, **132**, Suppl. 215.

Table 7.1 summarises the definition of aerobic fitness and shows its importance to both everyday living and specific health conditions. Tables 8.1 (p. 166) and 9.1 (p. 208) present the same position for muscular strength and joint mobility/flexibility, respectively.

DETERMINANTS OF AEROBIC FITNESS AND ADAPTATIONS TO AEROBIC EXERCISE

An individual's aerobic fitness or aerobic capacity is determined by a large number of interrelated factors, primarily by the individual's capacity to utilise oxygen. A person's maximum capacity to use oxygen is referred to as their $\dot{V}O_{2max}$, the maximum volume of oxygen that can be used in a minute. It is usually measured in litres of oxygen per minute ($l\,min^{-1}$) but is often related to the person's body weight ($ml\,kg^{-1}\,min^{-1}$). It should be emphasised that $\dot{V}O_{2max}$ refers to the amount of oxygen that a person can *use*, not simply the volume they can get in and out of their lungs. $\dot{V}O_{2max}$ can be assessed using sophisticated laboratory equipment, which measures oxygen consumption whilst working at maximum aerobic capacity on a cycle ergometer, treadmill or similar apparatus. However, because of the maximal nature of the exercise required, such assessments are not suitable for most individuals and therefore a number of submaximal methods are used to estimate aerobic fitness (see Chapter 6).

The physiological factors which determine a person's capacity to use oxygen include a number of 'central' factors which are involved with the delivery of oxygen to the muscles (lungs, heart and blood) and 'peripheral' factors associated with its use within the muscle.

1. Central factors:
   - The condition of the lungs, airways and muscles associated with breathing.
   - The oxygen-carrying capacity of the blood.
   - The condition of the heart.
   - The condition of the blood vessels.
2. Peripheral factors:
   - The capillary network within the muscles.
   - The amount of myoglobin in the muscle fibres.
   - The size and number of mitochondria within the muscle fibres.
   - Biochemical properties of the muscle fibres, such as the concentration of particular enzymes which are used in the aerobic production of ATP.

THE CONDITION OF THE LUNGS AND THE MUSCLES ASSOCIATED WITH BREATHING

The functions of the respiratory system are to get air (containing oxygen) into the body and to remove waste products, such as carbon dioxide. The gaseous exchange between the

Table 7.1 Aerobic fitness summary

What is aerobic fitness?	Why is aerobic fitness important for health?	Why is aerobic fitness important for active living?	How might aerobic fitness be improved by a structured exercise programme?	How might it be improved through everyday living?
The ability of the heart and lungs to deliver oxygen to the working muscles, and the capacity of the muscles to use that oxygen. This enables the performance of moderate-intensity activities without the accumulation of fatiguing waste products	Taking part in aerobic exercise significantly reduces the risk of coronary heart disease and many other diseases. Its importance is demonstrated by the emphasis given to aerobic physical activity in public health campaigns such as Active for Life. Aerobic exercise can also improve mental health and general well-being	All day-to-day activities such as walking to the shops or going up the stairs rely on the oxygen transport system either during the activity or afterwards during recovery. Poor levels of aerobic fitness have a significant effect on the mobility and independence of the individual. It should also be noted that good levels of aerobic fitness open up a range of opportunities such as participation in active leisure pursuits and sports	Structured aerobic exercise programmes are not limited to those which bear the name ('aerobics') but also include activities such as walking, jogging and swimming. The key is that the activity involves a large muscle mass being moved in a rhythmic manner over a prolonged period. Aerobic programmes are often prescribed in terms of their frequency, intensity and duration	Aerobic fitness can be improved by many day-to-day activities including taking the stairs instead of the escalator when shopping, parking the car at the far side of the supermarket car park and walking to the entrance and using a push lawn mower instead of a motorised version. Walking or cycling part or all of the way to work is another good means of developing aerobic fitness

air and the blood occurs in the small air sacs of the lungs (the alveoli). For an efficient gaseous exchange the airways must be unobstructed, the muscles associated with breathing need to work effectively and the lungs need a good blood supply. Any disorder that restricts these factors will inhibit the entry of oxygen into the body. However, unless a person is suffering from a specific respiratory disorder, this is not the major limiting factor which determines their aerobic capacity. Appropriate forms of aerobic exercise may enhance the respiratory process and promote an individual's capacity to get oxygen into the body and hence oxygenate the blood.

THE OXYGEN-CARRYING CAPACITY OF THE BLOOD

Oxygen is transported around the body by the blood. Via this system it is delivered to the various organs which need it, including the working muscles. Virtually all of the oxygen that is carried by the blood is transported by the erythrocytes (red blood cells). The oxygen combines with the haemoglobin within the erythrocytes to form oxyhaemoglobin. The oxygen-carrying capacity of the blood is therefore largely determined by the amount of haemoglobin in the blood. An increase in the number of erythrocytes (and hence the amount of haemoglobin) will enhance the delivery of oxygen around the body. Aerobic exercise increases these factors, thereby promoting the oxygen-carrying capacity of the blood and enhancing the delivery of oxygen to the muscles.

A point to note is that the adaptations to aerobic exercise include an increase in the fluid (plasma) component of the blood as well as the number of erythrocytes. In some individuals the fluid proportion increases by more than the cellular component, a feature referred to as *haemodilution*. Haemodilution decreases the individual's ratio of cell volume to total blood volume (the *haematocrit*) which is normally about 41–46%. However, this is not a negative response since their overall capacity to deliver oxygen is still enhanced by the increased number of erythrocytes, although when taking a 'blood test' it can sometimes be mistaken for mild anaemia, which it is not.

THE CONDITION OF THE HEART

The blood is pumped around the body by the action of the heart. One of the most significant chronic adaptations of the body to aerobic exercise is an increase in stroke volume (the amount of blood pumped out of each ventricle of the heart with each beat). As a consequence, the heart has to beat less often to deliver the same amount of blood to the muscles. It also means that for a given heart rate the heart will be able to pump more blood out of each ventricle each minute, resulting in an increased cardiac output (Q). Given that there is no change in the individual's maximum heart rate this means that the individual will have a higher maximum cardiac output (Q_{max}). The overall effect of this is a more efficient cardiovascular system: for the same heart rate the heart has a greater capacity to deliver more blood, and hence more oxygen to the muscles. In practical terms this means that when the muscles are working at a relatively high intensity they will be less dependent upon the anaerobic pathways for the production of ATP. The effect of this is to reduce the likelihood of fatigue. In the long term, training can also induce an increase in the size and strength of the heart, as well as improvements in the way in which it functions.

THE CONDITION OF THE BLOOD VESSELS

The blood is transported around the body via the blood vessels. Within the muscles there is an extensive network of minute blood vessels called capillaries, which are in close association with the muscle fibres and provide the site of gaseous exchange between the blood and muscle. Aerobic exercise can increase the size of this capillary network by increasing the number of effective blood capillaries in the muscle. The increased number of capillaries will greatly enhance the delivery of blood to the muscle fibres and thus increase the effective delivery of oxygen to and removal of waste products from the working muscle fibres.

Certain vessels, most significantly the arteries of the heart and brain, can become constricted by fatty deposits on the walls of the arteries (atheroma). Aerobic exercise can help to keep these blood vessels in good condition.

MYOGLOBIN IN THE MUSCLE FIBRES

Oxygen diffuses out of the blood and into the muscle fibres, a process enhanced by the presence of myoglobin within the muscle fibres. Myoglobin molecules have a great affinity for oxygen. They can therefore act as a temporary store for the oxygen within the muscle and enhance the extraction of oxygen from the blood. One of the adaptations to aerobic exercise is an increase in the amount of myoglobin in the muscle fibres. This enhances the muscle's ability to extract oxygen from the blood and effectively increases the muscle's oxygen supply.

CONDITION OF THE MITOCHONDRIA WITHIN MUSCLE FIBRES

Oxygen is ultimately used in the aerobic synthesis of ATP, specifically in the final stages of this process which occur in specialised organelles called mitochondria. Aerobic exercise increases both the size and number of mitochondria within a muscle fibre, increasing the muscle's capacity to use oxygen.

CENTRAL AND PERIPHERAL ADAPTATIONS

All forms of aerobic exercise will bring about central adaptations and will therefore enhance the body's overall capacity to deliver oxygen. The peripheral changes are, however, more specific and will occur only in the muscles being exercised. Thus, the specificity of the exercise needs to be considered. For instance, swimming will induce a number of central adaptations and peripheral changes to the muscles used while swimming; running may bring about similar central changes but will bring about peripheral changes only in the muscles that are primarily used during running. These subtle differences must be taken into account when considering the variety of exercises that should be included in an exercise programme: if an improvement is needed in a particular activity then the training exercises should be of the same mode. If, however, general health gains are sought then the choice of aerobic exercise is more likely to be determined by individual preference, physical capabilities and convenience because it is the general increase in physical activity which is important in reducing health risks. However, the inclusion of 'weight-bearing' exercise such as walking or exercise classes may be important if prevention of osteoporosis is a consideration.

PLANNING AN EXERCISE PROGRAMME FOR THE PROMOTION OF AEROBIC CAPACITY AND GENERAL HEALTH

As well as promoting an individual's physical capacity regular participation in aerobic forms of exercise is associated with the promotion of good health and a reduction in the risk of certain diseases. Some of the evidence in support of this is reviewed in Chapter 11. In summary, it appears that an individual's level of aerobic fitness is associated with a reduction in the probability of that individual suffering from a number of the diseases that are common in many Western societies (CHD, stroke, obesity, hypertension, type II diabetes and stress disorders) (Blair *et al.*, 1995). So when discussing exercises which will promote an individual's aerobic capacity it is important to remember that the same exercises are precisely those which are recommended for the promotion of general health. Therefore, they have implications for everyone, not just those with or trying to avoid a particular medical condition. Since aerobic fitness and the prevention of certain hypokinetic diseases are so intimately related they may be considered together, with the promotion of aerobic fitness being a major component in the more holistic development of 'health'.

As a general guideline many authorities advocate that for the development of aerobic fitness, and hence the promotion of health, an exercise programme should include at least 20 minutes of vigorous exercise three times a week. In this context the term 'vigorous' means a level of exercise which is sufficient to cause slight breathlessness but is not exhaustive. However, whether this level of intensity is essential is currently a matter of debate; significant improvements in health and reductions in the risk of disease have been obtained from relatively moderate levels of activity. Indeed, there is clear evidence (Blair *et al.*, 1995) that moderate activity significantly reduces the risk of diseases.

An exercise programme is more likely to produce optimal benefits if it is personalised according to an individual's goals and current physical condition. Individualising a programme requires personal contact with the participant and a degree of experience. However, there are basic guidelines to assist the exercise adviser in designing such programmes.

The aims of a programme may vary considerably, depending upon the age and circumstances of the individual. An exercise programme is likely to have a number of objectives, but it should also be dynamic. Hence, the aims and the content of the programme may alter with time, especially if the programme extends over a period of years.

The age of the participant may have a significant influence upon its objectives and hence its content. In people of 16–20 years an exercise programme may be oriented towards optimal growth and development, minimising the risk of disease later in life and initiating healthy lifestyle habits. These are the objectives behind the introduction of 'health-related fitness' into aspects of the school curriculum. These basic objectives can then be modified if the individual is suffering from certain physical or mental conditions, whether temporary, as in the case of rehabilitating from a fracture, or more permanent in the case of genetic disorders.

A programme for young adults who have reached physical maturity may concentrate on developing or maintaining physical capacity and reducing the risk of hypokinetic diseases such as obesity, atherosclerosis and diabetes. Again, these basic objectives must be individualised because of the diversity of conditions which the exercise adviser or therapist may encounter – from a general loss of physical fitness, a recent decline in physical capacity (for example if the participant has been bedridden following a fracture) or more debilitating and permanent conditions such as multiple sclerosis.

In older groups, in addition to the previously stated objectives the programme should be oriented towards preventing individuals from assuming too sedentary a lifestyle. The programme should help to maintain physical capacity (and thus independence) as a person ages, as well as reduce the risk of diseases such as osteoporosis.

A number of factors need to be considered when prescribing aerobic or activity-based exercise programmes:

1. The overall aims of the programme.
2. The kinds of activities that could be included.
3. How these activities may be integrated into a holistic programme.
4. The frequency, intensity and duration of the activities. These are described in more detail in Chapter 5 and will be discussed further later in this chapter.

OBJECTIVES AND A LIFESTYLE APPROACH

When devising an exercise programme it is first necessary to define the basic objectives of the programme and to consider the reasons for incorporating exercise into the lifestyle. The inclusion of exercise may have a physiological, social or psychological basis, although it is most likely that a combination of benefits will be sought.

The exercise adviser must remember that different types of activity convey different benefits in different settings and should therefore prescribe a balance of activities that will fulfil all the desired objectives. Careful consideration should also be given to the need for variety. A range of different activities will help to ensure that the participant receives a wider physical experience which may be valuable socially, psychologically and physiologically as well as helping to achieve a more comprehensive state of physical fitness. Variety will also help to alleviate staleness or boredom, which could prevent the participant from getting the most out of the programme and may even cause them to give up. A weekly programme could include walking or cycling to work and/or a number of formal exercise sessions in the gym where the emphasis could be on muscular strength or mobility and a number of 'social' sessions such as swimming or bowls (which, whilst having some physiological benefits, will also have psychological and social implications). In this way the programme may be devised to produce an optimal balance of physiological, social and psychological aspects, in accordance with the physical and mental needs of the participants.

Whatever the exercise prescribed, it will be of no benefit if the prescription is not followed. The psychological aspects of motivation and adherence are vital at all stages. The exercise adviser will be trying to establish 'active lifestyle' habits and a programme that achieves this will be more successful than one which may be more outstanding physiologically but which is adhered to for only a few weeks. Of course, some programmes are short term (such as specific rehabilitation sessions or the development of some particular aspect of physical capacity), but it is to be hoped that even after completing the programme the client would include some form of physical activity in their lifestyle.

THE PRINCIPLES OF EXERCISE APPLIED TO AEROBIC OR ACTIVITY-BASED EXERCISE PROGRAMMES

When devising an aerobically based exercise programme four basic factors need to be considered: the type, intensity, duration and frequency of the exercise.

Endorsement of the inclusion of aerobic type exercises into a person's general lifestyle or specific rehabilitation/recovery programme is based upon numerous research reports and support from various bodies including the Health Education Authority (UK), the American College of Sports Medicine and the American Heart Association.

TYPE OF EXERCISE

To increase aerobic capacity an exercise needs to put the cardiovascular system under an appropriate amount of stress by applying the principles of overload and specificity. Aerobic exercise has the characteristics of:

- primarily using the aerobic system to produce the required ATP;
- involving large muscle groups (such as the legs and/or arms) in rhythmic movements such as walking, swimming, cycling, jogging or arm ergometry;
- elevating the heart rate;
- elevating the rate and depth of breathing (pulmonary ventilation);
- being of an intensity which can be maintained for a prolonged period of time.

Examples of aerobic exercises include walking, jogging, swimming, cycling, rowing, skipping, aerobic dance, skating, cross-country skiing and arm ergometry. As well as improving aerobic capacity these forms of aerobic exercise are reported to be the most effective in reducing the risk of CHD, reducing high blood pressure, reducing body fat and improving blood lipid profiles. However, for a more complete overall physical fitness an exercise programme should also include activities that are designed to enhance or maintain muscular strength and joint mobility/flexibility. A comprehensive exercise programme should include additional exercises to supplement the aerobic components.

The choice of aerobic exercise to be included within an exercise programme is important because it must fulfil a number of sociological and psychological functions as well as be effective physiologically. Ideally the exercise should be enjoyable. This enjoyment factor is an important consideration for the social and mental well-being of the participant and to ensure that he or she adheres to the exercise programme. Adherence to an exercise programme is vital if it is to be effective, especially if it is hoped that the inclusion of exercise into a weekly routine represents a permanent positive change in lifestyles. Adherence can be promoted by choosing activities which fit in well with the individual's lifestyle, by considering time factors and the accessibility to facilities.

Whilst the general effects of the different types of aerobic exercise are similar, some forms of exercise may be less suitable than others for particular individuals. For example, obese individuals should avoid jogging because their weight can put excessive strain on their joints, causing overuse injuries – alternatives such as swimming or cycling may be preferable.

A number of team and racquet games also provide a good form of exercise. However, the effects of these activities can vary very considerably. They may be sociable and very enjoyable, thereby conveying some benefits but the level of activity required is often unsuitable for the individual's physical condition. In some cases the game may be too leisurely to convey the desired physiological benefits. This can occur in a social game of tennis where, due to the skill aspect, the players actually spend most of their time walking slowly or jogging short distances whilst their cardiovascular system receives very little benefit. The game may be tiring on the muscles but it may not be as aerobically beneficial as a brisk 20-minute walk or swim. Conversely, in some cases the intensity of a racquet game may be far too intensive, over-stressing the cardiovascular system – for example, someone who decides to play squash to get fit whereas they really should get fit before they play squash. The demanding nature of the game makes it highly unsuitable for some individuals, who would be better advised to adopt an alternative form of recreational exercise.

It can therefore be seen that factors such as age, skill, the opponent and the individual's own perception of exercise intensity will affect the nature of the exercise and hence its suitability for inclusion into an exercise programme. However, a combination of activities is likely to convey diverse benefits and the actual composition of the programme will depend upon the physiological, social and psychological needs of the participant.

When the various factors associated with each activity and its diverse benefits are taken into consideration, it is still possible to broadly categorise types of exercise into groups relating to their physiological and health-promoting effects.

Category 1

Very good, provided that the intensity and duration are appropriate. The intensity and duration of these activities can be prescribed and regulated fairly carefully, resulting in a bout of exercise which is predictable in terms of these factors. Category 1 exercises include walking, swimming, cycling, jogging, hill walking, exercise classes ('aerobics') and skipping.

Category 2

Good, but the aerobic benefits very much depend upon the level of skill of the participants and how vigorously they participate. The intensity and/or duration can be unpredictable and hence cannot be regulated very closely. Category 2 exercises include team games, racquet games, circuit training, dancing, martial arts and gardening.

Category 3

These activities are acceptable but tend to produce relatively small improvements in aerobic fitness. However, a client may be encouraged to incorporate them into their lifestyle because of the additional health benefits they convey and the current view that even moderate levels of activity are better being completely sedentary. Such activities include golf, bowls, yoga (primary benefit on suppleness) and weightlifting (primary benefit on strength).

INTENSITY OF EXERCISE

For aerobic exercise to be of benefit to the cardiovascular system it must provide an appropriate amount of overload to stimulate the desired beneficial adaptations. As a general guideline, exercise which makes the participant slightly breathless is likely to improve his or her aerobic capacity. Alternatively, the appropriate exercise intensity can be determined using either exercise heart rates or the participant's perceived exertion.

As a person's fitness level improves and their heart rate for a specific intensity declines, their perceived exertion should also fall by a corresponding amount. This means that as a person gets fitter, a certain exercise level will become easier. When embarking upon a programme for the sedentary and/or relatively unfit it is advisable to begin with exercise intensities at the lower end of, or even just below, the training zone. Significant improvements in the fitness of previously sedentary individuals have been reported when using relatively low exercise intensities. As with all forms of exercise, it is advisable to begin at a relatively easy level and gradually progress as the level of fitness improves.

Although attainment of a good level of aerobic fitness is important there are many other health benefits to be derived from a programme which includes aerobic activities. Almost any form of physical activity, even relatively low-intensity exercise below the level likely to generate substantial improvements in aerobic fitness, can be recommended for individuals who are currently very sedentary.

Determining intensity by heart rate

To be of aerobic benefit exercise needs to elevate the heart rate into what is known as the *training zone*. This intensity of exercise is also likely to make the participant slightly breathless. Exercising within the training zone will be of benefit to the cardiovascular system and is also reported to reduce the risk of certain ailments such as CHD, although it should also be noted that some health benefits can be gained from lower intensity exercise.

An individual's heart rate training zone may be calculated as follows. A person's maximum heart rate is estimated to be (with some variation):

220 minus age (in years)

and will therefore fall by approximately 1 beat min^{-1} year^{-1}. The maximum heart rate of an average 45-year-old person will be approximately 175 beats min^{-1} (220–45). However, there is some evidence to suggest that continued physical activity throughout life can minimise this reduction in maximum heart rate. As a consequence, the overall physical capacity of active individuals is less likely to decline as they get older.

When undertaking aerobic exercise for health most individuals should work well below this maximum rate. The upper end of the heart rate training zone is often put at approximately 85% of the maximum heart rate; the lower end is approximately 65% of the maximum heart rate. Therefore, for a 20-year-old woman with a maximum heart rate of approximately 200 beats min^{-1} (220–20), the heart rate training zone will fall between 130 and 170 beats min^{-1} (65–85% of 200). For the exercise to be effective this person's heart rate should reach at least 130 beats min^{-1} but should not exceed 170. The estimated training zone for someone of 50 will be between 110 and 145 beats min^{-1} (65–85% of (220–50)). The exact values for the heart rate training zones will vary slightly between different authorities but will be similar to those given here. A diagram of the heart rate training zone was presented in Figure 6.4 (p. 132). However, certain cardiovascular disorders may require modifications to the suggested training zones, and in some cases may make them inappropriate.

If exercise is to increase a person's aerobic capacity the heart rate should be maintained within the training zone for a prolonged period of time. Here, again, the exact value for the duration of the exercise may vary but most authorities recommend between 20 and 60 minutes per session. A minimum of 20 minutes is recommended for health benefits, with the longer sessions having the potential to promote greater adaptations in those who are relatively fit. There is currently some interest in the potential to gain benefits from accumulating exercise during a day via repeated short bouts. Depending upon the findings of current research the present recommendations of a minimum of 20 minutes per session may be revised during the next few years

The suggested exercise intensities and durations outlined here are for exercise programmes designed to promote a *general* increase in cardiovascular fitness and health; they are not specifically applicable to people 'training' for competitive sport. The objectives of these individuals may be somewhat different, as they strive for a peak of fitness which is specific to their sport and in doing so may push themselves extremely hard. These fit and competitive individuals may therefore elevate their heart rate in excess of the values recommended here. Although such efforts may be necessary in the pursuit of sporting excellence they are not necessary for people wishing to attain a level of fitness that is associated with good health.

It should also be noted that during the early stages of a training programme individuals should keep their heart rates at the lower end of the training zone. In addition, inability to get the heart rate into the suggested training zone should not cause undue concern; this may well be due to the muscles not being as fit (relatively speaking) as the cardiovascular system, which can cause 'local muscle fatigue' at relatively low heart rates and prevent the continuation of the exercise. Improvements will occur with continued training and the participant will eventually be able to elevate their heart rate into the recommended zones. As fitness improves, the heart rate at any given speed of swimming, cycling or walking/jogging will become slightly lower. Therefore, to continue the improvement the participant must jog, swim or cycle a little faster, or a little longer, thus applying the principle of progressive overload.

Determining intensity by perceived exertion

A further indication of the suitability of the exercise intensity can be obtained by using a scale of perceived exertion (Borg, 1970). With participants who are on medication such as beta-blockers (which suppress the heart rate during exercise) this becomes the major means of assessing exercise intensity since the exercise heart rate is no longer applicable. A table of perceived exertion may also prove to be of greater value when dealing with older participants (>60 years) since in this age group there is a great diversity in physical capacities. For example, this age group will include those who have a very good level of physical fitness, especially if they have always been active and individuals whose physical capacity is relatively poor due to illness, disability or a sedentary lifestyle.

A scale of perceived exertion commonly used to assess exercise intensity is that devised by Borg (Figure 5.1; p. 104). It can be used very effectively in conjunction with heart rates, especially during the early stages of a programme, to familiarise participants with feelings of perceived exertion, thereby enabling them to correspond their feelings with heart rates within their training zone. In this way they should quickly become familiar with how difficult a particular form of exercise should feel if it is to be of benefit to them. Patients for whom heart rate training zones are inappropriate could be advised to exercise at a perceived exertion of between 11 and 14.

A less quantitative means of assessing appropriate exercise intensity using perceived exertion is based upon the idea that, whilst exercising, individuals should become slightly breathless but still be capable of holding a conversation. This can easily be applied by the exercise adviser who can simply ask the subject how he or she is feeling whilst they are exercising: if the subject has difficulty in answering then he or she is working too hard.

DURATION OF EXERCISE

The traditional recommendation is for aerobic exercise sessions to last in the region of at least 20–30 minutes. The potential of shorter duration sessions repeated more often, such as three 10-minute bouts a day, is gaining interest, but as yet their efficacy remains uncertain. Even if some health factors may be improved via repeated short bouts of exercise, others will probably require a longer duration.

For non-steady-state activities such as team and racquet games, the situation is more complex due to the uncertainty of intensity and duration which tends to make exercise prescription less precise and more difficult to regulate.

To date many authorities continue to suggest that, for optimal health benefits, aerobic exercises should be undertaken for between 20 and 60 minutes per session, although the exact duration of each session will depend upon the type and intensity of the exercise and the fitness of the participant as well as the amount of time available. It is generally agreed that for those unfamiliar with exercise a lower intensity session of relatively long duration is preferable to one that is shorter but more intense. These suggested durations are exclusive of the time spent warming up and cooling down. In the early stages of a programme the participant may be unable to maintain 20 minutes of continuous exercise comfortably. A shorter duration may therefore be used as a starting point, or the session may be split up into several bouts of exercise interspersed with rest or periods of lower intensity exercise. For instance, a 20-minute swim could be split up into two 5-minute periods of brisk swimming, each being separated by 5 minutes of gentle swimming or rest. As previously indicated, four 5-minute walks, each separated by several hours, may also convey benefits, although the exact effects of exercise accumulation and which factors can benefit have yet to be elucidated.

FREQUENCY OF EXERCISE

The frequency of exercise sessions within a programme is likely to be determined by the physiological aspects of the participants' capability to exercise repeatedly and their need to recover, the accessibility of facilities and the amount of time that the individual can realistically spend exercising. This will be further complicated if a therapist needs to be present at all sessions because it may severely restrict the number of sessions that the participant can undertake in a week. Group-oriented activities will also depend upon the availability of fellow participants. The generally recommended frequency for aerobic exercise is 3–5 times a week.

For optimal health benefits, activity should be included on an almost daily basis. Activity could be as basic as walking or similar activities. In the context of formal exercise sessions it is generally considered that a frequency of three to five times a week provides optimal aerobic benefits for the amount of time spent exercising, although for the very unfit twice a week will still be beneficial, and is certainly preferable to no exercise at all. Exercising more than five times a week may convey further aerobic benefits but the relatively small additional benefits gained from the other two sessions may not be worth the extra commitment. Exercising with a greater frequency may also increase the risk of staleness or overuse injuries. Varying the type of exercises included within a weekly programme is likely to reduce such risk. When considering the frequency of exercise sessions within a programme other factors, such as the intensity and duration of the exercise, will also need to be considered. For instance, if an individual is exercising at a relatively low level and for relatively short durations, then an additional exercise session may be deemed to be worthwhile. Here again it must be emphasised that these suggested frequencies are for individuals desiring basic aerobic and health benefits and not for those such as competitive athletes seeking fractional improvements in performance.

A health-based exercise programme should also include rest days or days where the exercise is of a much lower intensity and duration. Individuals exercising three times a week should be advised to split up their three exercise sessions with a rest or 'easy' day between each. This helps the body to recover and helps to prevent staleness and/or overuse injuries, which can occur even in beginners using relatively low exercise loads if their bodies are not physically capable of coping with them. If, however, the exercise sessions are of a rela-

tively low intensity and are being undertaken for reasons other than the primary development of aerobic fitness, then the therapist/exercise adviser may advocate exercise every day (or even more than once a day in some cases).

The information given in this chapter should provide the basis for designing activity and aerobically based exercise programmes which will enhance the individual's physical capacity as well as conveying other social, psychological and health-oriented benefits. Participants who are taking medication (such as beta-blockers), have CHD or other forms of illness, or are recovering from an operation will often require modifications to the basic programmes outlined here. Such modifications are discussed in Chapter 11.

WARM-UP AND COOL-DOWN

The importance of warming up and cooling down is often forgotten with activity-based exercise. Whilst a warm-up may easily be included as part of the routine of a gym-based session it is often omitted in other surroundings. It is important to remember the principles of warm-up when participating in activities such as badminton, tennis, swimming or even gardening. A swimming session should commence with a few minutes of easy swimming, whilst a land-based activity could commence with a number of loosening exercises followed by a few minutes of gentle aerobic activity such as walking or gentle jogging if the intensity of the session is likely to be relatively high. This will gradually prepare the body for the forthcoming activity, which could be quite strenuous.

Similarly, a gentle cool-down should be included at the end of a session. This is important as there is often a tendency to end an activity session at the peak of exertion, especially if the activity has a competitive element, such as a game of badminton. The final phase of any session should thus involve a gradual reduction, rather than an abrupt cessation, of the intensity of the activity because it facilitates the removal of waste products from the muscles and allows the heart rate to return to its pre-exercise level (see p. 97).

EXAMPLES OF AEROBIC AND ACTIVITY-BASED EXERCISE PROGRAMMES

The programmes set out in this section illustrate exercise that may be included within an aerobically oriented exercise programme. Each programme suggests a number of starting points and the way in which the principle of progression can be applied. The programmes are illustrative only and therefore the exercise adviser/therapist may decide to make appropriate modifications to them or use a combination of different programmes. The central feature of each programme is the aerobic component, although activities such as swimming and cycling will also benefit muscular strength and joint mobility, especially if these components of fitness are relatively poor. If mobility and muscular strength are the primary areas of concern then the exercise adviser/therapist should include additional specific exercises for joint mobility and strength within the overall programme. The inclusion of these additional exercises will ensure a more comprehensive level of fitness in all participants.

The programmes presented include many levels and it is up to the exercise adviser/therapist and the participant to decide the level at which it is most appropriate to start. It may be necessary to commence at a very easy level to give the participant's body time to adapt to the physical demands it experiences and to provide motivation and positive feedback as the participant should be able to progress quite rapidly. Attempts to start at a level that is too demanding may reduce confidence and place inappropriate physical stresses upon the body.

Once the programme commences it is up to the exercise adviser/therapist and participant to decide how quickly to progress onto a higher level. Progress should be gradual if the body is to be given time to adapt to the increased exercise loads it is given. If progression is too rapid these adaptations will not occur fully and the body will be overstressed, resulting in unwanted aches and pains, which, if unheeded, could develop into overuse injuries. The final level that the participant attains will depend upon a large number of physiological factors, as well as motivation.

The most physically demanding levels illustrated here are not appropriate for most individuals. However, these levels of intensity, frequency and duration are included to illustrate how such levels may be attained gradually.

The walking and cycling activities can be incorporated into an individual's lifestyle by suggesting that they walk/cycle at least part of the way to work. This can also be the most effective way of ensuring that it becomes part of their regular routine.

A CYCLING OR CYCLE ERGOMETER PROGRAMME

Both the stationary cycle ergometer and the traditional bicycle provide useful forms of aerobic exercise. Each has its advantages and disadvantages and therefore it is up to the exercise adviser/therapist to decide which is the most appropriate.

The cycle ergometer is used in a consistent environment, which means that climatic factors will not affect the exercise. It is also isolated from other factors such as traffic and therefore the exercise will be performed in relatively safe surroundings. The consistency of the environment also makes the precise content of an exercise session easier to regulate. So, for many individuals the exercise ergometer presents a number of distinct and specific advantages. Indeed, for some participants, such as those with a poor level of motor co-ordination the cycle ergometer will be the only practical option, especially if they are unable to balance or cope with traffic. In particular, those suffering from disorders such as cerebral palsy may gain great benefits from the use of a cycle ergometer as it can help them to develop their motor control as they endeavour to pedal at a constant speed and maintain a constant pressure on the pedals. The duration of exercise on a cycle ergometer is more appropriately specified by time rather than a distance, although either may be used.

The major advantages of the traditional bicycle over the stationary ergometer are mobility and variation. When using a bicycle the participant is exposed to a changing and variable environment, which can make the exercise more enjoyable and will present a range of physiological challenges, such as hills. The independence offered by the bicycle may also provide appropriate social and psychological benefits. When using a bicycle all the safety aspects concerning the machine, lights, helmet, bright clothing and road safety must be considered. Whilst it is not within the realms of this text to discuss these specific details, it *will* be up to the exercise adviser, therapist and/or participant to be aware of such matters.

Using a bicycle to get to work should be considered and may be a viable means of becoming more active. This will help to make it part of the daily routine as well as saving time. Of course, it is not always feasible, and the prospect of cycling along an exhaust-filled city street may make it both inadvisable and unattractive. Cycling in the country with one's partner at the weekend is becoming more popular, and becoming more accessible as town and country planners respond with cycle track initiatives.

The exercise adviser/therapist must therefore consider the needs of the participant carefully before deciding the form of exercise that is most appropriate and how the exercise loads should be determined. If using the traditional bicycle, in the early stages of a programme the routes should be carefully worked out to ensure that the exercise is structured and appropriate for the participant's level of fitness. However, there are occasions when a 'random' cycle ride with no fixed route has its uses. If possible, the initial routes should be fairly short and flat. As the participant improves, the routes can gradually be made longer and a number of 'deliberate' hills included to increase the intensity of the exercise and, hence, the amount of overload. However, especially during the initial stages or early in a session, participants should not force themselves up hills and if they are tired of pedalling they should dismount and walk – the desired exercise intensity is that which makes them 'slightly breathless', not exhausted.

The cycling programme presented in this section is set out with various stages that can be used as starting points. Precisely at which stage the participant starts will depend upon his or her level of fitness and a few experimental sessions may be needed before an appropriate stage can be determined. Throughout the programme progression should be gradual and steady. If a stage is too difficult then the participant should go back one stage until an appropriate level is found. The times and distances given in the programme may be applied to either the cycle ergometer or the traditional bicycle. However, as with all programmes the exercise adviser will need to make appropriate modifications, especially in the bicycle programme where traffic may be a major consideration. The suggested times and distances for each stage are therefore given as alternatives; they are not target times for a specified distance.

CYCLING PROGRAMME WITH SPECIFIED TIME DURATIONS

In addition to the examples given here, where the duration and frequency of the exercise are increased, progression should be applied by increasing the intensity of the exercise. On the cycle ergometer this will involve increasing the resistance; on a bicycle it may involve cycling faster and/or including hills. In the more demanding sessions using the ergometer the exercise adviser/therapist may require the participant to work against a relatively high resistance for a couple of minutes, separated by phases of lower intensity exercise where the participant pedals against a relatively easy resistance. This will simulate the effects of going uphill. However, this form of 'interval' training is only for those who are considered to be aerobically very fit.

Stage 1:   10 minutes, 2–3 times a week
Stage 2:   15 minutes, 2–3 times a week
Stage 3:   15 minutes, 3–4 times a week
Stage 4:   15–20 minutes, 3–5 times a week
Stage 5:   20 minutes, 3–5 times a week
Stage 6:   20–30 minutes, 3–5 times a week
Stage 7:   30 minutes, 3–5 times a week
Stage 8:   35 minutes, 3–5 times a week
Stage 9:   40 minutes, 3–5 times a week
Stage 10: 45 minutes, 3–5 times a week
Stage 11: 50 minutes, 3–5 times a week.

CYCLING PROGRAMME USING DISTANCE TO DETERMINE THE DURATION

Stage 1:   2 miles, 2–3 times a week
Stage 2:   2.5 miles, 2–3 times a week
Stage 3:   2.5 miles, 3–4 times a week
Stage 4:   2.5 miles, 3–5 times a week
Stage 5:   3 miles, 3–5 times a week
Stage 6:   3.5 miles, 3–5 times a week
Stage 7:   4 miles, 3–5 times a week
Stage 8:   5 miles, 3–5 times a week
Stage 9:   6 miles, 3–5 times a week
Stage 10: 7 miles, 3–5 times a week
Stage 11: 8 miles, 3–5 times a week.

WALKING/JOGGING PROGRAMME

It is not essential for the participant to progress up to the jogging stages to gain the desired aerobic benefits: substantial improvements in aerobic fitness (and the associated health benefits) may be gained from brisk walking. Indeed, walking will be the preferred activity for the vast majority of individuals that an exercise adviser or therapist will work with, and jogging will be appropriate only for relatively fit individuals, most of whom will be in the younger age group.

For those individuals who do wish to jog it can be made into a social activity if people exercise in pairs or small groups and, without making the activity competitive, events such as 'fun runs' can be used as goals at various intervals in a programme. Competitive running is a specialist area of exercise and for those wishing to become involved in the sport local running clubs will be able to supply the required advice and support. In this context the therapist should also be aware of the growing number of 'disabled' runners who run not just for the exercise but also to participate in competitive sport. Even relatively severe disabilities such as blindness and amputation will not preclude some individuals from these competitive activities. Blind athletes run with the assistance of a 'guide' and are able to compete in all events from 100 m to the marathon, while those lacking limbs may run with the aid of specially designed artificial limbs. So, therapists should not automatically preclude any disabled person from jogging or running. For further advice, therapists should contact the relevant sporting associations for the disabled.

In the context of the walking/jogging programme presented in this section the principles already discussed apply: participants should commence at a relatively easy stage and progress gradually until they reach the desired level. Attempting to do too much will overstress the body, causing minor aches and pains which, if not heeded, may result in overuse injuries. Specific conditions may cause the therapist to begin the prescribed programme at an easier level than that presented here, and appropriate modifications may be needed throughout the programme. If progressing from an initial walking programme it is acceptable to move onto a jogging programme without going through all the walking stages, provided that the progression is gradual and well within the participant's capabilities. In the following list, stage 20 illustrates a form of intensive training called 'interval training'. This is an advanced form of training and is likely to be appropriate only for those wishing to run competitively.

The terrain used for the walking/jogging programme may be streets, paths, tracks, woods or parkland, and is likely to be dictated by convenience. Comfortable footwear should be used for the walking programme and if progressing onto the jogging stages specific jogging or training shoes should be worn. These are a good investment even for the walking stage as they help to cushion the impact especially if walking on hard surfaces.

Stage 1: Walk 0.5 mile, 2–3 times a week
Stage 2: Walk 1 mile, 2–3 times a week
Stage 3: Briskly walk 1 mile, 2–3 times a week
Stage 4: Briskly walk 1.5 miles, 2–3 times a week
Stage 5: Briskly walk 2 miles, 3 times a week
Stage 6: Walk 2 miles, varying the pace between brisk and fast walking, 3 times a week
Stage 7: Walk 2 miles, gradually increasing the amount of 'fast' walking, 3–4 times a week
Stage 8: Walk 2.5 miles, varying the pace between brisk and fast walking, 3–4 times a week
Stage 9: Gradually increase the distance walked and/or the frequency of walking sessions each week.

Those with a good basic level of fitness, and who are familiar with exercise, may wish to start a basic jogging programme.

Stage 10: Try a mixture of brisk walking and jogging. For instance, walk 100 m then jog 100 m, walk 100 m and so on for 2 miles. Repeat 3–4 times a week

Stage 11: As for stage 9 but gradually increase the amount of jogging, 3–4 times a week
Stage 12: Walk for half a mile then jog continuously for 1 mile, then walk for half a mile
Stage 13: Walk for half a mile then jog continuously for 1.5 miles, 3–4 times a week
Stage 14: Jog for 2 miles, 3–4 times a week
Stage 15: Jog for 2.5 miles, 3–4 times a week
Stage 16: Jog for 3 miles, 3–4 times a week
Stage 17: Jog for 3.5 miles, 3–4 times a week
Stage 18: Jog 3–4 miles, 3–4 times a week
Stage 19: Gradually increase the distance and frequency of the runs, perhaps by half a mile per run each week
Stage 20: On some of the runs try a mixture of fast and slow running, (200 m fast, 200 m slow, 200 m fast and so on). The fast runs should be done only when the participant is properly warmed up.

SWIMMING PROGRAMME

Swimming is an excellent form of exercise and can be used to improve strength and joint mobility as well as aerobic fitness. It is especially good for those who are overweight or injured as the water will help to support the body. Since pools vary in size and the participant's technique will greatly influence how fast they can swim, it is not possible to prescribe a detailed swimming programme with suggested distances. However, outlined here are a set of guidelines and suggested progressions.

The times given are for the total amount of time spent on brisk swimming, not just time in the pool! For instance, if 6 minutes brisk swimming is the target, the participant could split this into six 1-minute swims with several minutes of rest or easy swimming between each. The brisk swimming should be preceded by several minutes easy swimming as a warm-up. Therefore, although the target times may be only 3 minutes, these are 3 minutes of brisk swimming and the session could also include about 15 minutes of easy swimming. The participant should progress up the stages at their own rate and only when they feel ready to do so. As with the running programme, the final stages represent fairly demanding exercise sessions which will be appropriate only for fit competent swimmers and should not be considered as a 'goal' for the vast majority of individuals who will gain the desired benefits at the lower stages.

Stage 1: 3 minutes, 2–3 times a week
Stage 2: 5 minutes, 3–4 times a week
Stage 3: 7 minutes, 3–4 times a week
Stage 4: 9 minutes, 3–4 times a week
Stage 5: 11 minutes, 3–5 times a week
Stage 6: 13 minutes, 3–5 times a week
Stage 7: 15 minutes, 3–5 times a week
Stage 8: 17 minutes, 3–5 times a week.

Those with a good level of fitness, and who are familiar with regular exercise, may wish to start at stage 9. At all stages it is possible for the participant to determine the exercise intensity by deciding how fast to swim.

Stage 9: 20 minutes, 3–5 times a week
Stage 10: As for stage 9 but gradually decrease the amount of rest until the participant can swim for 20 minutes continuously
Stage 11: 20 minutes, swim two slow lengths then one fast, two slow, one fast (and so on), 3–5 times a week
Stage 12: 20 minutes, swim alternate fast and slow lengths, 3–5 times a week
Stage 13: It is now up to the participant to increase gradually the amount of time spent swimming and the number of fast lengths undertaken.

ACTIVITY-BASED EXERCISE

The cycling, walking/jogging and swimming programmes given here provide illustrations of exercise for which the physical require-ments of the session can be fairly closely defined and regulated. Thus the intensity and duration, as well as the type of exercise, may be determined before and during the session. Alternative activities, such as team or racquet games, can be more variable in their intensity and duration. Although the type of exercise in these activities may be fairly predictable its intensity may vary depending upon the skill of the player, the opponent(s) and the com-petitiveness of the game. For example, golf courses vary in length and steepness: walking the course rather than using a buggy (golf cart) makes a significant difference to the activity; likewise carrying the golf clubs rather than using a trolley makes it more demanding, but care should be taken to avoid straining the back. Similarly, the exact type, intensity and duration of exercises that con-stitute 'aerobics' (a term generally used to describe a form of exercise to music) vary considerably. Some forms will be of a rela-tively low intensity, others will be high intensity; some will include exercises that are unsuitable for some individuals, others may provide an ideal exercise session. These alter-native activities can provide a valuable form of exercise *provided that* they adhere to the desired principles of exercise and are appro-priate for the individual. Participating in these activities has social and psychological as well as physiological implications which are discussed more fully elsewhere in this text.

When deciding upon the activities to pre-scribe the exercise adviser/therapist must consider the needs of the participant. Physio-logically this includes the type of exercise and the demands it places upon muscular strength, joint mobility/flexibility and cardio-vascular system. He or she must then consider the amount of overload that a particular activ-ity places upon the individual and whether it is appropriate and likely to bring about the desired improvements in physical fitness. Tennis is clearly more strenuous than bowls, but that does not necessarily mean that it is better for everyone; squash, for example, tends to be even more strenuous and can be too strenuous for some individuals but appropriate for others. The intensity and duration of the exercise must be sufficiently strenuous without overstressing the individual. For example, to derive aerobic benefits from a game of badminton it should be fairly continuous, make the participants slightly breathless and, if applicable, elevate their heart rates into the training zone for much of the session, which should last a minimum of 20 minutes.

The exercise adviser also needs to ensure that the activity being considered is not likely to cause any injury through overstretching or excessive pressure on the joints. Here again the suitability of different activities will depend upon the individuals and their physical capabilities. It is also important to ensure that the principles of warm-up and cool-down are observed.

In summary, whilst local resources and clubs may provide a useful setting for these activities it is the exercise adviser who must judge their suitability and apply any restrictions or modifications that they feel are necessary. Appropriate modifications to the rules may be devised in accordance with the individuals' capabilities and the setting within which they are performed. In the context of such activities or training those confined to wheelchairs provide no exception and suitable modifications to most activities can produce a viable alternative which may be enjoyed by all, as well as conveying the desired physiological, psychological and social benefits.

REFERENCES

Blair, S.N., Kohl, H.W., Barlow, C.E., Paffenbarger, R.S., Gibbons, L.W. and Macera, C.A. (1995). Changes in physical fitness and all-cause mortality: a prospective study of healthy and unhealthy men. *Journal of the American Medical Association*, **273** (14), 1093–1098.

Borg, G.V. (1970). Perceived exertion as an indicator of somatic stress. *Medicine and Science in Sport and Exercise*, **14**, 377–387.

COMPONENTS OF AN EXERCISE PROGRAMME 2: MUSCULAR STRENGTHENING EXERCISES

8

Table 8.1 summarises the definition of strength and shows its importance to both everyday life and specific health conditions. It can be compared with Tables 7.1 (p. 148) and 9.1 (p. 208), which present the same information for aerobic and joint mobility/flexibility respectively.

THE PHYSIOLOGICAL DETERMINANTS OF STRENGTH

Muscular strength is determined by a number of factors:

- the size of the muscle
- the structure of the muscle (whether it is fusiform, pennate, etc.)
- the proportion of the different types of muscle fibres within the muscle
- biochemical and histochemical properties of the muscle fibres
- neurological factors
- co-ordination, which should produce efficient movement that optimises the action of the muscles, producing the desired amount of force for the minimal amount of effort
- whether the individual is suffering from a particular disease or disorder affecting their neuromuscular system and/or have simply lost the strength of their muscles through disuse.

MUSCLE SIZE

If all other factors are equal, a larger muscle will contain more contractile filaments, which means that the muscle can generate more force and hence express greater strength. An exception to this is seen in muscular dystrophy where fatty deposits are laid down in the muscle as the contractile fibres degenerate. This can cause the muscle to maintain (or even increase) its size but lose its strength due to the loss of contractile filaments.

MUSCLE STRUCTURE

All muscle fibres contract in the same way, as described by the sliding filament model of muscle contraction (See Chapter 2). However, the precise alignment of the contractile fibres within muscles can vary considerably and this has a profound effect upon the amount of force they can generate. Muscles in which the fibres run parallel to the main axis (fusiform) are capable of a considerable amount of shortening, whereas those in which the fibres are aligned at an angle to the long axis (pennate) can pack more into the same volume of muscle, thereby resulting in a stronger muscle but one which cannot shorten as much as a fusiform muscle.

Table 8.1 Summary of muscular strength

What is muscular strength?	Why is muscular strength important for health?	Why is muscular strength important for active living?	How might muscular strength be improved on a structured programme?	How might muscular strength be improved through everyday living?
Muscular strength can be defined as the ability to overcome resistance	A good level of muscular strength enables the individual to perform basic everyday tasks without undue fatigue. It is also needed to maintain good posture and, particularly in elderly people, can prevent falls and other accidents. Keeping the joint structures in good condition may also limit musculoskeletal injuries and instability. Overall it can help the individual to cope with the physical demands of their lifestyle and maintain independence	Independence within the community can often depend upon the strength of the individual to get out of a chair unaided, to climb stairs or to carry their shopping home. Strength is also needed to carry and lift children and even to drive cars that do not have power steering	Muscular strength is often gained through resistance programmes which incorporate working against body weight (e.g. circuits), water (swimming) or weights (e.g. gym work). These exercise programmes are often prescribed in terms of sets, repetitions and resistance. A common misconception is that all forms of resistance work will lead to big gains in muscle mass. This is not true: most improvements in strength occur without substantial increases in muscle mass	The home and garden provide many opportunities for resistance sessions. Two tins of beans can take the place of dumbbells and pushing a wheel barrow or turning soil can act in the same way as a gym workout. Many forms of exercise that use body weight as a resistance can be learned from an exercise leader at a leisure centre and used at home

TYPES OF MUSCLE FIBRES WITHIN THE MUSCLE

Although all muscle fibres have the same basic structure they vary in physiological, biochemical and histochemical properties, which are largely dictated by the neurological innervation they receive. Certain kinds of fibre are stronger; others have greater endurance properties. Muscle fibres can be classified into two broad categories: type 1 fibres, also called red fibres or slow-twitch fibres, and type 2 fibres, also called white fibres or fast-twitch fibres. Type 1 fibres are smaller than type 2 fibres but possess a better blood supply. They are therefore weaker than the type 2 but have greater endurance properties. Type 1 fibres have a greater capacity to produce ATP aerobically whilst type 2 fibres are more biased towards the anaerobic production of ATP. Therefore the composition of a muscle will affect its strength and endurance. In general, it is suggested that a greater proportion of type 1 fibres will give the muscle more endurance qualities, whilst a greater proportion of type 2 fibres will give it greater maximal strength. However, the relative proportions of these fibres are only one aspect in the determination of these properties and appropriate exercises can increase both the maximal strength and endurance capacities of the muscle.

BIOCHEMICAL AND HISTOCHEMICAL PROPERTIES OF MUSCLE FIBRES

These factors are related to the fibre type. Variations exist within the broad categories of type 1 or type 2 fibres: for example, type 2 fibres may be subclassified into type 2a, type 2b and type 2c, and different categories of type 1 muscle fibres have different aerobic (endurance) and anaerobic (maximal strength) limits. Through exercise it may be possible to slightly alter the properties of muscle fibres without altering the category into which they are placed. The possibility of converting one type or subcategory of fibre into another remains an area of debate and research interest.

NEUROLOGICAL FACTORS

Muscle fibres are stimulated to contract by motor neurones. The force, and hence the strength of a muscular contraction is determined by the number of fibres that are recruited into the contraction. If the process of stimulation or recruitment is altered then the strength of contraction will be affected. When a person performs strengthening exercises the strength will increase without any apparent change in the muscle fibres because the nervous system has adapted to recruit the existing fibres in a more effective manner. Conversely, the strength of a muscle may be adversely affected by neuromuscular diseases such as motor neurone disease, myasthenia gravis and cerebral palsy, which all result in an inhibition of effective motor unit recruitment and hence reduce the strength of contraction.

CO-ORDINATION

Neuromuscular co-ordination should result in an efficient movement that optimises the action of the muscles, producing the desired movement for the minimal amount of effort. For efficient and effective movement an appropriate and co-ordinated balance of neurological inputs is required. Complex movements often need to be learnt and can, with practice, become automatic. Such movements are usually very efficient, but in disorders such as stroke, in which certain neurological motor areas have been damaged, basic movement patterns may need to be relearnt. In other disorders there may be an imbalance between the excitatory and inhibitory impulses being sent to the motor neurone. If the inhibitory inputs are too weak or the excitatory inputs too strong hypertonic spasticity can result (the muscles which should relax and lengthen during a movement remain tense). As a result the limbs possess a degree of rigidity. This will cause much of the force being generated by the concentrically contracting muscle(s) to be resisted by their antagonist(s), which should have relaxed to permit the movement. The overall effect of this is to impede or prevent the desired movement.

EFFECTS OF EXERCISE ON MUSCLE TONE AND STRENGTH

Appropriate exercises can have beneficial effects upon many of the factors that determine muscular strength. If the muscles are weak and lack tone, exercises can improve the muscle's strength, endurance and tone and may help to develop the individual's co-ordination and muscular control. However, certain aspects of the muscle cannot be altered by exercise. These include the overall organisation of the muscle fibres within a muscle and factors which are constrained by biological limitations to change and growth.

A well designed exercise programme can develop muscular strength by affecting a number of physiological factors to a greater or lesser extent. The precise adaptations of the muscles to an exercise programme will depend upon the individual, the type of exercise, the intensity of the strengthening exercises and the number of repetitions performed and will therefore vary from those associated with the development of maximal strength to those associated with endurance. As a general rule, an exercise session which includes high-intensity exercises will stimulate adaptations that are oriented towards the development of maximal strength. Exercise sessions that include exercises of a lesser intensity, but which are performed for a greater number of repetitions, will stimulate adaptations that are in accordance with the development of muscular endurance. In the context of health-related exercise programmes, whilst an exercise programme may be biased towards

the development of maximal strength or muscular endurance, these fitness components are related along a continuum and are not completely isolated from each other.

Exercises that are used to develop muscular strength and/or endurance are also likely to have beneficial effects upon hypotonic muscles by improving the general physical properties and general tone of the muscle fibres.

MUSCLE SIZE

The size of an individual muscle is determined by the number and sizes of fibres within the muscle. Muscle fibres are made up of smaller units (myofibrils), which are in turn composed of contractile filaments of actin and myosin (Figures 8.1 and 8.2). Appropriate exercises will increase the number of contractile filaments and myofibrils within a muscle. This increase will result in the muscle possessing a greater capacity to develop tension and force, which will make it 'stronger'. An increase in the number of myofibrils within the muscle fibres will also cause an increase in the size of the muscle fibres (hypertrophy). As a consequence, there will be an overall increase in the size of the muscle. There is therefore a link between muscle size and strength, although size is not the only factor determining strength.

The increase in muscle size through fibre hypertrophy is generally accepted amongst physiologists. However, there is also some controversial evidence to suggest that some of the observed increases in muscle size may be attributable to an increase in the number of fibres (hyperplasia). The nature of the investigations into this subject makes the collection of conclusive data difficult and many authorities discount the possibility of a significant increase in the number of fibres, stating that the number of fibres in a muscle are fixed before birth and cannot be altered by exercise. This topic is therefore an area of debate and requires further research.

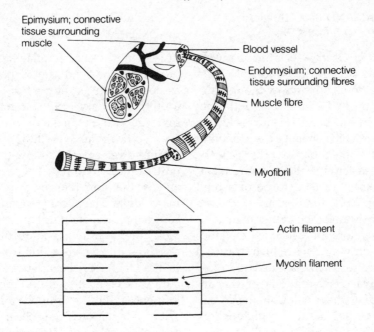

Figure 8.1   Skeletal muscle

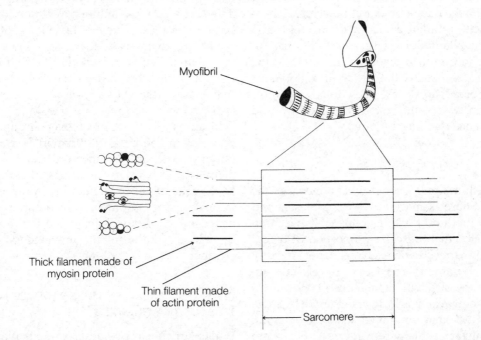

Figure 8.2   Alignment of thick and thin filaments

HISTOCHEMICAL AND BIOCHEMICAL PROPERTIES OF THE FIBRES

Whilst there is a clear association between muscle size and strength it is possible for a muscle to increase its strength without a significant alteration in its size. This improvement is caused by biochemical changes within the muscle fibres which enhance the capability to generate ATP anaerobically. This is to be expected because activities that require maximal muscular strength tend to be of a high intensity but of short duration and therefore are predominantly anaerobic rather than aerobic. There is therefore an associated development of the energy systems which are used during the exercise. Such changes are linked with the relative concentrations of the enzymes that mediate the reactions in the energy systems, and the abundance of high-energy molecules such as phosphocreatine.

Exercise programmes that are oriented towards the development of muscular endurance will stimulate a balance of anaerobic and aerobic adaptations within the muscle, in accordance with the energy demands of the exercise. Similarly, the resultant adaptations to the blood supply are likely to be a compromise between the maximal strength and endurance qualities required.

FIBRE COMPOSITION

Strength-training exercises can increase the muscle fibre's capacity to develop tension and hence produce a stronger force. It has been suggested that a greater proportion of type 2 fibres in a muscle will result in greater strength. Strength-training exercises can certainly increase the strength capabilities of all muscle fibres; however, it is further suggested by some authorities that continued maximal strength training may actually convert type 1 fibres into type 2 fibres, or type 2c fibres to type 2b. This process is referred to as 'fibre type conversion', which is again an area of controversy and debate that requires further research.

NEUROLOGICAL FACTORS AND CO-ORDINATION

Muscle fibres are stimulated to contract by motor neurones. A motor neurone and its associated muscle fibres form a motor unit. Motor units vary in the strength of stimulus that is required to make the muscle fibres contract: some require very little stimulus and are therefore referred to as low-threshold motor units; others require a far stronger stimulus and are therefore referred to as high-threshold motor units. The overall strength of a muscle's contraction depends upon the recruitment of these motor units. If more motor units are recruited into a contraction it will be stronger. It has therefore been suggested by some authorities that strength training significantly influences the recruitment of motor units. These adaptations may occur in the central nervous system, and there is some evidence that the improved recruitment is caused by a reduction in the inhibitory action of the central nervous system. The effects of this would be to increase the ease with which motor units can be recruited. This also helps to explain the observed increases in strength (which are often very significant) without an apparent increase in muscle size.

In terms of the ease of movement and the economy of effort, co-ordination is also an important factor. An unco-ordinated movement will be wasteful in terms of the force being generated by the muscles. Appropriate exercises can improve co-ordination and increase the effective strength of the muscles by making the resultant movements more efficient.

PLANNING EXERCISE PROGRAMMES FOR MUSCULAR STRENGTH

Whenever an exercise programme is planned the following factors must always be remembered: (1) the body takes time to respond and make its adaptations to the exercise; (2) not all parts of the body adapt at the same rate.

In the context of strength training this has specific implications. If the tendons and muscles are overstressed too often they will be damaged. Therefore, strength training should commence at a relatively low intensity and build up over a period of weeks.

The initial stages of a programme should involve exercises that use relatively light resistances and are repeated a moderate number of times. For example, a session could consist of three sets of 6–9 exercises with each set involving 12–20 repetitions of each exercise. This would produce a total of 36–60 repetitions of each exercise. This type of session should enable the body to become 'familiar' with the exercises and begin to initiate some training adaptations. Over a period of weeks the intensity and/or volume of the exercise session can be increased gradually by increasing the resistance, the number of repetitions, the number of exercises, or by progressing onto more demanding versions of the exercises.

If general muscular tone and a combination of maximal strength and muscular endurance are required, then three sets of 12–15 repetitions may be advocated for each exercise, making a total of 36–45 repetitions for each exercise. If, however, the development of maximal strength is of primary concern, then the programme must incorporate a gradual increase in the intensity of the exercises coupled with a corresponding decrease in the number of repetitions. For example, a programme could progress to sessions where the participant performs three sets of six repetitions, with heavy resistances. Conversely, if the development of muscular endurance is of primary concern then the programme may progress towards three sets of 30 repetitions.

When making progressions it is important to increase the number of repetitions or the amount of resistance *gradually* because the tendons as well as the muscles need to adapt to the exercise. The muscles may generate the force, but the force is conveyed to the bones via the tendons. Tendons are often slower to adapt than muscles, which can mean that,

even though the muscles may be capable of more work, the tendons may not. Increasing the exercise loads when tendons are in this vulnerable condition makes them prone to overstress and overuse injuries. Hence, even if the strength of the participant improves quite rapidly, progress must be gradual if it is to continue without the risk of injury.

It should also be noted that the participant's progress may not be linear and that in practical terms everyone has a maximum potential. Often an individual will find that after some initial improvements their level may 'plateau' for a while before further improvements. Such plateaux may become longer and more difficult to overcome as the participant gets closer to their physical potential. Indeed, the closer a person gets to their maximum potential the more difficult it will be for them to make further improvements even with substantial increases in the amount of exercise. Such limitations to growth and development are determined by basic biological factors; psychological factors may also be involved.

When commencing a strength-training programme an initial assessment of strength may help to indicate the type and intensity of exercises that would be suitable. The exercise adviser should produce a draft of the proposed exercise sessions, which the participant should then attempt. During the initial session the exercise adviser may to need to modify the proposed programme in accordance with the participant's capabilities (increase or decrease the number of repetitions, alter the variations of the exercise, and even adjust the number of exercises included within a session). When drafting the initial session it is always advisable to underestimate the participant's capabilities. The successful completion of the session, with a subsequent increase in its content, will provide positive feedback whereas failure to complete the session could be disheartening. Modifications to a session should also take account of the participant's condition one or two days after the exercise;

those who are unfamiliar with exercise often suffer from stiffness in the 24–48 hours immediately following exercise, even if they did not find it too demanding at the time. This is known as the 'delayed onset of muscular soreness' (DOMS) and is a common occurrence. Stiffness indicates overexertion, and it may be necessary to reduce the content of the exercise session slightly until the necessary physiological adaptations to the exercise have occurred and post-exercise stiffness is no longer experienced. While this method of designing a session may appear to be somewhat unsystematic, the exercise adviser will soon become experienced at judging a participant's capabilities and the exercises that are suitable. This experience, coupled with adherence to the following basic guidelines:

- commence at a level that is well within the participant's capabilities
- adhere to safety aspects such as warm-up
- react appropriately if the participant experiences pain or discomfort with any exercise

should ensure the design of effective and safe exercise sessions.

COMPONENTS OF A STRENGTH-TRAINING SESSION

As with all forms of exercise, a strength-training session should commence with a warm-up. Typically this would include some loosening and aerobic exercises, such as cycling on an ergometer for 5–10 minutes, to prepare the muscles. The aerobic work should be followed by a series of stretching exercises that incorporate exercises for all the major muscle groups likely to be used during the session. The exact duration and content of the warm-up will depend upon the relative importance of aerobic fitness and mobility exercises. For those wishing to develop mobility, a longer period of time may be spent stretching, while those who need to develop their aerobic fitness and stamina may spend longer on the aerobic component. As a final

stage of the warm-up individuals can perform some light strength-based exercises, using much lower resistances than they will go on to use during the main part of the session – for instance, biceps curls with half the normal weight or 'half press-ups'. This final part of the warm-up will specifically prepare the muscles for the more strenuous exercises that follow.

The main part of a strength-training session can be composed of different types of strengthening exercises, such as:

- 'body resistance' or circuit-training exercises
- free weights
- multigyms
- exercise machines
- assisted exercises and/or partner work.

An exercise session could concentrate purely on one form of strength training but more commonly it will include a mixture of the different types. The individual exercises within a session are likely to work the muscles concentrically, eccentrically and isometrically. A single exercise can work many different muscle groups in different ways. The duration of any exercise within the session may be determined by time, repetitions, or, with more experienced participants, by perceived exertion when training to their maximum. The recovery period between exercise sets can be determined by a fixed time interval, the general feelings of the participant or simply by convenience, as when working in pairs or sharing pieces of equipment. The strength-training aspects of the session can be interspersed with other forms of exercise, such as supplementary work on the exercise cycle or additional stretching exercises, if desired. This can help to keep the participant warm and provide the muscles with an 'active' recovery if necessary.

The main part of the session should be followed by a cool-down period. This will commonly include a few minutes of gentle aerobic exercise and further gentle stretching.

The cool-down will help to reduce the risk of stiffness the following day.

In the following sections the different types of strength-training exercises that can be incorporated into a strength-training programme will be considered. The relevant safety aspects and organisational methods used for each type of training will be discussed separately under each heading and specific points associated with particular exercises will be included with the description of how to perform it.

CIRCUIT-TRAINING AND BODY-RESISTANCE EXERCISES

Circuit-training and body-resistance exercises do not require any sophisticated equipment because they use either the person's own body weight as a form of resistance or simple apparatus such as mats and benches. They also have the advantage of being very 'functional' – that is, when performing the movement all the relevant stabilising and supporting muscles must be recruited and hence are exercised in an appropriate manner, along with those causing the movement. Muscular control and co-ordination can also be incorporated into the work.

In general terms, most circuit training exercises can be broadly categorized into one of four groups, according to which area of the body they predominantly exercise:

1. The legs
2. The trunk
3. The upper body
4. General conditioning.

This is, of course, a gross simplification because most exercises will involve all parts of the body. In addition to the obvious work being performed by the prime movers other muscles throughout the body will be working as fixators and stabilisers. For example the press-up may be classified as an upper-body exercise since it predominantly and obviously uses the arms, but press-ups also require a considerable amount of isometric work from the abdominal muscles, which are used to keep the body in a rigid position throughout the exercise.

SESSION ORGANISATION

With all forms of circuit training, diagrams of the exercises are useful. The participants or exercise adviser should keep progress cards which record the number of repetitions they perform for each exercise. The exercise adviser may like to modify the organisational versions suggested here in accordance with their own experience and resources. For example, instead of simply walking to the next exercise station it may be appropriate to encourage the participants to gently jog on the spot or complete one lap of the room during the recovery period between each exercise. However, this will depend upon the fitness of the individuals concerned.

Exercise sequence and spatial organisation

In an exercise session the component exercises are usually performed in a sequence that gives the muscle groups alternate periods of exercise and rest. Therefore the exercises should be organised into a sequence which works the lower body, trunk, upper body, lower body, trunk, upper body, and so on. For each body part there are a number of possible exercises: these can be graded from easy to difficult and it is up to the exercise adviser to determine which versions are appropriate for each participant. The duration aspect within a session can be organised so that the participant completes a predetermined number of repetitions of each exercise before moving on, or may work for a set time before progressing around the circuit. Similarly, the amount of recovery may or may not be specified.

When specific equipment is needed (e.g. a mat for sit-ups or a bench for step-ups) it should be situated so that a minimum amount of movement is required between the apparatus or 'exercise stations'. This arrangement is not only convenient but it becomes more important if a number of individuals are exercising at the same time: appropriate spatial organisation will minimise the possibility of people colliding or interfering with each other as they move around the room. Likewise, apparatus should not be situated where it is possible for a person to fall over it and the safety considerations for each exercise should be followed at all times. The following section discusses the incorporation of strengthening exercises into a circuit but they can also be undertaken in a less structured manner along with other exercises. Therefore this section aims to present general guidelines for the use of such exercises rather than setting out fixed, inflexible 'rules'.

DETERMINING TRAINING LOADS

In an ideal situation it may be possible to give each participant an individual 'circuit training fitness test' from which the type of exercises and number of repetitions can be determined. This could involve the participant attempting a relatively easy version of the exercise, and if 30 repetitions are completed with relative ease the participant may then be asked to attempt a more difficult version. In this way the appropriate variation of an exercise can be determined. Having established this, it is necessary to determine the appropriate number of repetitions. This may be found by asking the participant to repeat the exercise until they begin to struggle or feel undue local muscular fatigue. In order for any exercise to convey benefits it must 'stress', but not overstress, the body, as this can lead to injury. In the early stages of an exercise programme the exercise adviser should always be cautious with the participant's capabilities. Minor adjustments to the number of repetitions can then be made during the first few sessions as the participant becomes familiar with the exercises. Increasing the number of repetitions in the early stages also has a positive psychological effect.

By following these general guidelines the appropriate variation of each exercise, and a suitable number of repetitions to be completed, may be determined. This should result in a circuit containing 5–12 different exercises that will appropriately stress the participant whilst he or she remains within his or her capabilities. During an exercise session the participant may complete each circuit one, two or three times depending upon their physical capacity. The advantage of this form of exercise programming is that it is very personalised. It also enables the exercise adviser to closely monitor progress and make appropriate adjustments to the programme. Having performed an initial assessment the results can be used to monitor the progress of the participant and provide positive feedback.

CIRCUIT TRAINING FOR GROUPS

While an individualised programme may be highly desirable there are occasions when constant individual attention is not feasible (if, for example, the exercise adviser is dealing with a number of individuals but is only able to provide exercise facilities on limited occasions). In this situation they are likely to be involved with group sessions. Group sessions have the advantage of making the activity more sociable and, as such, do not preclude the use of initial 'fitness assessments' for all individuals. The organisation of such sessions may involve a room being made available at particular times with individuals arriving, exercising and leaving when convenient. In these circumstances, to prevent organisational difficulties, individuals should visit each exercise station in the same sequence even though they may not be doing exactly the same type of exercise. If the amount of space is limited and the participants numerous, this could result in queuing for exercise stations – especially if, for instance, there is only one mat for sit-ups. To prevent this more specific temporal organisation may be necessary. This can be achieved by allocating each participant a certain time at each station, during which they will complete the predetermined number of repetitions, and then move on to the next station. The person organising the session will have to provide instructions on when to start exercising, when to stop and when to move on. By doing so he or she will ensure that all participants move between stations and commence each exercise at the same time. With this form of organisation there may be an additional slight pause between individuals completing their repetitions and being asked to progress to the next station (suggested intervals are 30 or 40 seconds exercise time with 30 seconds to change stations). In practice, this will depend upon the type of circuit being undertaken and the individuals involved.

With more advanced and 'fitter' individuals a variation on the above theme can be used, in which they do not perform a set number of repetitions but exercise for a given duration. Individuals may exercise for 20 seconds and then be given 40 seconds of recovery, during which time they change stations. To make it more difficult a ratio of 30 seconds to 30 seconds may be used but this is only likely to apply to the fitter exercisers.

There may be circumstances in which the exercise adviser is unable to assess all the participants individually. As an alternative he or she may set out graded circuits, which are often designated by colours such as yellow, red, blue and black. The different levels of circuit may vary in the type of exercises they include and/or the number of repetitions advocated. For instance, a yellow circuit may be the easiest circuit, which would involve the participants performing relatively few repetitions (say 6–12) of the easier versions of the exercises, whilst a black circuit may incorporate much higher repetitions (30–40) of the more difficult variations. The red and blue circuits could incorporate exercises of intermediate difficulty and/or an intermediate number of repetitions. Cards can be produced stating the number of repetitions required at each station for each circuit. These should be placed by each station to remind the exercisers what to do. A problem may be encountered with this form of organisation if a participant's capabilities vary considerably over different bodily areas. For instance, if their legs were 'fitter' than their arms, they may be very capable of performing the leg exercises of the black circuit but may only be able to perform the suggested arm exercise variations and repetitions given in the yellow circuit. This emphasises the value of individualising an exercise programme whenever possible.

EXAMPLES OF BODY-RESISTANCE AND CIRCUIT-TRAINING EXERCISES

As with most forms of strength-training exercises these exercises will require a combination of eccentric, concentric and static work involving many different muscle groups. Therefore where an exercise is classified as 'exercising' a particular muscle group it should be remembered that, although this may be the major site of activity, other muscles will undoubtedly be involved.

ABDOMINAL EXERCISES

Knee raises

This exercise predominantly involves the hip flexors but can be used as a prelude to 'sit-ups' if the participant's abdominal muscles are particularly weak. The participant sits in a chair and raises one knee by flexing the hip and then slowly lowers the leg to the starting position before repeating the exercise (Figure 8.3). This may be performed using one leg at a time or with both legs together.

Sit-ups

The degree of difficulty of a sit-up may be altered by varying the position of the hands and arms. With all basic sit-ups the participant

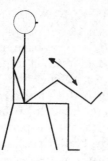

Figure 8.3

should sit on a mat (for comfort and protection of the back) with the hips and knees flexed at about 90°. Flexion of the hips and knees (as opposed to doing sit-ups with 'straight legs', hips and knees extended) should prevent any back problems. All movements should be performed in a slow and controlled manner: this includes both the upward concentric phase and the lowering or eccentric phase. With all variations of the sit-up the feet should be free and not hooked under a support. Use of a support makes the exercise somewhat easier, slightly alters the nature of the exercise by affecting the relative demands placed upon the muscle groups involved and may cause undue strain on the thigh muscles and hip flexors. Similarly, whilst sit-ups on an incline, with the feet elevated and hooked under a support may be suitable for 'athletic' individuals involved in hard training they are not recommended those of a lesser physical capacity.

Version 1

The participant lies on the mat with their hips and knees flexed and their hands resting comfortably on their thighs (Figure 8.4). The body is then raised and the hands moved so that each one touches the corresponding lower leg just below each kneecap. During the movement the arms should be kept virtually straight with the elbows being only slightly flexed so as to minimise the amount of trunk movement (flexion). From this point the body is then gently lowered so that the shoulders

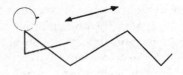

Figure 8.4

touch the mat and in doing so the hands slide back up the thighs to their starting position. The movement can then be repeated. With this exercise it is unnecessary to flex the trunk more than specified since the abdominal muscles perform most of the 'work' involved in a sit-up during the early phases of flexion and would perform very little additional work if the trunk was made to flex further.

Version 2

The participant lies on the mat with their hips and knees flexed and their arms crossed over their chest so that each hand touches the opposite shoulder (Figure 8.5). The trunk is flexed and raised so that it is almost vertical, then slowly lowered so that the shoulders once again touch the mat. The trunk movement is virtually identical to that described in the Version 1, but the exercise is made more difficult by the positioning of the hands and arms.

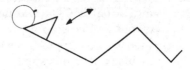

Figure 8.5

Version 3

The participant lies on the mat with their hips and knees flexed and their hands touching their ears (Figure 8.6). The trunk movement performed in this exercise is identical to that described in Versions 1 and 2 but the exercise is made more difficult by the positioning of the hands and arms. With this exercise the hands should be touching the ears and not

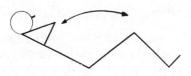

Figure 8.6

clasped behind the neck, which could cause unwanted strain in this region.

Version 4

The participant lies on the mat with their feet elevated and resting free on a chair or bench (Figure 8.7). While this exercise may not look very spectacular the elevation of the feet makes the movement considerably more demanding on the abdominal muscles. Therefore, when initially performing this exercise the hands should be placed on the thighs and moved to touch just below the kneecap as the trunk is flexed (as in Version 1). Further progression may then be achieved by repositioning the arms across the chest as in Version 2, or by placing the hands just behind the ears as in Version 3.

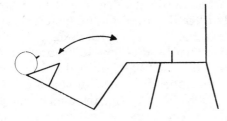

Figure 8.7

Twisted sit-up

The 'twisted sit-up' is a simple variation of the sit-up and involves a small amount of trunk rotation as well as flexion.

Version 1: rotation to alternate sides

The participant lies on the mat with their hips and knees flexed and their hands touching

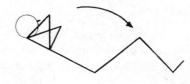

Figure 8.8

their ears (Figure 8.8). The trunk can then be flexed and rotated so as to bring the right elbow close to the left knee (at this stage there is no necessity to make the elbow touch the knee). The body is then slowly lowered back to the starting position and the movement is repeated, rotating in the opposite direction so that the left elbow is brought close to the right knee. The exercise may be repeated as desired.

Version 2: Rotation to one side

The right hand is positioned so that it is touching the right ear whilst the left elbow and lower arm are positioned flat on the mat in line with the trunk. The participant then flexes and rotates the trunk so that the right elbow is brought towards the left knee (Figure 8.9). In doing this the left elbow will need to be flexed but the lower arm should remain on the mat. The participant then slowly lowers the body back to the starting position and the movement is repeated. This exercise therefore involves repeated flexion and rotation to the left. To exercise the muscles of the opposite side of the body the positions will need to be reversed such that the left hand is positioned by the left ear whilst the right arm is positioned on the mat. The body can then be flexed and rotated to the right.

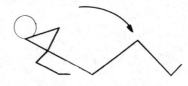

Figure 8.9

Crunches

This is a more advanced form of exercise, requiring good co-ordination, which exercises the hip flexors as well as the abdominal muscles.

Version 1

The participant starts by lying flat on their back on the floor. The hips and knees are then flexed, bringing the knees towards the head. At the same time the trunk is flexed by raising the head and back off the floor. In this position the participant should be able to touch both knees with their hands (Figure 8.10). The hips, knees and back are then extended to return to the starting position.

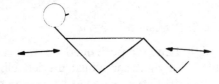

Figure 8.10

Version 2

This involves the same movements as Version 1 but during the second phase of the movement, when the knees, hips and back are extended, they are not fully lowered back onto the floor but are kept just a few inches off the ground (Figure 8.11). This requires constant work from the abdominal and other muscles in order to maintain the body position throughout the set. This exercise may be performed quite rapidly (up to a rate of about one cycle per second) but is not suitable for those who have weak abdominal muscles.

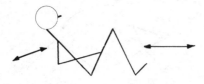

Figure 8.11

BACK-STRENGTHENING EXERCISES

It is the opinion of many authorities that in most people the constant use of the back muscles prevents them from becoming 'weak'. One of the primary functions of the back muscles is the maintenance of posture, and in this context they are used isometrically. Many exercises (such as press-ups and the military press), when performed correctly, will exercise the back muscles isometrically and thus no further exercises may be required. While many exercise programmes may appear to concentrate upon the abdominal muscles (which are often weak), they do not neglect the back muscles, as these are usually strengthened by other exercises already included in programme. However, should the exercise adviser wish to include specific back-strengthening exercises, there are several to choose from.

Back extensions

Care should be taken with this exercise; it should not be undertaken by those suffering from back complaints. The participant lies face-down on a bench with their hips level with the end of the bench, and their upper body extending over the end (Figure 8.12). In this position the participant flexes at the waist so that their head is close to the ground. The lower body will be horizontal on the bench with the upper body at 90° to it and the head close to the floor. During the exercise the participant's feet should be held down by a fixed support or partner. The participant then clasps

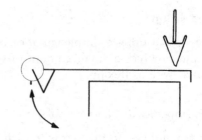

Figure 8.12

their hands behind their head and raises their upper body so that it becomes parallel with the floor and level with the lower body. Slight hyperextension may be permissible, provided that it does not cause any back discomfort. The participant then slowly lowers their upper body so that their head once again almost touches the floor before repeating the movement. The exercise involves both concentric and eccentric contractions of the back muscles. Whilst this exercise may be used for strengthening the back muscles, it should be omitted if it causes discomfort. Additional back-strengthening exercises are presented in the section on free weights (p. 202).

UPPER BODY EXERCISES

Press-ups

Press-ups are primarily aimed at the musculature of the upper body, arms and shoulders. However, the activity also requires postural muscles, such as back and abdominal muscles, to work in order to maintain body position. Therefore, such exercises may statically exercise these muscle groups as well as dynamically exercising those more obviously involved in the movements.

Version 1: press-ups against the wall

These exercises provide a basic beginning for the press-up movement. The participant stands with their arms outstretched and the palms of their hands flat against the wall at shoulder height, and then moves their feet back approximately half a metre and lowers their hands about half a metre down the wall. This will cause the participant to lean in towards the wall slightly and forms the starting position (Figure 8.13). The participant then flexes their elbows and leans forwards until their face almost touches the wall. Throughout the movement the body should be kept fairly rigid, with the lean coming from the flexion of the ankles, not the back. The

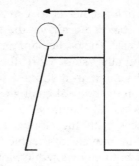

Figure 8.13

participant then straightens their elbows by pushing against the wall and returns to the starting position. The movement can be repeated as required.

Version 2: kneeling or half press-ups

The participant kneels on the floor with their knees positioned slightly behind, rather than directly underneath, their hips. In this position the participant may elevate their feet slightly and cross them if it is found to be more comfortable (Figure 8.14). The participant then flexes their elbows and lowers their upper body until their face almost touches the floor. The elbows are then extended by pushing against the floor in order to return to the starting position. Throughout the movement the body should be kept fairly rigid so that it pivots where the knees are touching the ground and the back does not bend.

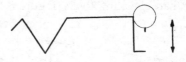

Figure 8.14

Version 3: press-ups with the upper body elevated

This exercise represents an intermediate version between Version 1 and the full press-up described in Version 4. To perform this movement the participant needs to use a step or similar fixed object: the higher the step, the easier the exercise. The participant places their hands flat on the step with their body extended out behind in a straight line. This should position the body at an angle of about 45° to the horizontal (Figure 8.15). The exercise commences with the elbows extended, and the press-up movement is achieved using the flexion of both elbows, which lowers the body, followed by extension of both elbows, which raises it. Throughout the movement the body, should be maintained in a straight line so that it pivots about the ankles and feet without any flexion of the back.

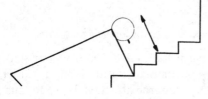

Figure 8.15

Version 4: press-ups flat on floor

This exercise may be described as the 'classic' press-up position. Exercise advisers will find that few of their female participants will reach this stage; indeed it is likely to be beyond many men. The movement sequence is the same as that described in Version 3 but the participant keeps their hands on the floor rather than elevating them (Figure 8.16).

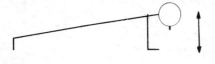

Figure 8.16

Version 5: press-ups with the feet elevated

This is an advanced press-up which will be achieved only by those who possess a strong, well developed musculature. In this version

the feet are elevated on a bench or chair whilst the hands are positioned on the floor (Figure 8.17). Elevating the lower body makes the exercise considerably more difficult, with the degree of elevation influencing the degree of difficulty: the higher the feet, the more difficult the exercise becomes.

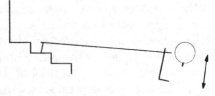

Figure 8.17

Bench dips

Version 1

The participant places their hands at the back of a bench or fixed object, extending their feet out in front and flexing at the waist. The feet should be placed flat on the ground and the knees slightly flexed (Figure 8.18). The exercise commences with the elbows extended; the participant then flexes the elbows and lowers their body until it almost touches the floor. The elbows are then extended, pushing against the bench to raise the body back up. Throughout the movement the emphasis should be upon elbow flexion and extension, keeping flexion of the trunk to a minimum and the back relatively straight.

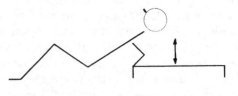

Figure 8.18

Version 2: bench dips with feet elevated

In this version the basic movement sequence is identical to that in Version 1 but the participant's feet are elevated on another bench (Figure 8.19). This permits a greater degree of body lowering, and hence elbow flexion, which makes the exercise more difficult. In this position it should be possible to lower the body sufficiently for the elbows to be flexed at 90° and hence the upper arms, which extend behind the body, will be parallel to the floor.

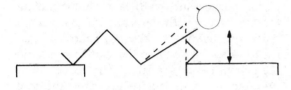

Figure 8.19

Bench raises

This exercise requires some basic apparatus such as a bench and wall bars which are commonly found in exercise areas. One end of the bench is securely hooked over the wall bars at approximately shoulder height. The participant holds the other end level with their shoulders; this forms the starting position. From this position the participant raises the bench above their head, fully extending their elbows. The bench is then lowered back down to the starting position, carefully controlling the movement with eccentric contractions (Figure 8.20). Throughout the movement the back should be kept straight: back hyperextension indicates overexertion and the exercise may need to be modified accordingly. Some individuals will prefer to keep their feet flat on the floor throughout the exercise, others may wish to remain on the balls of their feet, keeping their heels off the ground throughout. Having to push with the legs or rising up and down on the feet indicates that the bench is too heavy. The degree of difficulty may be altered by changing the weight of the bench or, with a strong participant, by using just one arm (in exceptional cases the participant may use two benches, one for each arm). In these circumstances great care is needed

when lifting and lowering the bench from the floor at the beginning and end of the exercise set. The back must be kept straight and the participant should always look directly ahead at the wall. When using two benches they may be raised together or worked in opposition (one being elevated as the other is lowered).

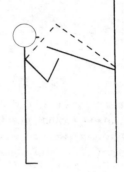

Figure 8.20

Bench curls

This exercise uses the same apparatus as the bench raises but with the bench attached to the wall bars at elbow, rather than shoulder, height. The participant commences the exercise in almost the same position as the bench raises but with the bench grasped with an underhand grip. During the first phase of the movement the bench is lowered by extending the elbows until they are fully extended. The elbows are then flexed to return the bench to shoulder height (Figure 8.21). This exercise primarily works the elbow flexors (bench raises primarily work the elbow extensors).

LEG EXERCISES

Owing to the involvement of the large muscle groups of the legs and the relatively long duration of some of these exercises, leg exercises such as step-ups, step-overs, ski jumps, astride jumps and bench jumps may convey benefits to the participant's cardiovascular system as well as enhance leg strength. These

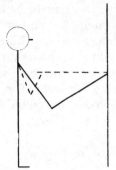

Figure 8.21

benefits will be most pronounced if the exercises are of an intensity that permits a relatively long duration and are repeated a number of times within an exercise session.

Step-ups

Version 1

Step-ups may be performed in a number of different ways. Firstly, they may use a low bench or step with the participant stepping up with one foot, and up with the other, then down with one foot and down with the other – following the cycle 'up, up, down, down, up, up, down, down'. This can be performed to a set rhythm, such as 20 steps per minute. A consistent stepping rhythm may be achieved using a metronome set at 80 beats per minute. Each beat will correspond to one component of the four-stage cycle (up, up, down, down). When performing this exercise the participant should change their leading leg at intervals – every fifth, tenth or fifteenth step, depending upon the individual and the duration of the exercise. During the exercise the participant should fully extend both knees when stepping onto the bench. The degree of difficulty may be altered by adjusting the height of the step or by changing the rate to make it slower or quicker as desired. A rhythm of 30 steps per minute (120 beats per minute) is fairly brisk.

Version 2

The exercise may be modified to put greater emphasis on the use of the quadriceps muscles. This can be achieved by using a step which is slightly higher than the participant's knee (two benches usually suffice) (Figure 8.22). The bench(es) should be placed next to a wall or support as this will reduce the risk of the participant overbalancing and falling forward. During the exercise the participant places one foot on the bench(es) and uses that leg to raise the body so that both feet are on the bench. He or she should try to minimise the amount of assistance given by the foot that was on the floor. The foot that was initially on the bench is then lowered so that the opposing foot is left on the bench. From this position the exercise is repeated. During the exercise the participant always has one foot on the bench, and with each step it alternates between the right and left foot. The exercise adviser should ensure that the participant straightens both legs when standing on the bench. The exercise should be performed slowly and precisely since a rapid rate will cause the lower leg to 'bounce' back up when it hits the floor and will remove the emphasis from the hip and knee extensors of the upper leg.

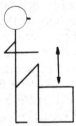

Figure 8.22

Step-overs

This requires the use of a low bench or step. The participant stands with one foot on the bench and one foot positioned on the floor behind the bench, raises their back foot and steps over the bench so that the foot is now on the floor in front of the bench (Figure 8.23). Throughout this movement the other foot remains on the bench. The participant then brings the foot on the floor in front of the bench back over the bench and places it on the floor behind the bench, again keeping one foot on the bench. Throughout the exercise one foot remains firmly on the bench whilst the participant steps over and back across the bench with the other. During the exercise the non-stepping leg should be extended as the other foot is brought across the bench. After the desired number of repetitions the legs should be swapped so that the other leg becomes the 'stepping leg'.

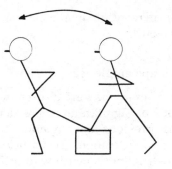

Figure 8.23

Side leg raises

Version 1: single leg raises

This exercise primarily involves the abductor muscles of the legs. The participant lies on their side in a comfortable position with their legs extended and their upper body 'propped' up by their arms to provide support and stability. From this position the participant then raises and lowers the leg which is uppermost (Figure 8.24) (if lying on their right side this will be their left leg, if lying on their left side it will be their right leg). This movement involves the concentric contraction of the abductor muscles in raising the leg and eccentric contraction of these muscles in

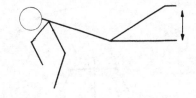

Figure 8.24

controlling its lowering. The participant must remember to change sides in order to exercise both legs.

Version 2: double side leg raises

This exercise is similar to the previous one with the participant starting the exercise in the same position. However, during the exercise he or she attempts to raise and lower both legs at the same time (Figure 8.25), working both the abductor and adductor muscles. When lying on their right side, raising and lowering the legs will work the abductor muscles of the left leg and the adductor muscles of the right, with the raising movement requiring concentric contractions and the lowering phase requiring eccentric work. Lying on the left side will exercise the abductor muscles of the right leg and the adductor muscles of the left.

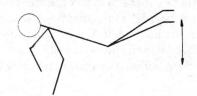

Figure 8.25

Ski-jumps

This exercise may be performed over a white line or two white lines positioned approximately 30–45 cm apart. The participant stands on one side of the white line(s) with their feet approximately 30 cm apart and their ankles, knees and hips slightly flexed. He or she then

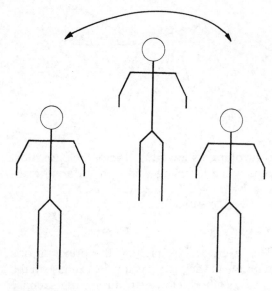

Figure 8.26

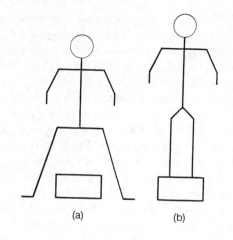

(a)   (b)

Figure 8.27

fatigued, may result in the person tripping over the bench.

Bench jumps single leg

This is a more advanced exercise which, although not significantly more demanding than the previous one, requires a greater degree of co-ordination. The participant faces along the length of a bench with their feet on the floor, one on each side of the bench.

One foot is then placed on the bench whilst the other is kept on the ground. This forms the starting position (Figure 8.28). In a rapid movement the participant then places their other foot on the bench and the first foot on

takes off with both feet and jumps sideways (in the frontal plane) across to the other side of the line(s) slightly flexing their ankles, knees and hips on landing. After landing the participant immediately jumps back in the same manner to the starting position (Figure 8.26). The exercise involves repeated two-footed sideways jumps back and forth across a line or lines. There is no need to flex the ankles, knees and hips beyond that which is sufficient to cushion the landing and to provide sufficient power for take off. Indeed, assuming a 'deep squatting' position may cause knee problems.

Astride bench jumps

The participant begins by facing along the length of a bench with the feet positioned on the floor, one on each side of the bench (Figure 8.27a). He or she then jumps up, and places both feet simultaneously on the bench (Figure 8.27b), and immediately jumps back down to the starting position. This exercise involves repeated jumps on and off the bench. A fairly good level of co-ordination is required for this activity; lack of co-ordination, especially if

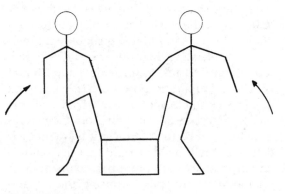

Figure 8.28

the ground. The movement is then repeated by moving the foot that was on the ground onto the bench whilst at the same time moving the other foot from the bench to the floor. In effect, they rapidly hop from one leg to the other with one foot on the floor and the other on the bench.

Bench clears

This is an advanced exercise which can be very demanding and requires good co-ordination. It is similar to the astride bench jumps. The participant begins in the same manner, with both feet positioned astride the bench (Figure 8.29a). When jumping up the feet are brought together to touch in the air (Figure 8.29b) and are then moved apart rapidly so as to land astride the bench in the starting position, rather than on the bench. During this exercise the bench is not touched. It is a fast exercise which requires good co-ordination as well as strength. Alternatives may be used instead of a

bench since, clearly, if the person becomes fatigued he or she may stumble on the bench.

GENERAL CONDITIONING EXERCISES

Many of the above exercises will involve muscle groups other than those specifically stated. Some of them, if performed rapidly, will also require a good level of cardiovascular fitness. Indeed, if organised appropriately, circuit-training exercises may be used as a means of developing cardiovascular fitness along with aspects of muscular strength and endurance. The following exercises are more advanced general exercises which can be incorporated into a circuit session for those who are considered to be 'fit' and capable of more demanding activities. The exercises tend to involve a combination of the major muscle groups to a greater or lesser extent.

Sprint starts

This exercise commences in the press-up position (Figure 8.30a). From this preliminary position the hip and knee of one leg are flexed to bring the leg under the body with the knee almost touching the chest (Figure 8.30b). This forms the starting position: from this position the flexed leg is rapidly extended and at the same time the extended leg is rapidly flexed and brought up to almost touch the chest. This motion is repeated, with the legs flexing and extending in opposition to one another. During this exercise the person's weight tends to be over their hands, which makes it tiring on the arms and shoulders (which are working statically), as well as the leg muscles (which are working dynamically).

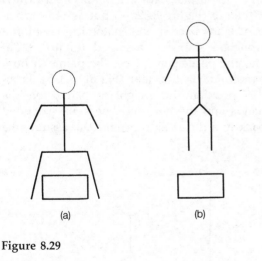

(a) (b)

Figure 8.29

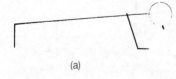 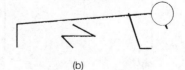

(a) (b)

Figure 8.30

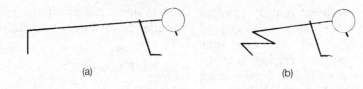

(a)   (b)

Figure 8.31

Burpees

This exercise is similar to the 'sprint start'. It commences in the 'press-up position' (Figure 8.31a), from which both hips and knees are rapidly flexed to bring the knees under the body and close to the chest (Figure 8.31b). The legs are then rapidly extended in a thrusting movement which extends the hips and knees to return them to the starting position. Throughout the exercise the palms of the hands remain on the floor and, as with the 'sprint starts', much of the person's weight is taken over the hands.

Star-jumps

The participant starts in the anatomical position, feet slightly apart and hands by their sides (Figure 8 32a), and jumps into the air, opening their legs (abduction) and at the same time bringing their arms over their heads, again using an abduction movement (Figure 8.32b). The participant then lands in

this position, with their feet slightly wider than shoulder width apart and their hands over their head (Figure 8.32c), and jumps into the air again, this time adducting both arms and legs (Figure 8.32d) to land back in the anatomical position. This activity may be performed quite rapidly and hence involves jumping with the simultaneous abduction of the legs and arms followed by a second jump which is accompanied by the simultaneous adduction of the arms and legs.

Jumping jacks

This exercise is a combination of the star-jump and the burpee. The star jump is performed as before (Figure 8.32a–c) but as the participant lands back in the anatomical position a crouched stance is assumed (Figure 8.33a) and the participant places the palms of both hands flat on the floor (Figure 8.33b). From this position the weight is placed on the hands and the hips and knees are extended back in a thrusting movement to assume the

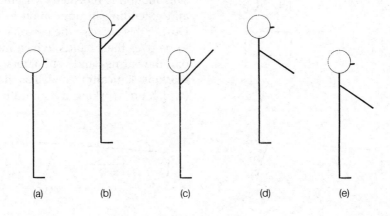

(a)   (b)   (c)   (d)   (e)

Figure 8.32

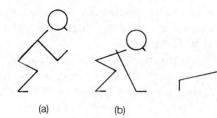

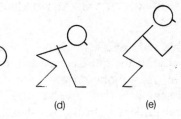

(a) (b) (c) (d) (e)

Figure 8.33

'press-up position' (Figure 8.33c). The movement is then reversed, hips and knees flexing rapidly to once again put the participant into a crouched position (Figure 8.33d) from which to commence a star jump (Figure 8.33e) and the cycle is repeated. These movements should be performed in a smooth, continuous manner, producing a fast co-ordinated action. Overall it is a rapid and demanding exercise which is suitable only for the physically fit – and even these individuals are unlikely to achieve many repetitions.

Leg cycling

This exercise can be performed in a number of different ways and in so doing may convey different benefits. The starting position involves the participant lying flat on their back flexing both knees and hips to bring the knees towards the chest. If the exercise is to be performed slowly (conveying benefits to leg muscle strength, muscle control and abdominal muscle strength), participants should raise themselves up and support their upper body on their elbows, which will help to prevent any unwanted strain on the back (Figure 8.34). The participant commences the exercise by slowly extending the knee and hip of one leg until it is fully extended, then slowly flexing it whilst the opposite leg is extended. This movement is repeated in a slow controlled cycling motion. As a preliminary version of this exercise the extended leg may touch the floor during each cycle; however, as the participant progresses both legs should remain elevated throughout the exercise.

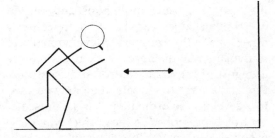

Figure 8.34

If more aerobic benefits are sought, this exercise should be performed at a faster rate but with a reduced amount of leg extension.

Shuttles

This is a simple running exercise which can be incorporated into any exercise session. It involves running or jogging from one side of the room to another for a specified number of repetitions or time (Figure 8.35). It is physically demanding and places overload on the cardiovascular system. When doing this exercise care should be taken to ensure that participants do not collide with each other, equipment or the wall. As a variation, the exercise could involve hopping rather than jogging.

Figure 8.35

THE USE OF MULTIGYMS AND EXERCISE MACHINES

Multigyms and exercise machines provide the opportunity for the muscles to work through a given range of motion against a resistance. These machines often involve the use of levers and pulleys with the resistance being provided by weights. When such equipment is first introduced into an exercise programme it is important for the participant to become fully familiar with the exercises by beginning with relatively light resistances. Even so, exercises such as the military press may be too difficult for many – indeed, if the participant is relatively weak it is often advisable to start them with alternative forms of exercise before undertaking this form of training. If the participant is rehabilitating from an injury it is important for the muscles to be capable of moving the limbs with ease before resistance is applied because, if the muscles are too weak, they may be overstressed by resistance training. Any exercise session is unlikely to involve the sole use of exercise machines or multigyms but will incorporate a combination of activities such as circuit training, dumbbells and exercise machines.

Another point that the exercise adviser should be aware of is the fact that some novice exercisers will find a fitness gym full of exercise machines and (possibly) fit athletic bodies very daunting. Therefore some reassurance and additional support will be required during their initial sessions until their confidence develops.

The exercise adviser should also remember that exercises using multigyms and related exercise machines can be used in contexts other than the primary development of muscular strength. Since the exercises require a degree of muscular control and co-ordination and are relatively safe, they may be used to develop co-ordination and muscular control. If prescribed in the correct way these exercises can convey great benefits to individuals with neuromuscular disorders such as cerebral palsy or similar disabilities where movement patterns are difficult to perform or need to be relearnt.

The equipment used with these types of strengthening exercises can be in the form of a single exercise station or a 'multigym', which combines a number of exercise stations that can be used concurrently by different exercisers. Other, more sophisticated, exercise machines that involve the use of hydraulics and accommodating resistances will be discussed later. Exercise machines can convey certain advantages and disadvantages over other means of strength training.

1. Advantages:
   - The amount of resistance can be adjusted very precisely by altering the amount of weight used
   - The muscles may be worked through specified ranges of motion
   - As with other forms of strength training, the exercises involve a combination of concentric, eccentric and isometric work
   - Because the movement of the weights is limited there is no necessity for assistants or 'spotters', who are essential for the safe use of free weights.
2. Disadvantages:
   - The machines determine the precise movement during the exercise, which can be a slight disadvantage when compared with free weights. For example, with multigyms, where both sides of the body are being exercised together, it may be possible for one side to perform more of the work
   - The controlling and guiding influence of the machine means that the individual's muscles do not have to work as hard to control the movements as they would with free weights. Therefore the stabilising and controlling action may not be developed as effectively.

However, for those involved in general strengthening exercises (rather than weight training for competition), the advantages of safety and convenience often far outweigh the disadvantages.

ORGANISATION OF A WEIGHT-TRAINING SESSION USING EXERCISE MACHINES

An exercise session involving the use of exercise machines should always commence with a warm-up that involves some form of aerobic activity and loosening/stretching exercises. If the participant is relatively strong, and hence the resistances being used are relatively high, then a few repetitions using light resistances can make up the final phase of the warm-up before heavy resistances are attempted. This will ensure that the body is fully warmed up and prepared for the stresses that the exercise will place upon it. The main part of the session is likely to involve a combination of exercises using exercise machines, free weights such as dumbbells and traditional body resistance exercises such as sit-ups and press-ups, thereby producing a varied combination of activities. As with almost any exercise session the final phase should involve a gentle aerobic cool-down and stretching exercises, which will gradually return the body to its 'resting state' and help to reduce the likelihood of stiffness the following day.

SAFETY ASPECTS OF EXERCISE MACHINES

For many makes of equipment, in order to produce the desired resistance it is first necessary to select the desired weight by inserting a 'selector key'. In some machines the selector keys will be attached to the equipment as permanent fixtures, in others they may be removable. If the keys are removable it is important that only the manufacturer's recommended and specifically designed key is used. It may thus be useful to purchase spares or to provide each user with an individual key for personal use during the session. On no account should substitute keys such as nails or screwdrivers be used – these present a potential hazard to both user and machine. Substitute keys can become wedged in and may even damage the machine. This could require maintenance work or dismantling of the machine to remove the offending 'key'. In addition, substitute keys may not be strong enough to take the stresses placed upon them by the weights; consequently they can break and injure the user.

All exercise machines require regular maintenance, from a weekly lubrication of moving parts to a yearly overhaul and safety checks. Both are important for the safety of users, the smooth operating of the machine and the general condition of the equipment. The manufacturer's handbook will usually provide guidance on the nature and frequency of maintenance.

It is also important for all exercise machines to be carefully positioned to allow free access and ease of movement when performing the exercises. Where appropriate they should be securely and expertly fixed to the wall or floor. In all cases equipment should be situated so as to minimise the possibility of people colliding with it or being too near to each other whilst exercising, as this would present a safety hazard as well as an inconvenience.

DETERMINATION OF 'TRAINING LOADS'

When commencing a muscular strengthening exercise programme it is important to start gradually with light resistances. Therefore, in the initial stages the exercise adviser will need to determine appropriate resistances for each exercise. This usually involves setting a fairly light resistance and then seeing if the participant can perform the exercise 15 times with a moderate amount of exertion. If he or she finds this easy the weight should be increased; if the resistance is too difficult the weight should be reduced. This means that a number of minor adjustments are required during the first few sessions. Therefore it is important that the exercise adviser keeps comprehensive records (including details of the exercise, weights used and number of repetitions performed) for all the individuals they are working with.

Once the programme has commenced a record should be kept of each session as this will help to determine when the participant is ready to progress. It will probably be necessary to stay at the initial training load for at least six sessions before gradual progression can be considered. As he or she progresses, the participant should remain at the new level for a number of weeks. To ensure gradual progression it is desirable to increase just one or two exercises at a time in each session, making each successive session slightly more demanding. However, each individual exercise may remain constant for six or more sessions before being once again increased. Advisers will find the assessment of initial workloads and the determination of appropriate progressions easier with experience as they become more familiar with the activity.

EXAMPLES OF MULTIGYM AND EXERCISE MACHINE EXERCISES

These descriptions refer to the exercises that are being performed at a single isolated station or at one of the stations of a multigym. Owing to the complexity of muscle action it is sometimes inappropriate to specify which muscles are being worked by a particular exercise. It is often more appropriate to refer to the movement and relate it to the many muscle groups that could be involved in the activity, such as arm extension or knee flexion.

EXERCISES FOR THE LOWER BODY

Leg press

The participant adjusts the seat so that when sitting with their feet resting on the foot-plate, their hips and knees are flexed at approximately 90° (Figure 8.36a). Flexing the hips and knees further will make the exercise more difficult. It is therefore important to note the seat position as well as the amount of weight being used. Some machines will provide more than one possible foot position and, as this will also affect the degree of difficulty of the exercise, it should be noted in the exercise programme. Since this exercise tends to use levers the foot position that provides the longest lever will provide the easiest version of the exercise, while the selection of a foot position which gives a shorter lever will make the exercise more difficult.

When performing the exercise the participant should ensure that their feet are securely positioned on the correct foot placement. The participant then pushes against the foot-plate, extending their hips and knees and thereby lifting the weights (Figure 8.36b). This action should be smooth and controlled, not jerky or erratic. It is especially important to control the movement near the point of full knee extension. If the movement is too rapid, the legs will become fully extended but due to the momentum of the movement the weights may continue to rise slightly. The weights will then fall under the influence of gravity and in doing so will exert additional force on the

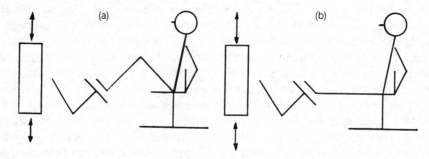

Figure 8.36

participant's legs, which, with the knees fully extended, are not in a position to absorb this additional force. Therefore, in order to protect the joints from this unwanted stress the movement must be controlled at all times. Following full extension the weights are lowered by flexing the hips and knees, again by a controlled movement using the leg extensors to regulate the movement via eccentric contractions. The weights being lowered should not be allowed to touch the remaining weights of the stack but should be held about 3 cm above them and the movement repeated. This requires good eccentric control of a movement which involves muscular co-ordination as well as strength. This exercise may be performed using one leg at a time rather than with both legs together.

The controlled eccentric phase of the exercise places a considerable amount of overload on the muscles. In those unfamiliar with the exercise this can result in muscle soreness 24–48 hours later due to microtrauma and slight inflammation within the muscle, which will fade within a few days. Therefore, as with all forms of exercise, it needs to be gradually introduced into a programme.

Calf press

The calf press may be performed at the same station as the leg press. The starting point for the calf press is at the point of full extension of the leg press. At this point the knees should be fully extended but the ankles will be flexed. From this position the participant then extends and flexes their ankles, which will cause a slight rise and fall of the weights (Figure 8.37).

Push backs

This exercise may be performed at the 'leg press' station of some multigyms. The exercise is performed in a standing position with the participant facing away from the machine. The participant stands on one leg, flexes the knee of the other leg and places the sole of that foot on the foot-plate of the machine (Figure 8.38). Then, holding onto the machine or another object for support, the participant pushes back with their leg, extending the hip and knee and thereby raising the weights. The weights are then carefully lowered by controlled flexion of the hip and knee (using eccentric contractions of the extensor muscles). As with the leg press, the lowered weights should not be allowed to touch the remaining ones but should be held just above them, from where the movement can be repeated. When performing this exercise it is important that the foot of the leg performing the work is placed firmly on the foot-plate and does not slip. With some multigyms the angle and positioning of the foot-plate makes this difficult, which could allow the foot to slip off the plate and the foot-plate to hit the

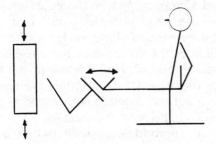

Figure 8.37

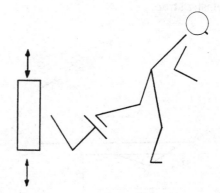

Figure 8.38

back of the legs. For reasons of safety, it is thus inadvisable to undertake this exercise with machines that are not specifically designed for it.

Hamstring curls

This exercise is performed with the participant lying face down on a bench, legs extended and ankles hooked under a padded bar to which the weights are attached. From this position the participant repeatedly flexes and extends the knees (Figure 8.39). The flexion causes the weights to rise due to the concentric activity of the knee flexors, the lowering action is regulated by the eccentric activity of the knee flexors. The movement should go to full flexion and, as with the previous exercises, should be smooth and controlled. A variation of the exercise could involve the use of one leg at a time. This could be valuable if one leg is weaker than the other, as the stronger leg tends to do most of the work when both legs are used.

If the appropriate exercise station is not available then an alternative exercise may be performed using a strong elasticated strap. One end of the strap is attached to the participant's ankle whilst the other is connected to a wall or similar fixed object. The participant lies face down with one knee slightly flexed, and attempts to fully flex this knee whilst working against the resistance provided by the elastic strap.

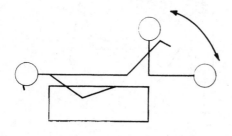

Figure 8.39

Knee extension

This exercise is usually performed using the same bench as used for hamstring curls. In this exercise the participant sits at the end of the bench with their knees flexed so that the legs hang vertically over the end of the bench and the ankles are hooked behind a padded bar to which weights are attached. From this position the participant extends their knees, working against the resistance of the weights (Figure 8.40). Upon reaching full extension the weights are lowered by the controlled flexion of the knees and the movement repeated. As with many of these exercises the knee extensions can be performed either on both legs at the same time or on each leg separately, as desired.

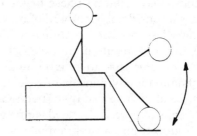

Figure 8.40

Adductor pulls

The station for this exercise is not commonly found, either separately or as part of a multi-gym. The participant performs the exercise in a standing position with one ankle attached to a cord. Commencing with the leg abducted, he or she then adducts this leg (which is attached to the machine). Pulling the leg towards the midline of the body raises the weights and causes the adductors to work against a resistance (Figure 8.41). During this exercise the participant may require some support in order to maintain his or her balance.

If an appropriate exercise station is not available this exercise may be performed using a strong elasticated strap. One end of

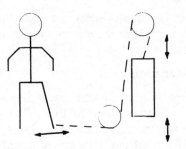

Figure 8.41

the strap is attached to the participant's ankle whilst the other is attached to a wall or similar immovable object. The adduction movement therefore works against the resistance of the strap.

Knee raises

Although this is really a 'body resistance' exercise, an exercise station for knee raises is sometimes incorporated into a multigym. To commence the exercise the participant lifts and holds their body in position above the ground using arm rests and handles. The exercise therefore requires a considerable amount of upper body isometric strength and endurance. The exercise starts with the hips and knees extended. The participant flexes their hips and knees, raising the knees as high as possible towards the chest then lowers them by a controlled extension of the hips and knees (Figure 8.42).

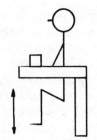

Figure 8.42

EXERCISES FOR THE UPPER BODY

Bench press

The participant lies face up on the bench with the bar positioned so that it is approximately level with their chin. It is important that during this exercise the participant does not arch their back – it should be kept firmly on the bench at all times. To ensure this, and to provide a comfortable position from which to perform the exercise, the feet may be placed either one on each side of the bench with the soles flat of the floor or together, with the soles of the feet flat on the bench. The latter position may be more comfortable for many people, especially those who are not very tall and find foot placement on the floor awkward. To commence the exercise the participant grasps the bar and pushes upwards, extending the elbow in a controlled movement (Figure 8.43). Once both elbows have been fully extended the bar is gently lowered using eccentric contractions of the elbow extensors until the weights almost touch the remaining weights in the stack. The extension movement is then repeated. This exercise therefore involves aspects of control as well as concentric and eccentric muscular work.

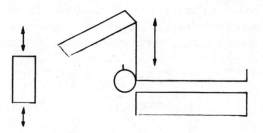

Figure 8.43

Military press

In muscular terms this exercise is similar to the bench press but it is performed from a seated rather than a lying position. The participant sits on a stool facing the exercise machine or multigym. In this position the bar should be positioned just above shoulder height and slightly to the front, ensuring that when the exercise is performed the participant pushes upwards and slightly away from their body. This helps to prevent the back from arching during the exercise. For this exercise taller participants may place their feet flat on the floor whilst others may place them firmly on the rungs of the stool (if present). These positions should provide the individual with a firm stable base from which to push. The participant grasps the bar firmly and pushes up and slightly away from their body, extending the elbows in a controlled movement (Figure 8.44). When the elbows are fully extended the bar is then gradually lowered so that the weights being used almost touch the weights remaining in the stack. From this position the exercise is repeated.

As with most of the exercises described in this section, the military press includes elements of control, concentric and eccentric muscular activity. During the exercise the back should not be arched, but should be kept straight. Arching the back indicates that the exercise is too strenuous and that the weight or number of repetitions should be reduced to prevent undue stress on the back. The military press thus not only exercises the arm and shoulder muscles but also requires the back

muscles to work isometrically in order to maintain posture throughout the movement.

Shoulder press

In terms of the muscles used, the shoulder press is very similar to the military press. However, the shoulder press is performed with the participant facing outwards, away form the machine rather than towards it. The individual commences the exercise with the bar level with their shoulders, then pushes directly up, or up slightly behind, Figure 8.45). This alignment and movement can cause some individuals to arch their backs when performing the movement. It is therefore less preferable than the military press for most participants and, owing to the overall similarity of the two exercises, it may be omitted from most programmes.

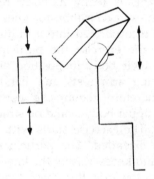
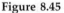

Figure 8.45

Biceps curls

This exercise involves the use of weights and a pulley system. The participant faces the machine and holds the bar with arms down and elbows extended (almost in the anatomical position). To get into this starting position the weights may need to be lifted slightly if the cable to which they are attached is relatively short. Care should be taken in getting into this position. Firstly, the participant should face the machine and then flex their

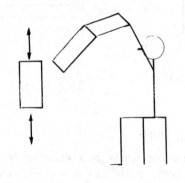

Figure 8.44

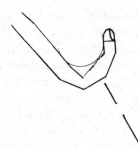

Figure 8.46

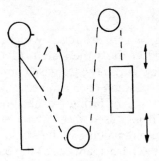

Figure 8.47

knees and hips in order to crouch down and reach the bar which will be resting on the floor. From this position the participant will grasp the bar using an underhand grip (Figure 8.46) and straighten their back, looking up directly ahead whilst doing so. The participant then stands up by straightening their hips and knees, *not* by bending their back (which should be kept straight throughout the movement). This means that the weights are lifted into the starting position by the action of the legs and not the back. Lifting with a curved back or using the back to lift rather than the legs can put too much stress on the back. With some machines it is possible to alter the length of the wire; if this is possible the wire should be adjusted so that the weights being used are lifted about 5 cm above the others when the participant assumes the starting position. Once in the starting position the exercise may commence. The participant flexes their elbows, raising the weights whilst keeping their upper arm and elbows close to their body and as still as possible (Figure 8.47). This ensures that the movement is caused by the elbow flexors rather than the shoulder flexors. Throughout the movement it is important that the back is kept still and not hyperextended to assist the movement. Any back movement may make the exercise easier but puts unwanted stress on the back and should be avoided. During the exercise the shoulder muscles will be used

statically to hold the shoulder in position. If, however, the exercise adviser wishes the participant to use their shoulder flexors dynamically then some shoulder flexion may be incorporated into the lifting action, but again the back should remain static throughout. The weights are lowered by extending the elbows. The downward movement is controlled by the eccentric contraction of the elbow flexors.

Reverse curls

Reverse curls provide a slight variation of the biceps curl. For the reverse curl the movement is performed with an overhand grip (Figure 8.48). In all other respects the movement and safety considerations are identical to those described for the biceps curl.

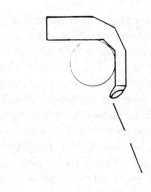

Figure 8.48

Chinning

Chinning is an exercise which may be performed at the same station as the biceps and reverse curls. The exercise commences in the same position as the reverse curl: using an overhand grip, facing the machine with the weights being used already raised slightly above those remaining in the stack. From this position the participant raises the bar directly upwards so that it almost touches their chin (Figure 8.49). This is achieved by simultaneous abduction of the upper part of the arms at the shoulder joint and flexion of the lower arms at the elbow joint in the frontal plane. The bar is then lowered using the reverse movement and the exercise is repeated.

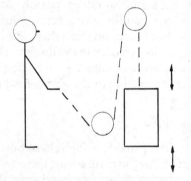

Figure 8.49

Seated row

The seated row may be performed at the same station as the biceps curls and chinning exercises. The basic movement is similar to that of chinning. However, this exercise is performed in a seated rather than a standing position. To get into the starting position the participant sits down and places their feet against the foot placement provided. The knees and hips should both be flexed. The participant then takes hold of the bar with an overhand grip and extends their elbows. He or she then straightens their back into a vertical position whilst continuing to hold the bar in front of them with extended arms. At this point the cable or chain attached to the weights should be slack. The participant then pushes against the foot placements to straighten their hips and knees whilst keeping their back straight and upright. This will push the body away from the machine, causing the wire to tighten, and should result in the weights rising slightly. During this phase it is important to keep the back and arms straight so that the initial lifting of the weight off of the stack is caused by the action of the legs. If the wire is too slack it may need to be adjusted so that the weights are lifted slightly off the stack. This forms the starting position (Figure 8.50).

From this position the participant pulls the bar towards their chest using an arm action similar to that described for chinning; however, in this case the arm movements will be in an oblique plane, with the overall bar movement being upward and outward towards the participant's chest. The weights should then be carefully lowered using a reverse movement and held just above those remaining in the stack. Throughout this exercise it is important to ensure that the back is kept vertical and is not used dynamically. Flexing and extending the back during this exercise may place unnecessary stress on the back. This exercise works the back muscles statically as well as dynamically exercising the arm and shoulder muscles.

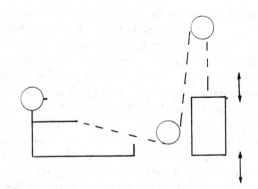

Figure 8.50

Lats pull-downs

This exercise is for the arms and upper back. It derives its name from one of the muscle groups involved, the latissimus dorsi. There are a number of variations of this exercise, which may be performed kneeling on one knee, on both knees or even seated. Participants should select the position they find most comfortable. The exercise uses the station commonly called the 'lats bar'. The bar is suspended overhead and is pulled down using a combination of the shoulder muscles and elbow flexors as well as the forearm muscles (which are involved in holding the bar). To get into the starting position the participant holds the bar with an overhand grip, with the hands positioned towards the ends of the bar (the hands will be approximately 60 cm wider than shoulder width apart). From this standing position the participant then assumes a kneeling or seated position whilst keeping their arms extended above their head and bending their knees to lower their body (Figure 8.51). Owing to the length of the pulley this will raise the weights slightly. This two-stage movement into the starting position is preferable to one in which the participant immediately assumes a kneeling position with flexed arms, as this makes the weight more difficult to control and may put unwanted strain on the back.

In the starting position the pulley should be directly above the participant's head. If the participant is positioned too far from the machine the exercise will be awkward to perform. The participant pulls the bar down behind their head so that it almost touches the back of their neck, thereby raising the weights. The weights are then lowered by slowly extending the arms using eccentric contractions to control the movement. Once the arms are again fully extended the movement can be repeated.

Upon completion of the desired number of repetitions the participant extends their arms above their head and then slowly stands (if performing the exercise from a kneeling or seated position), keeping their arms extended until the weights are lowered to the stack. This movement is preferable to the participant standing up with their arms flexed, which makes the weight more difficult to control and could place unwanted strain on the back.

As a variation, the participant can pull the bar down in front of their body until it is level with the chest or until the weights almost reach the top of the machine. As a further variation the participant could pull the bar down alternately behind and in front of their head.

Triceps pushdowns

This exercise uses the same station as the lats pull-down. The triceps pushdowns are performed in a standing position with the participant holding the bar with an overhand grip (as shown in Figure 8.48) and their hands approximately 45–60 cm apart. To get into the starting position the bar must be pulled down so that the elbows are positioned close to the body just above their hips. The elbows are fully flexed with the bar being held at approximately shoulder height. From this starting position the participant then extends their elbows, pushing the bar down whilst keeping their elbows close to their body just above

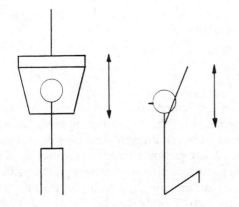

Figure 8.51

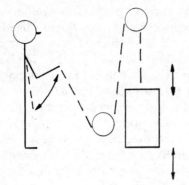

Figure 8.52

their hips (Figure 8.52). Once the elbows are fully extended the bar is slowly returned to the starting position by flexing the elbows, controlling the movement with eccentric contractions. Again the elbows should remain close to the body and when full elbow flexion is reached the movement can be repeated.

The exercise involves elbow flexion and extension with the minimum amount of shoulder movement. Shoulder movement (flexion and extension) will make the exercise easier, therefore it may be modified depending upon whether the exercise adviser wishes the participant to use their shoulders or to limit the dynamic aspects of the exercise to primarily elbow extension. Upon completion of the desired number of repetitions the weights are lowered back onto the stack by allowing the bar to rise above the participant's head, again controlling the movement with eccentric contractions.

Chins

Chins are a body-resistance exercise but are included in this section because stations for performing this exercise are commonly included in most multigyms. Chins require good upper body strength and are therefore only likely to be appropriate for individuals who are exceptionally strong. The 'chinning bar' is fixed to the multigym several feet

above head height (as an alternative bars fixed to the wall can be used). To perform the exercise the participant reaches up and holds the bar with both hands. Shorter individuals may need to be lifted into this position, or use a chair. The bar is held with the hands positioned so that they are slightly wider than shoulder width apart. An overhand or underhand grip may be used and indeed may be changed to provide a variation of the exercise. The exercise commences with the arms extended and the participant holding onto the bar with their feet above the ground. For comfort some individuals prefer to cross their feet as they are suspended in mid air (Figure 8.53a). The participant then raises their body using their shoulder and arm muscles so that their chin is raised slightly above the bar (Figure 8.53b). They then slowly lower their body until their elbows are again fully extended. The movement can be repeated for the desired number of repetitions.

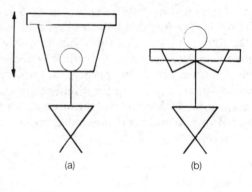

(a)   (b)

Figure 8.53

Dips

Like the 'chins', dips are a body resistance exercise for which a station is often incorporated into a multigym. The dips described in the earlier section on body resistance involved the participant having their feet on the ground or on another object, thereby supporting some of the participant's weight. The dips described here involve the feet being off the ground and therefore all the participant's weight being supported by their upper body. This makes it a much more advanced exercise which is suitable only for those with good upper body strength. The participant commences the exercise holding the bars with their elbows extended and feet elevated (Figure 8.54a). From this position the body is lowered (by elbow flexion and shoulder hyperextension) using eccentric contractions until the upper arm is parallel to the floor (Figure 8.54b). In this position the elbows should be positioned behind the body, flexed at right angles with the lower arms in a vertical position. The body is then raised back into the starting position by extending the elbows and flexing the shoulders. For the duration of the exercise some participants slightly flex the knees and cross their legs because they find it makes the exercise more comfortable.

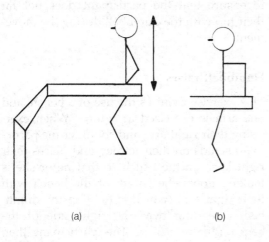

(a)   (b)

Figure 8.54

USE OF DUMBBELLS

Dumbbells can be used in a large variety of resistance exercises to develop muscular tone, local muscular endurance and muscular strength. Dumbbell exercises are usually very simple and safe. Some dumbbells are fixed weights whilst others can be adjusted by adding or removing weights. Dumbbells should be stored in a rack for easy access and should be replaced immediately after use to reduce the risk of someone falling over them. Although dumbbells tend to be relatively light (1–10 kg each) care should still be taken when lifting them from the stack, especially the heavier ones. When preparing to lift a dumbbell from the stack or off the ground it is important to always bend the knees, keep the back straight and look up. The dumbbells should then be lifted by straightening the legs and assuming the anatomical position. From this position the individual may walk to the area in which they are going to perform the exercise and carefully, without any hurried movements, assume the starting position for the exercise. Equal care must be taken when returning the dumbbells to their storage area.

DUMBBELL EXERCISES

Biceps curls

The participant begins the exercise in the anatomical position. From this position the elbow is flexed and the dumbbell bought up to shoulder height in a smooth and controlled movement. It is then carefully lowered back to the starting position, controlling the movement with eccentric contractions of the elbow flexors (Figure 8.55). Throughout the movement the upper arm should be kept close to the body and shoulder movement should be minimal. In addition to this the back should be kept straight and still (the back should not be used dynamically to assist with the movement). Biceps curls may be performed in a variety of ways:

- The arms may be worked separately, with one arm completing its full set of repetitions before the other one is exercised.
- The arms may work alternately, with one arm completing one full cycle of the exercise whilst the other remains in the starting position, the roles then being reversed. This means that each arm completes one

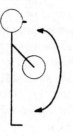

Figure 8.55

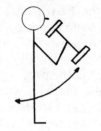

Figure 8.56

repetition and then rests whilst the other arm completes one repetition (and so on) for the desired number of repetitions.

- Both arms work together in parallel, raising and lowering the dumbbells in synchrony.
- Both arms work at the same time but in opposition: one arm raises its dumbbell using concentric contractions whilst the other arm is in the process of lowering its dumbbell using eccentric contractions.

There is little difference in the effectiveness of each of these variations so the choice of which version to use will depend upon individual preference.

Running arms

The arm action used in this exercise is similar to that when a person is walking or running. From the anatomical position the arms are pronated so that the palms are facing the thighs and both elbows are flexed at 90°. This is the starting position. From this position the arms are moved with a running/walking action and are therefore moved in opposition with one moving back as the other moves forwards (Figure 8.56). On completion of the forward movement the dumbbell may reach shoulder height, whilst on completion of the backward movement the upper arm may be flexed at the shoulder so that it is not quite parallel to the ground. Care should be taken to ensure that the participant does not hit their hip with the dumbbell during the movement.

Dumbbell raises

This exercise requires the use of a bench, and one arm is exercised at a time. When exercising their right arm and shoulder the participant stands on their left leg and places their right knee on the bench so that he or she is looking down the length of the bench with their right arm (which is holding the dumbbell) extending over the right side of the bench (Figure 8.57a). The participant then

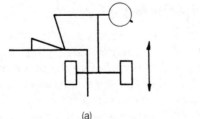
(a)

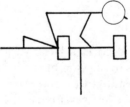
(b)

Figure 8.57

flexes their back to approximately 60° and places their left hand on the bench for balance. This then forms the starting position. From this position the dumbbell is raised by flexing the right elbow and extending the right shoulder so that the dumbbell is brought up to the height of the right hip (Figure 8.57b). The dumbbell is then lowered using the reverse movements and the exercise repeated for the desired number of repetitions. To exercise the left side the positions are reversed.

Triceps pullovers

During this exercise one arm is worked at time. In this example the movements are described for the right arm – therefore to exercise the left arm the roles need to be reversed.

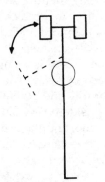

Figure 8.58

To get into the starting position the participant stands in the anatomical position. The right arm, which is holding the dumbbell, is pronated so that the palm faces their right thigh. The arm is then fully flexed at the shoulder (keeping the elbow extended) until the dumbbell is held vertically overhead (Figure 8.58). The left arm is then moved to hold the right elbow in position. From this starting position the right elbow is flexed so that the dumbbell is lowered behind the head until it is level with the neck and extended to raise the dumbbell back to the starting position.

Dumbbell flies

This exercise is performed with the participant lying face upwards on a bench with their feet firmly positioned flat on the floor or on the bench. He or she holds a dumbbell in each hand and abducts both arms to 90° to their body and parallel to the floor or slightly hyperextended in the transverse plane (Figure 8.59a). From this position both dumbbells are slowly raised so that the arms are held vertically, directly above the chest (Figure 8.59b). This movement could be described as shoulder flexion in the transverse plane or as an anticlockwise rotation of the right arm and clockwise rotation of the left arm in the transverse plane. The arms are then lowered back to the starting position using the reverse movements.

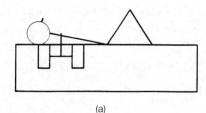

(a)

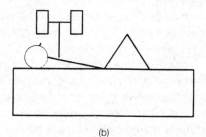

(b)

Figure 8.59

THE USE OF FREE WEIGHTS

For many of the available exercises which have been described for exercise machines there are similar versions using 'free weights'. However, exercises that use free weights require the participants to not only work with a resistance (provided by the weight) but to be in complete control of the movement. Exercise machines provide some degree of control over the movement of the weights (the advantages and disadvantages of this were discussed earlier). Exercise machines provide an extra safety dimension because the weights can only move in a very limited direction (up and down the stack) and the participant's control of the movement is limited to the speed of the movement up and down. Exercises that use machines are therefore less likely to cause injury because losing control of the weights will only cause them to fall onto the stack. Using free weights the participant has to control not only the speed of movement but also the direction, which makes the exercise more difficult. The additional control needed with free weights may require the fixator muscles to work harder than when performing the equivalent movement on an exercise machine. This may be desirable in some cases but if the participant loses control of the weights they could be injured by struggling to regain control or dropping them. Although free weights have certain advantages over exercise machines they have the potential to cause injury if the participant has a poor technique, becomes fatigued or drops them through carelessness.

When using exercise machines for exercises such as the bench press, leg press and military press it is possible for one side of the body to do more work than the other. Free weights require both sides of the body to work equally hard in moving the weights and controlling the movement. Therefore, if one side of the body is stronger than the other it may be desirable to use free weights. Alternatively, each side of the body could be exercised separately.

It should also be remembered that exercises using free weights often require the assistance of a helper or 'spotter', especially in exercises such as the bench press. The spotter will assist if the participant becomes too fatigued during the exercise or the weight becomes too heavy, and will also assist with the initial movement of the weight off the stand and its replacement after the desired number of repetitions. A spotter is important to ensure the safe use of free weights.

Additional safety considerations associated with the use of free weights include ensuring that all weight 'collars' are firmly secured to prevent the weights from falling off the bar. On a final note of safety, it is very easy for free weights to be left around the exercise areas after use. This is not only untidy but also presents a serious safety hazard as someone can easily trip over them and fall. Free weights must always be returned to their storage area after use, and strong matting should be used in the exercise area to protect the floor. A mirror is also a standard inclusion in most exercise areas as it can help the participant to ensure that he or she is using the correct technique for each exercise. The relative factors of safety, control, and potential bias must therefore be considered when setting an exercise programme, and the exercise adviser should select the free weights and/or exercise machine exercises accordingly.

In some cases ankle or wrist weights can be used as an alternative to the heavier free weights. Examples of such exercises include the leg extension and hamstring curl which are described in this section. During these exercises the overall movement is the same and the relevant sections should be referred to for details.

EXERCISES USING FREE WEIGHTS

Bench press

This exercise uses the same movements as the multigym bench press (Figure 8.43). However, it requires the presence of an assistant or 'spotter' to ensure that the exercise is performed safely. It also requires a set of stands which are positioned on each side of the bench to support the weight before and after the exercise. As the movement of the weights to and from the stand requires good control and co-ordination, the spotter is therefore likely to assist with this aspect of the exercise, especially if the participant is fatigued.

Squats

This exercise also requires the use of stands and a 'spotter'. This is an advanced strength-training exercise and is therefore not likely to be appropriate for those requiring basic exercise therapy. The stands are positioned so that the weights bar is situated just below shoulder height. The participant then stands under the bar with their knees slightly flexed, supporting the bar on the back of the neck (Figure 8.60). For comfort, additional padding should be positioned between the neck and the bar (a folded towel will often suffice). The participant's hands are positioned towards each end of the bar to provide optimum control and balance. From this position the participant extends their knees and lifts the bar off the stands. They then move forward a few paces to get clear of the stands. The exercise can then commence.

The participant should stand with their feet slightly wider than shoulder width apart and from this standing position assume a slight squatting position (not a deep squat) by flexing the hips, knees and ankles whilst keeping the back straight and looking forward directly ahead. For most individuals the knees should be flexed no more than 90° because additional flexion will place unwanted strain on the knee. With this exercise a mirror is useful. If the participant stands in front of the mirror, he or she can ensure that they keep their head up throughout the exercise. From the semi-squatting position the participant extends hips, knees and ankles to return to the starting position. During this exercise the heels of both feet may be elevated by getting the participant to stand with their heels on a block of wood (2–4 cm high) whilst the balls of the feet remain flat on the floor. This appears to help some individuals keep their back straight and their head up. The exercise should be performed slowly and in a controlled manner without bouncing (as this puts strain on the knees). When the desired number of repetitions have been completed the participant is guided back to the stands by the spotter and assisted in returning the weights bar to the stands.

'Good morning' exercises

As previously stated, many of the exercises described in earlier sections will strengthen the back. However, these exercises can be prescribed for those who already have relatively strong back muscles but wish to develop their strength further. It is not an exercise for

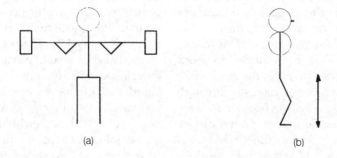

(a) (b)

Figure 8.60

beginners, who will probably develop their back strength sufficiently through other exercises such as press-ups and the military press. The starting position (Figure 8.61a) is the same as for the squats, though much lighter weights are used. From the starting position the back is flexed 30–45° (Figure 8.61b). This should be done slowly and should not go so far that the participant feels stretch on the hamstrings. From this flexed position the participant slowly extends the back and straightens up into the starting position before repeating the movement. Throughout the exercise the movement should be slow and controlled, without bouncing. Upon completion of the exercise the participant returns the weights to the stands with the assistance of the spotter.

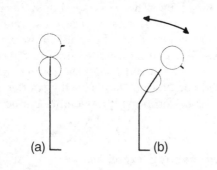

(a)　　(b)

Figure 8.61

ISOKINETIC AND OTHER FORMS OF ACCOMMODATING RESISTANCE WORK

As previously discussed, a feature of most exercises is that the muscles experience different degrees of difficulty during the different phases of the movement. This means that the muscles may be required to work quite hard during one phase of the movement yet work at a much lower intensity through the remainder. The consequences of this are that an optimal training effect occurs at one point of the range of movement but that limited benefits are attained at other points. Accommodating resistance work endeavours

to overcome this problem by altering the amount of resistance experienced at different phases of the movement. This should produce a more effective training effect throughout the entire range of movement, rather than at isolated points. This accommodating resistance may be achieved through the use of specific 'isokinetic' machines, accommodating resistance machines that use cams, hydraulics and pneumatics, or with the aid of a partner.

ISOKINETIC MACHINES

The term 'isokinetic' means 'same speed'. Isokinetic machines incorporate a 'speed governor' and can be programmed to work at a specific speed, usually measured in units of degrees per second and can range from 0° (isometric) to in excess of 450° per second. When the speed is set it means that regardless of the amount of force exerted by the muscles against the machine, the movement will always proceed at the designated speed. The advantages of this are that the muscles can be made to exert their maximal force throughout the entire movement, thereby ensuring a training effect at all phases of the motion.

Most isokinetic machines have the attachments required to exercise all the major joints through the common ranges of movement: extension, flexion, abduction and adduction of both the upper and lower limbs. Whilst basic isokinetic machines may be confined to concentric actions, more advanced versions have the capacity for eccentric as well as concentric work. A feature of isokinetic devices is that the participant is strapped to the machine to isolate a particular joint movement. This has certain advantages in ensuring exercise specificity, but it must be remembered that for more complex actions the co-ordination of many joint movements is required, and the co-ordinated movements of many joints cannot be produced with the restrictions of an isokinetic machine. Consequently whilst most of the movements described for multigym exercises can be produced using an isokinetic device, the exercise adviser should be aware of the possible need to develop these into functional activities by additional exercises. A specific advantage of isokinetic devices is their capacity to control the speed of a movement and thereby provide a degree of additional safety. This has particular implications for rehabilitation programmes, when an exercise may initially be prescribed at a slow speed but will then be increased over a period of weeks.

In addition to their use as training devices isokinetic machines have a diagnostic use as they can record the strength of the muscles during different phases of a movement. This can be used to assess whether a muscle is significantly weaker at any particular phase of movement and/or whether the strength ratio of different muscles is appropriate or unbalanced (see Chapter 6).

Isokinetic machines are becoming more widespread in hospital rehabilitation, sports injury and specialist exercise facilities, although their cost makes their use prohibitive in many exercise studios. Those utilising isokinetics should receive specific instructions on their use both as a diagnostic tool and as an exercise facility. For further details on the use of isokinetic machines see Baechle (1994), Maud and Foster (1995) and Chan *et al.* (1996).

ACCOMMODATING RESISTANCE MACHINES (CAMS, HYDRAULICS AND PNEUMATICS)

Accommodating resistance machines provide the range of exercises available with standard exercise machines whilst incorporating an element of accommodating resistance. The rationale for doing this is to provide the muscles with a training effect throughout the full range of movement. This is achieved in the design of the machines which use hydraulics or cams. Cams alter the leverage of the machine during the range of movement. This compensates for the problems that occur with standard exercise machines when the training effect on the muscles may be minimal during the 'easier' phases of the movement. The shape of the cams endeavour to overcome this by shortening the leverage during the phases of the movement which would normally be easier, thereby making it more difficult and producing a stronger training stimulus at these points in the movement.

Other accommodating resistance machines use hydraulics, creating a partial isokinetic effect. Their design incorporates the use of a piston which pushes liquid through an orifice of adjustable diameter from one compartment to another as the machine is used. The greater the force applied by the participant the greater the resistance offered by the machine. A similar principle is utilised in machines which use pneumatic (gas) resistance. However, unlike true isokinetic machines, the speed at which the movement occurs will be influenced by the strength of the person using it. Whilst these machines do not have a true isokinetic effect, they do make some adjustments to account for the limitations of standard exercise machines.

ACCOMMODATING RESISTANCE PARTNER WORK

A form of accommodating resistance work can easily be incorporated into a programme if the participant is able to exercise with a partner (or their exercise adviser) who will apply the required resistance instead of a machine. Accommodating resistance can be applied to virtually any dynamic muscular movement and therefore only one specific example is given in this text to illustrate its application. An advantage of including accommodating resistance exercises in a programme is that movements which normally occur under the influence of gravity (and hence require very little muscular activity) can be made more difficult and the exercise used to work certain muscle groups which could be neglected by many other exercises.

ACCOMMODATING RESISTANCE EXERCISE

Knee extensions

The participant sits on a bench with their knees flexed at 90° so that their lower legs hang vertically over the edge of the bench. One leg is exercised at a time. The movement for the exercise is the same as that used in the knee extension exercise (see Figure 8.38): the participant simply extends one knee so that the leg is straightened. However, during the exercise their partner places a hand on the ventral side of the participant's ankle and pushes, thereby resisting the movement (Figure 8.62). The pressure applied by the partner should not be so great as to prevent the movement but should be sufficient to retard its speed considerably. Throughout the exercise the participant should push as hard as possible throughout the full range of

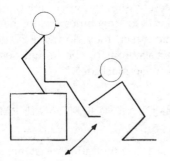

Figure 8.62

movement and the exercise adviser or partner should provide resistance throughout, thereby keeping the speed of movement consistent and making the muscles work hard throughout the full range of movement.

Accommodating resistance may be simply applied to other movements such as knee flexion, elbow flexion and extension and shoulder movements (and indeed virtually any body movement that requires concentric muscular contractions).

ASSESSMENT OF MUSCULAR STRENGTH

The assessment and monitoring of muscular strength can be an important aspect of many exercise programmes, both in the determination of suitable training loads and to monitor the effectiveness of an exercise programme. A fuller rationale for assessments and some examples are presented in Chapter 6.

REFERENCES

Baechle, T.R. (1994). *Essentials of Strength Training and Conditioning*. Champaign, IL: Human Kinetics.

Chan, K., Maffulli, N., Korkia, P. and Li, R.C.T. (1996). *Principles and Practice of Isokinetics in Sports Medicine and Rehabilitation*. Hong Kong: Williams and Wilkins.

Maud, P.J. and Foster, C. (1995). *Physiological Assessment of Human Fitness*. Champaign, IL: Human Kinetics.

COMPONENTS OF AN EXERCISE PROGRAMME 3: FLEXIBILITY AND JOINT MOBILITY

9

Table 9.1 summarises the definition of joint mobility/flexibility and shows its importance to both everyday life and specific health conditions. Tables 7.1 (p. 148) and 8.1 (p. 166) present the same information for aerobic fitness and muscular strength, respectively.

THE DETERMINANTS OF JOINT MOBILITY

Joint mobility is the amount of movement available at a joint or over a range of joints. Each joint is structured to permit certain kinds of movement and prevent others. This has the overall effect of enabling effective movement whilst at the same time providing stability. For instance, the structure of the knee joint permits flexion and extension movements in one plane but largely inhibits all other movements. In contrast, joints such as the hip and shoulder permit a far greater variation of movement, including flexion and extension in various planes, abduction and adduction, rotation and circumduction.

The amount of movement permissible at a joint depends upon the shape of the bones, the joint capsule and associated ligaments and the muscles and tendons associated with the joint.

In general, each joint permits specific types of movement which are characteristic of that joint. For example, all 'normal' knee joints move in the same manner, as do all hips. However, some individuals have more mobility at a particular joint or joints than others.

This is because the exact structure of the joints varies between different individuals.

When attempting to develop an individual's mobility it is appropriate to try to alter some of the factors associated with the joint but inadvisable to affect others. For instance, the shapes of the bones at the joint, and structures such as the ligaments and the joint capsule, which play an important role in joint stability, should not be altered through exercise. The ligaments are structured to permit movement in the 'desired' plane(s) of motion but to restrict movement in undesired plane(s). In the knee the lateral, medial and cruciate ligaments permit flexion and extension of the knee but restrict excessive twisting or sideways (abduction and adduction) movements. If ligaments are overstretched, as occurs in a sprain, the joint loses stability, making it less effective and more vulnerable to further damage. The structures that flexibility and mobility exercises seek to stretch are the muscles, particularly the connective tissues within them (Figure 9.1) and, to some extent, the tendons. Muscles and tendons that are 'short' or 'tight' will restrict movement at a joint. By lengthening them and reducing their 'tightness', mobility (or the potential for movement) will be increased. Appropriate mobility or 'loosening' exercises also promote the production of synovial fluid, thereby helping to lubricate the joint, and some stretching exercises help to strengthen the muscles associated with the joint. Finally, a programme of

Table 9.1 Summary of joint mobility/flexibility

What is joint mobility/flexibility?	Why is joint mobility/flexibility important for health?	Why is joint mobility/flexibility important for active living?	How can joint mobility/flexibility be improved by a structured exercise programme?	How can joint mobility/flexibility be improved through everyday living?
Joint mobility/flexibility is the range of movement possible at a joint or over a series of joints	Poor joint mobility/flexibility may be related to back pain and other types of musculoskeletal problems. Stretching before and after strenuous exercise may reduce the risk of injury and muscular stiffness. Rehabilitation programmes for a range of musculoskeletal injuries often include stretching exercises	Poor joint mobility/flexibility reduces the ability of the individual to perform basic tasks around the home; for example, reaching a high shelf may become a problem and decorating may become difficult. Very poor levels of joint mobility/flexibility may hinder personal hygiene and grooming – for example, combing the back of the head and washing	Stretching exercises are often built into the warm-up and cool-down phases of an exercise class. Flexibility can also be gained through participation in yoga and t'ai chi classes. The key is to find a programme that incorporates exercises that take the joints through a full range of movement and which the individual enjoys and will stick to	Stretching can be done whilst watching television, making a cup of tea or before and after gardening. Long-distance drivers may also find it helpful to stretch when they stop at motorway services and at the end of their journey. Children should be encouraged to stretch at the start and end of every PE lesson

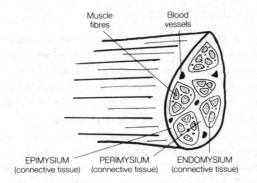

Figure 9.1 The connective tissue within a muscle

stretching exercises may also be a means of relaxation – stretching exercises are often used as a means of combating 'stress'.

In a therapeutic setting, mobility exercises are likely to be used in conjunction with other forms of therapy such as joint manipulation and 'accessory glides', which are commonly used by physiotherapists.

THE JOINTS OF THE BODY

Central to the topic of flexibility and mobility exercises are the joints of the body. It is therefore essential for the health professional who is seeking to maintain or develop an individual's flexibility to have a good understanding of joints and their structure. Such an understanding will provide greater insight into the objectives of the exercises listed and the limitations that are placed upon individuals by their basic anatomy and physiology. It should also enhance the health professional's ability to devise effective and safe stretching programmes.

The human body contains over 200 joints or articulations. Joints may be classified by the amount of movement they permit as:

● synarthrodial (no movement);
● amphiarthrodial (slight movement); or
● diarthrodial (freely moveable).

Alternatively, they may be classified by structure as:

● fibrous: suture, syndesmosis, gomphosis;
● cartilaginous: synchondrosis, symphysis; or
● synovial: ball and socket, hinge, gliding, condyloid or ellipsoidal, saddle, or pivot.

Fibrous and cartilaginous joints may be synarthrodial or amphiarthrodial; synovial joints are diarthrodial. The following sections on joint structures and actions will use both forms of classification, depending upon which is most appropriate.

SYNARTHRODIAL JOINTS

These joints permit no movement. Examples include the fibrous sutures of the skull and the cartilaginous epiphyseal plates. The sutures of the skull are formed by bones which have irregular jagged edges that fit together and are held firmly in place by fibrous tissue. The synchondroses are cartilaginous joints, which include the epiphyseal plates and the connection between the first rib and sternum. An epiphyseal plate is an area of hyaline cartilage which is found between the epiphysis and diaphysis of a growing bone. It is only present in those who have not reached full physical maturity. Like other synarthrodial joints, a synchondrosis permits no movement in normal circumstances; however, a severe blow may damage it and cause the cartilage to move. This can result in growth deformities unless corrected. During the normal course of growth and development the hyaline cartilage of an epiphyseal plate is replaced by bone, and this replacement is complete when growth ceases.

AMPHIARTHRODIAL JOINTS

These joints permit a very limited amount of movement between the bones. Amphiarthrodial joints may be fibrous or cartilaginous. Examples of fibrous amphiarthodial joints, where the bones are connected to each other via fibrous tissue, are the mid and interior tibiofibular joints and the articulations between the shafts of the radius and ulna. These fibrous joints are classified by structure as syndesmoses. In cartilaginous amphiarthrodial joints the bones are separated by a disc of fibrocartilage. This type of joint includes the symphysis pubis and the joints of the vertebral column.

DIARTHRODIAL JOINTS

These joints permit movement in certain directions, the exact extent and direction of movement depending upon the shape of the bones and other factors such as the joint capsule, ligaments and muscles associated with the joint. Synovial joints are diarthrodial and will be discussed in some depth later in this section.

FIBROUS JOINTS

Fibrous joints permit little or no movement and, as the name would imply, the bones are held together by fibrous tissue with no joint capsule. Fibrous joints may be subclassified as sutures, syndesmoses or gomphoses. A suture is a synarthrodial joint in which the ends of the bones are held firmly together by fibrous connective tissue, examples are the sutures of the skull. Gomphoses are also synarthrodial, having a 'peg and socket' structure. Examples include the articulations between the teeth and jaw bones (maxilla and mandible). Syndesmoses are fibrous joints which permit a small amount of movement; they are therefore functionally classified as amphiarthrodial. Like the bones in a synarthrodial fibrous joint (sutures) the bones in a syndesmosis are connected by fibrous tissue but are not held together quite as tightly, which permits a small amount of movement. Examples of syndesmoses include the articulations between the radius and ulna and between the tibia and fibula.

CARTILAGINOUS JOINTS

In a cartilaginous joint the bones are held together by cartilage. Cartilaginous joints that permit no movement (synarthrodial) are classified structurally as synchondroses whilst those that permit a small amount of movement (amphiarthrodial) are classified structurally as symphyses. Synchondroses include the epiphyseal plate and the articulation between the first rib and sternum; symphyses include the joints between the vertebrae. These were discussed under the headings of synarthrodial joints and amphiarthrodial joints, respectively.

SYNOVIAL JOINTS

The joints which most concern the exercise adviser in the development of movement are the diarthrodial joints of the body and the amphiarthrodial joints of the vertebral column. Diarthrodial (freely movable) joints are structurally classified as synovial joints because of the presence of synovial fluid within a joint capsule. The generalised structure of a synovial joint is illustrated in Figure 9.2. The following characteristics are common to all synovial joints:

- there is a space between the articulating bones called the *synovial cavity*;
- a *synovial membrane* lines the joint cavity and secretes the *synovial fluid* into it;
- the synovial fluid within the cavity lubricates the joint;
- a *joint capsule* surrounds and encloses the joint;
- smooth, hard-wearing *articular cartilage* covers the articulating ends of the bones (this is usually hyaline cartilage but in a few cases is made of fibrocartilage).

Also associated with synovial joints are ligaments, which provide the joint with additional strengthen and stability. Ligaments permit movement in certain directions but restrict movements that would damage the

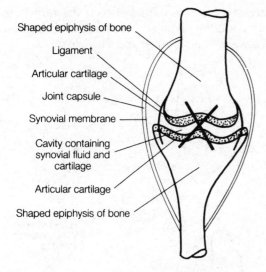

Shaped epiphysis of bone
Ligament
Articular cartilage
Joint capsule
Synovial membrane
Cavity containing synovial fluid and cartilage
Articular cartilage
Shaped epiphysis of bone

Figure 9.2 A generalised synovial joint

joint or make it unstable. Other structures associated with synovial joints are the *bursae*: fluid-filled sacs between the moving structures and the joint itself which prevent excessive friction and damage to tissues around the joint. The bursae prevent a muscle or tendon from being damaged and worn as it continually rubs past the joint. Synovial joints may also contain discs of fibrocartilage. These discs are known as *menisci* and provide the

joint with additional stability – as in the case of the lateral and medial menisci of the knee.

There is a great deal of variation in the precise structure of the synovial joints of the body. They are therefore subclassified according to their structure and the amount of movement they permit as:

- ball and socket;
- hinge;
- gliding;
- condyloid or ellipsoidal;
- saddle;
- pivot.

In some cases other slight movements may also be possible. For instance, although the knee and elbow are primarily considered as hinge joints, a slight amount of rotation is possible. Therefore these categorisations are to some extent generalisations.

Ball and socket joints

The ball-shaped end of one bone fits into a socket formed by the other bone(s) of the joint (Figure 9.3). This kind of joint permits an extensive amount of movement in many planes including flexion, extension, abduction, adduction, rotation and circumduction. The hip and shoulder are ball and socket joints.

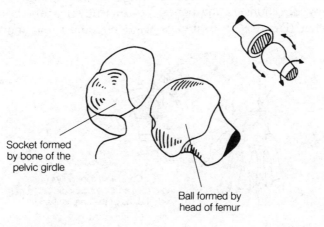

Socket formed by bone of the pelvic girdle

Ball formed by head of femur

Figure 9.3 A ball and socket joint

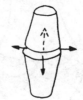
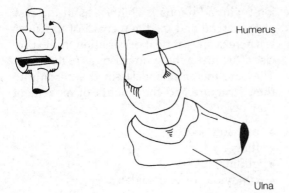

Figure 9.4   A hinge joint

Hinge joints

This name can be slightly misleading as the joint does not have a pin extending through it (as in the case of a true hinge). However, like a hinge these joints primarily permit movement in just one plane. The structure of a hinge joint involves the convex surface of one bone fitting into the concave surface of another (Figure 9.4). Hinge joints include the knee joint, elbow joint and the first and second joints of the phalanges which permit the flexion and extension movements of the fingers and toes.

Gliding joints

Gliding joints permit a limited amount of movement in many directions as the bones slide past each other (Figure 9.5). Examples

are seen in the joints between the tarsals of the foot, the carpals of the hand and the joint between the sternum and clavicle.

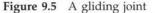

Figure 9.5   A gliding joint

Condyloid or ellipsoidal joints

In a condyloid or ellipsoidal joint an oval or ellipsoid-shaped head (condyle) of one bone fits into a shallow elliptical cavity of another (Figure 9.6). The structure of the joint enables extension/flexion, abduction/adduction and circumduction movements. Such joints

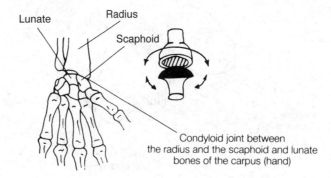

Figure 9.6   A condyloid or ellipsoidal joint

include the wrist and the metacarpal/phalangeal joints (between the fingers and the metacarpals of the hand).

Saddle joints

The carpometacarpal joint of the thumb provides the one human example of a saddle joint. The bones are shaped like a saddle so that they are convex in one direction and concave in another (Figure 9.7). This shape permits a considerable range of movement – including flexion, extension, abduction, adduction and circumduction.

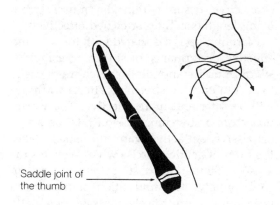

Figure 9.7   The structure of a saddle joint

Pivot joints

A pivot joint consists of a hole (fossa) in one bone into which fits the bony process of another (Figure 9.8). Pivot joints enable rotations. An example is the joint between the ulna and radius, where the rounded head of the radius rotates within a concave notch of the ulna, enabling rotation of the forearm.

SESAMOID BONES

The exact functions of some sesamoid bones remains unclear; they may serve a number of specific functions with respect to movement. In general, sesamoid bones are found within the tendons of some muscles where they alter

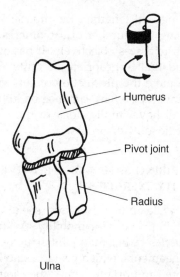

Figure 9.8   A pivot joint

the angle of pull of the muscles and make the action of the muscle more efficient. The patella (knee cap), which is situated within the patellar tendon, is a sesamoid bone. The positioning of the patella also provides the knee joint with a degree of physical protection from trauma.

THE EFFECTS OF MOBILITY EXERCISES

The aim of mobility exercises is to increase or maintain the range of movement at a joint or over a range of joints without losing any of the joint's stability. In a carefully designed programme the musculature around a joint can also be strengthened with appropriate exercises. This will provide the joint with a greater degree of stability and an increased capacity for movement. Joint flexibility should not be developed at the expense of overstretching the ligaments and therefore flexibility exercises should concentrate on increasing the length of the *muscles*. This is primarily achieved through lengthening the connective tissue that extends throughout the muscles and forms the attachments to the bones. It is suggested by some authorities that stretching will lengthen the muscle fibres by increasing the number of sarcomeres. This is difficult to assess objectively. It has also been reported that appropriate mobility exercises can promote the production of synovial fluid at a joint and thereby enhance its lubrication. This will have implications in the treatment of specific joint disorders.

PRESCRIBING SAFE AND EFFECTIVE MOBILITY EXERCISES

Mobility/flexibility exercises seek to retain and/or improve joint mobility by stretching the muscles rather than joint structures, such as the ligaments, which provide stability. It is therefore important that the joints are stretched correctly by employing the correct technique and ensuring that the joints are stretched only when they are in the correct alignment. To be effective, stretching exercises need to be of the correct type, which usually means gentle loosening exercises and prolonged static stretching rather than vigorous ballistic stretching movements.

Loosening exercises involve slow, controlled movements that mobilise a joint and enhance its range of movement. Provided that all loosening exercises are performed at a slow, controlled speed they will not overstretch or damage the joint.

Static stretching exercises produce an effective lengthening of the connective tissue by holding the muscle in a stretched position for a prolonged period. This inhibits the muscle's stretch reflex, causing the muscle fibres to relax and lengthen further, producing a greater amount of stretch on the surrounding connective tissues. However, not all static stretches are necessarily safe, and those which are incorrectly performed will convey a risk of injury. Incorrect alignment of the joint when it is being stretched can result in overstretching of the ligaments; correct alignment will allow a safe and effective static stretch. Details of the precautions needed are given with each of the exercises presented in this chapter.

In general, vigorous ballistic stretching should be avoided because it conveys a greater risk of injury than static stretching. This is due to the dynamic nature of the exercises, during which the momentum of the movement can force the joint beyond its safe limits and can damage the ligaments, tendons and muscles associated with the joint. Ballistic stretching is also less effective than static stretching; again, due to the ballistic nature of the movement, which initiates the muscle's 'stretch reflex'. The overall effect of the stretch reflex is to cause the muscle fibres to contract, and tense the muscle. This prevents the connective tissue within the muscle from being lengthened and stretched effectively.

Warming up is associated with the safe and effective performance of stretching exercises. Warm muscles and joints stretch more easily than cold ones, so stretching after a warm-up will be safer and more effective. The warm-up before a stretching session may be active or passive. An active warm-up usually takes the form of gentle exercise which elevates the muscle temperature, a passive warm-up could involve the application of heat via a heat lamp, warm towels, massage or a bath. In some cases an active warm-up will be preferable as it can be more effective in raising the temperature of deep muscles. In practice both are useful and the choice of warm-up is likely to depend upon the condition of the participant.

INTRODUCTION TO FLEXIBILITY EXERCISES

As with most forms of movement, different vocabularies may be used by different authorities. In this chapter flexibility exercises will be considered under four headings:

1. Loosening exercises
2. Ballistic stretching
3. Static stretching
4. Proprioceptive neuromuscular facilitation (PNF).

The static stretching, PNF and loosening exercises are all advocated by this text. Concerns regarding the use of ballistic stretching are discussed on pp. 214 and 231.

Joint mobility/flexibility exercises may be undertaken either as a separate session or may be incorporated into a more diverse session designed to develop a number of aspects of physical capacity. Such sessions will therefore involve other activities, together with the flexibility exercises that are often included as part of the warm-up phase of an exercise session. Inclusion of joint mobility/flexibility exercises in a warm-up is strongly recommended because they will develop flexibility and are likely to enhance the effectiveness of the session and reduce any risk of injury (which may occur if the muscles are unprepared for strenuous activity). During the initial stages of a warm-up, gentle loosening exercises are strongly recommended to mobilise the joints and prepare the body for activity. At this time gentle static stretches are also effective, provided that the stretches *are* gentle and not forced. Once the muscles have warmed up a greater degree of stretch may be applied by repeating the static stretches in a more concerted manner.

Sessions that include flexibility work may have the following format:

1. Flexibility specific session:
   - possible passive warm-up (if an active warm-up is not to be included later);
   - gentle loosening exercises;
   - gentle static stretching;
   - active warm up to elevate muscle temperature (if this is being used rather than a passive warm-up);
   - intensive stretching exercises: this forms the major content of the session;
   - gentle loosening exercises to cool down.
2. Flexibility as an element within another session:
   - gentle loosening exercises;
   - gentle static stretching;
   - active warm-up to elevate muscle

temperature and prepare the body for the activity;
- further loosening and static stretching;
- major content of the session, which may be aerobic, strength or activity based (or a combination), and during which additional flexibility exercises may be incorporated to provide a recovery from the strenuous elements of the session as well as being of value in their own right;
- cool-down, which should include flexibility exercises.

GENERAL CONSIDERATIONS FOR STRETCHING EXERCISES AND STRETCHING ROUTINES

It is important that the joints involved are moved through their 'normal' range of movement and not forced out of their natural alignment. Moving a joint into an 'unnatural' position can overstretch the ligaments of the joint, making it less stable. Comments relating to joint position are given with the details of each exercise

The loosening and stretching exercises presented in this chapter represent a comprehensive selection which may be used to stretch most of the major muscle groups of the body and hence develop the mobility of most of the major joints of the body. The number of exercises used in a session, the duration for which the static stretches are held and the number of repetitions of each exercise will depend upon the client's circumstances. Factors such as the amount of time available and the condition of the participant will have a major influence in dictating the design of the session.

Therapists and exercise advisers may select any number of stretches from those presented in this chapter, according to the aims of their session. They may choose to follow a general routine that includes all the main joints or focus upon a specific problem area. The practised and experienced exercise adviser/therapist will be able to modify certain stretches according to individual needs, and thus develop an extensive repertoire of stretching/ joint mobility exercises. There are a number of exercises that may be used to stretch the muscles associated with any particular joint and the choice of variation to use must be left to professional judgement because people vary in their anatomical make-up – some individuals may find one particular exercise very effective whilst another may prefer a variation of that exercise. Therefore, the overall stretching routine will be developed through the experience and knowledge of the exercise adviser/therapist in conjunction with the participant's own perception of the ease and effectiveness of the exercises.

It is usual to produce a list or chart of the exercises which may be ticked off as each one is completed. In this way no stretch is likely to be forgotten. Progression should also be included in the exercise programme; recording the time for which each stretch should be held, together with the type and number of stretches included in each session, will help to demonstrate progression. It will also aid the exercise adviser/therapist in ensuring that progression is steady and logical rather than random. Regular monitoring at intervals of 4–6 weeks also provides positive feedback for both the participant and assessor, informing them of the effectiveness of the exercises.

As with all forms of exercise, flexibility work needs to be frequent. Ideally a stretching/ loosening routine should be repeated daily, with particular conditions necessitating several sessions a day. Therefore the participant should be encouraged to incorporate the exercises into a regular routine, even if they are unable to attend their gym frequently or if their therapist is unable to see them so often.

LOOSENING EXERCISES

Loosening exercises should be conducted in a slow and controlled manner. The emphasis is on a slow, gentle stretch without forcing the joint. Each exercise should be performed about six times on each limb and, where appropriate, should be repeated in both directions (i.e. clockwise and anticlockwise). The specific factors to be considered with each exercise will be presented with details of the exercises.

Loosening exercises are an important aspect of flexibility work. They often involve slow, controlled circumduction movements at joints such as the ankle, hip, wrist and shoulder. They may be active/non-assisted or passive/assisted. In assisted loosening exercises the assistance comes from either the participant or their instructor. For example, a greater range of movement may be produced at the ankle joint if the movement is assisted with the hands. Loosening exercises may be used as part of a warming-up process before static stretching or some other form of activity.

Other loosening exercises involve gentle swinging actions of the arms or legs. These are similar to the ballistic actions condemned in the previous section; however, these exercises are to be performed well within a participant's normal range of motion for that joint and participants should not attempt to increase their range of motion by swinging close to the range they are able to attain when performing static flexibility exercises. It should also be emphasised that these loosening exercises should be performed in a controlled, *gentle*, manner and should not be fast or vigorous. They should be performed as a 'loosening' activity within a session rather than as a specific attempt to develop a permanent increase in mobility at a specific joint.

EXAMPLES OF LOOSENING EXERCISES

Ankle circling

The participant sits on the floor and slowly circles one foot in a clockwise direction. The movement should be slow and the emphasis should be upon trying to make the circle as large as possible (Figure 9.9). The movement

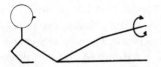

Figure 9.9

should be repeated in an anticlockwise direction before performing the exercise on the other ankle. This exercise may be active or passive and may be assisted by the participant or therapist using their hands. The movement should be repeated 6–12 times in each direction for each ankle.

Wrist circumduction

This exercise for the wrists is equivalent to that previously described for the ankles. Whilst keeping the forearm relatively still the wrist should be slowly circumducted in a clockwise direction, trying to describe as large a circle as possible (Figure 9.10). The movement should be performed 6–12 times in both directions for both wrists. Again the exercise may be active or passive and assisted depending upon the requirements of the participant.

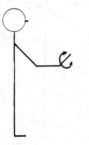

Figure 9.10

Shoulder circumduction

The participant stands or sits in a position which will not impede their arm movements. In this exercise both shoulders may be exercised at the same time with one arm mirroring the movements of the other. The movement

Figure 9.11

is a circumduction of the shoulders, during which the arms describe as large a circle as possible (Figure 9.11). During the movement the arms should be brought in front of the body so that they cross, and the movement should be repeated 6–12 times in both directions for both shoulders.

Hip circumductions

For this exercise the participant should hold on to a support for balance. He or she stands on one leg and flexes the hip and knee of the other leg, raising the knee until it is approximately at the same height as the hip (Figure 9.12). The circumduction movement moves the knee towards the midline of the body and then away in a circular movement. During this movement the amount of flexion of the knee will vary. The movement should be repeated 6–12 times in each direction for each hip.

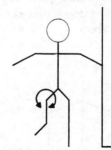

Figure 9.12

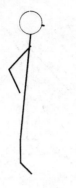

Figure 9.13

Heel raises

The participant stands with their feet approximately shoulder width apart then raises both heels off of the ground, putting the weight over the balls of the feet (Figure 9.13). The heels are then slowly lowered back down to the ground and the movement repeated. The exercise may be repeated 10–20 times – or more if it is being used as a loosening exercise before some other activity such as jogging.

Shoulder shrugs (shoulder elevation and depression)

In this exercise the participant starts with their shoulders in a comfortable and relaxed position. They then elevate their shoulders as high as possible (keeping their arms in a relaxed position by their sides), hold the position for about 5 seconds and then lower the shoulders (shoulder depression) as far as they can go, once again holding the position for about 5 seconds (Figure 9.14). The exercise may be repeated about six times. A similar

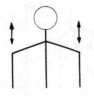

Figure 9.14

exercise could involve a more continuous movement of the shoulders without holding the end positions, or even clockwise and anti-clockwise rotations of the shoulder joints (in the sagittal plane) with the arms kept by the sides.

Arm swings (together and in opposite directions)

This exercise is similar to the shoulder circum-duction exercise. However, in this exercise the arms are primarily moved in the sagittal plane in a circular motion (if the participant is viewed from the side; Figure 9.15). Initially this exercise may be performed using one arm at a time, with the movement being repeated in both clockwise and anticlockwise directions 6–12 times. The exercise may also be performed with both arms working together in the same direction (mirroring each other's movements) or with the arms moving in opposite directions; this last variation will require a greater degree of co-ordination.

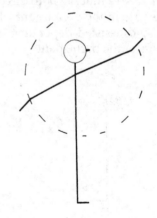

Figure 9.15

Leg swings

This is a dynamic exercise: therefore the swings should be gentle and performed well within the participant's normal range of static flexibility. Also, it should be performed only after appropriate static hamstring flexibility

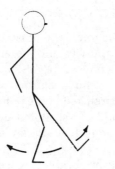

Figure 9.16

exercises have been used to stretch out the muscles. The participant stands on one leg using a support for balance. The other leg is then gently swung backwards and forwards in a relaxed manner, keeping the extent of the movement well within the participant's range of static flexibility in both directions (Figure 9.16). During the swinging movement the knee may be naturally flexed. The movement may be repeated 6–12 times for each leg.

Spinal and hip rotation

The participant stands with their feet approximately shoulder width apart and rotates their upper body in a circular motion (in the transverse plane) (Figure 9.17). The extent of the

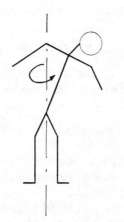

Figure 9.17

movement may be enhanced by using the hips in a similar rotatory action. The movement should be performed slowly and repeated 6–12 times in both clockwise and anticlockwise directions.

STATIC STRETCHING

In all examples of static stretching the stretched position should be reached in a slow and controlled manner, without jerking or bouncing. The stretched position should be held for a minimum of 6–15 seconds, after which the stretch should be gently extended and held for a further 6–15 seconds. If desired, this process may be repeated two or three times more for each exercise before returning to the starting position. Each stretching exercise should be repeated the prescribed number of times. During the initial exercise sessions the static stretches should be held for a minimum of 6–10 seconds, but as the participant becomes more familiar with the exercises the stretches can be held for longer, up to a minute for each stretch.

Some muscles extend over more than one joint and to achieve an effective stretch on these muscles the position of both joints must be considered. Examples of such muscles include the gastrocnemius and the hamstring group. If the stretches are being used as part of a warm-up before some other activity time may dictate that each static stretch will be held for only 6 seconds and repeated just once or twice. If, however, the stretches are being used to specifically develop or maintain joint movements than a more extensive stretching routine should be undertaken, with each static stretch being held for longer and repeated several times. Throughout such a session the participant should keep warm, and therefore, in addition to the participant wearing warm clothing, the exercises may be interspersed with other activities.

Static stretching exercises may be considered under three sub-headings: active or non-assisted stretching; passive or assisted stretching; and proprioceptive neuromuscular facilitation (PNF).

ACTIVE OR NON-ASSISTED STRETCHING

In active or non-assisted stretching the stretch on a relaxed muscle is achieved through active contraction of the participant's own muscles (with the stretched muscle being antagonistic to those contracting and therefore, by definition, being relaxed and lengthened during the stretch). Active stretching can also help to develop the strength of the muscles that are contracting to place their antagonists in their stretched position.

PASSIVE OR ASSISTED STRETCHING

In this form of stretching the stretch on a muscle is achieved with the assistance of some external force or object. The therapist or exercise adviser may apply a gentle force which stretches a muscle further than the participant could achieve on their own, or a stationary object, such as a wall, may be used to increase the amount of stretch; another way of increasing the stretch is for the participant to assist the stretch, for example by using their arms to pull their legs further into, and hold them in, a stretch that they would be unable to do unaided. It is usually possible to achieve a greater degree of stretch with passive/assisted stretching than with active/non-assisted stretching.

PNF

PNF is a more advanced form of stretching which can be used to develop muscular strength as well as flexibility. It works on the basis that a muscle can be stretched further if it first undergoes a maximal static contraction. PNF may be active or passive; the difference between the two will be discussed, together with the exercises, later in this section.

THE PHYSIOLOGY OF STATIC STRETCHING

Static stretching is a most effective way of stretching muscles and, because it is static, it does not convey the risks associated with ballistic stretching. During a static stretch a muscle is stretched to the point where the participant can feel the stretch, and perhaps even slight discomfort, but the stretch should not be so great as to cause pain. The muscle spindles (a type of proprioceptor) will detect the stretch and send signals to the central nervous system via sensory neurones. Impulses are sent back to the muscle from the central nervous system, causing some of the muscle fibres to contract. This causes a certain amount of tension to develop within the muscle, preventing it from being stretched further. However, if the stretch is held for at least 6 seconds the Golgi organs (other proprioceptors situated at the muscle–tendon junction) send signals to the central nervous system that inhibit this stretch reflex. After about 6–10 seconds the tension in the muscle is reduced and the muscle may be stretched a little further without pain or risk of damage. This cycle may be repeated several times to produce an effective stretch on the muscle. The primary effect is to stretch the connective tissue within the muscle. In this way the connective tissue between the muscle fibres, and in some cases the tendons, are effectively stretched, thereby increasing the range of movement permissible at the joint.

PRACTICAL STATIC STRETCHING

For effective static stretching the following sequence of events and considerations should be followed.

1. The muscles should be warmed up and relaxed.
2. The muscles should be moved *slowly* to the point of stretch (to minimise the stretch reflex).
3. The stretch should be held for at least 15 seconds (for effective stretching and to inhibit the stretch reflex).

4. The stretch should then be slowly increased.
5. Steps 3 and 4 should be repeated a number of times before allowing the limb back to its resting state.
6. The participant should try to keep the stretched muscles as relaxed as possible throughout the exercise.
7. The therapist or exercise adviser should talk to the participant throughout the exercise to try to ensure that he or she remains relaxed and does not tense up the muscles.
8. The stretch must not be forced. It is therefore important for the participant to inform the person assisting them of the amount of stretch being experienced.
9. When applying a force to assist the stretch care must be taken not to overstretch the muscles.

A key aspect of static stretching is the holding of the end position which enables the initial stretch reflex to be inhibited. The stretch reflex is also one of the reasons why vigorous ballistic stretching is not recommended as a means of developing joint mobility.

When undertaking any of the exercises in this section remember that the stretched position should be reached slowly and then held. These exercises are a combination of active and passive exercises, many of which can be modified into an assisted form if necessary. With assisted stretches good communication is required between the participant and the person they are working with to ensure that the correct amount of stretch is achieved. Also, while certain exercises are reported to stretch the same muscle groups, the participant may find some exercises more effective than others and different stretches to be effective in different regions of the same muscle group. For instance, a number of stretches are designed to stretch the muscles of the hamstring group but the participant may find that one causes more stretch at the distal end of the muscle group (near the knee) whilst another more effectively stretches the proximal end (near

the hip joint). The effectiveness and region of stretch will vary between individuals.

EXAMPLES OF STATIC STRETCHING EXERCISES

Achilles and soleus stretch

The participant stands with one foot approximately one metre behind the other; they then flex the knee of their back leg whilst keeping the foot flat on the floor (this exercise will stretch the Achilles tendon and the soleus muscle of the back leg). During the exercise the knee of the front leg will also have to be flexed slightly and a support such as a wall or table may be used for balance (Figure 9.18). Hold the stretch for the desired duration and repeat on both legs.

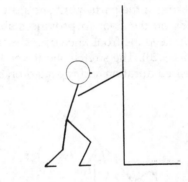

Figure 9.18

Gastrocnemius stretch

The participant stands approximately one metre away from a support such as a wall, places their hands on the wall for support then takes a step back with one foot. They place the sole of their back foot flat on the floor and keep the knee of their back leg fully extended. To achieve this the knee of the front leg will need to be flexed slightly (Figure 9.19). They should feel stretch in the gastrocnemius: if not they should move further away from the wall and/or tilt their hips forwards towards the wall. The stretch should be held for the desired duration and repeated on both legs.

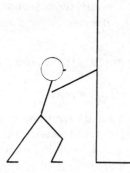

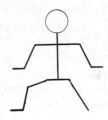

Figure 9.21

Figure 9.19

Hip flexor stretch

The participant kneels on one knee, then moves their hips forwards slowly until stretch is felt in the hip flexors of the back leg. When doing the stretch the participant should place their hands on the floor to provide stability and should keep the front knee over the front foot (Figure 9.20). The stretch should be held for the desired duration and repeated on both legs.

Figure 9.20

Adductor stretch 1

The participant stands with their feet apart, approximately half a metre wider than shoulder width. They then rotate one leg outwardly so that one foot faces forwards whilst the rotated foot faces to the side. The forward-facing foot should be kept flat on the ground and the corresponding knee extended. They then flex the knee of the sideways facing foot and gently lower their body until stretch is felt in the adductor muscles of the extended leg (Figure 9.21). When flexing the knee and low-

ering the body it may be necessary to move the feet further apart for comfort, and further adjustments to foot positioning may be needed to attain the ideal position, with the flexed knee being positioned directly above the outwardly rotated foot. The stretch should be held for the desired duration and repeated on both legs.

Adductor stretch 2

This is performed in a seated position. The participant sits as illustrated with the soles of their feet touching and their elbows resting gently on their thighs (Figure 9.22). This may produce an initial stretch, which can be enhanced by the participant pushing down on their thighs with their elbows.

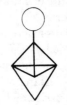

Figure 9.22

Hamstring stretch 1

This is most likely to be performed as an assisted stretch. The participant should lie on his or her back and flex one hip, raising their leg and keeping the knee extended. Alternatively, the leg could be raised by their

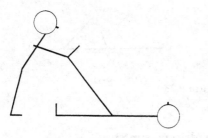

Figure 9.23

adviser or partner (Figure 9.23). The leg should be eased forward by further flexion of the hip until the point of resistance or slight discomfort is reached. Stretch should be felt in the hamstrings and the position should be held for the desired duration before lowering the limb. When performing this stretch with a partner good communication is required to ensure that the correct amount of stretch is applied. The participant may be able to perform this stretch alone by looping a short piece of rope or clothing around the foot and pulling it to achieve the stretch. An advancement of this stretch is described in the section on PNF (p. 230).

Hamstring stretch 2

The participant places one foot on an elevated object approximately 0.5 m high (a chair will usually suffice). Keeping the knee of the elevated leg extended, he or she places their hands on the thigh of the elevated leg (Figure 9.24). They then flex forwards from the hips, trying to keep their back straight, and slide their hands down towards the ankles of the

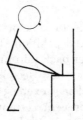

Figure 9.24

elevated leg, without curving their back too much. If the stretch is felt directly behind the knee rather than in the main body of the muscles the stretch should be repeated with a slightly flexed knee, which should produce the desired stretch.

Hamstring stretch 3

This is a variation of hamstring stretch 2 and is performed from a kneeling position on the floor. The participant kneels on one knee and extends the other leg in front of them then places their hands on the thigh of the extended leg (Figure 9.25). From this position they flex at the hips and slowly slide their hands down the extended leg towards their foot. In performing this stretch the participant should attempt to keep their back straight in order to ensure that the stretch occurs in the hamstrings and does not stress the back.

Figure 9.25

Hamstring stretch 4

This is a variation of Stretch 2 and is performed in a seated position on the floor (Figure 9.26). When performing this stretch both legs may be extended, or one may be flexed with the foot positioned next to the knee of the extended leg. As with the other variations, the emphasis is on stretching the hamstrings without putting

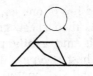

Figure 9.26

stress on the back. This may be ensured by keeping the back relatively straight and bending from the hips.

Hamstring stretch 5

A pile of books or mats is placed on the floor. The participant stands behind the stack and then bends down to place their hands flat on the top. To do this the knees must be flexed (Figure 9.27). Whilst keeping their hands flat on the pile the participant tries to stand up by slowly extending their knees. This should produce a gentle stretch in the hamstrings. If the participant can fully extend their knees whilst keeping their hands on the mats or books, he or she should try the exercise with a smaller pile or even with their hands flat on the floor. Although similar to the more traditional 'stand and touch the toes' exercise, this stretch is preferable because the muscles are being stretched by the action of other muscle groups rather than by gravity. The 'touching the toes' exercise is now avoided by many authorities because it can put unwanted strain on the back.

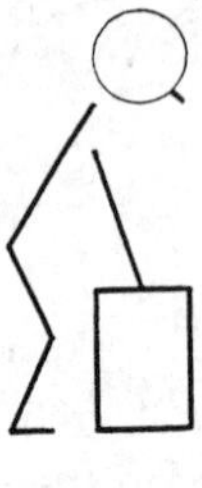

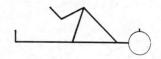

Figure 9.28

Quadriceps stretch

The participant stands on one leg whilst fully flexing the knee of the other leg. They grasp the ankle of the flexed leg and hold it close to the buttock, ensuring that the knee is in the correct alignment and is not twisted or rotated (Figure 9.29). To apply additional stretch the participant should extend the hip joint whilst continuing to hold onto the ankle. To do this it will be necessary to lean forward slightly in order to maintain balance. This should produce a stretch in the quadriceps muscle. Since the quadriceps extends over two joints the hip must be extended and the knee flexed in order to achieve an effective stretch over the whole muscle group.

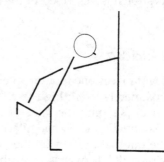

Figure 9.29

Figure 9.27

Hamstring stretch 6

The participant lies on their back with their head resting gently on the floor. They then flex the knee and hip of one leg, bringing the knee up towards their chest, grasp the knee with both hands and gently pull the knee towards their chest, keeping the other leg fully extended and flat on the floor (Figure 9.28). Stretch should be felt in the hamstrings.

Back stretch

The participant should lie on their back on the floor in a relaxed position. They then try to push their lower back into the floor and hold the position for a few seconds (Figure 9.30). This is a general back exercise which may help to reduce or prevent certain forms of back pain. It can also help to develop the strength of the back muscles and back mobility.

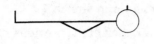

Figure 9.30

Upper back and shoulder stretch

The participant kneels on the floor as illustrated (Figure 9.31). They stretch their arms out in front of their head and place their hands on the floor. When performing this stretch the participant should not sit back on their heels but should lean forwards. The hands should be moved forwards along the ground until a stretched position is reached. Stretch should be experienced in the upper back and shoulders.

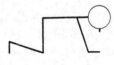

Figure 9.31

Lower back and hip stretch

The participant should lie on their back in a relaxed position. To stretch the left side the left arm should be abducted at right angles to the body with the palm touching the floor. The left knee should then be flexed at 90° and the left foot crossed over the right knee (Figure 9.32). The left leg is then grasped in the right hand and pulled across the right leg in an adduction movement, easing the left

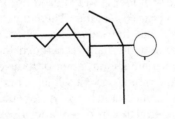

Figure 9.32

knee across until stretch is felt down the lateral side of the left hip and lower back. The stretch may be enhanced by turning the head to the left whilst performing the stretch. To stretch the right hip and right side the positions are reversed.

Abductor stretch

To stretch the left abductor muscles the participant sits on the floor and crosses their left leg over their right, placing the left foot just to the right of the right knee (Figure 9.33). The participant then turns the body to the left as far as it will go and places their right elbow on the lateral side of the left knee (the lateral side being the side which is furthest from the midline of the body when standing in the anatomical position). He or she then uses their right elbow to push the left knee further to the right until they feel a stretch in the abductor muscles down the left side of the body. As with the previous stretch, the positions must be reversed in order to stretch the muscles down the right side of the body.

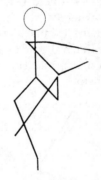

Figure 9.33

Side stretch

To stretch the left side of the body the participant abducts or flexes their left arm so that it is raised above their head, and turns the palm of the hand so that it comfortably faces inwards. They then laterally flex to the right,

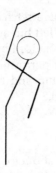

Figure 9.34

and stretch should be felt down the left side of the body (Figure 9.34). The position should be held for the desired duration and the positions reversed in order to produce the stretch on the right side of the body.

Shoulder and arm stretch 1

The participant should clasp their hands in front of their body and flex their shoulders to raise their arms above their head. The hands should remain clasped together and, if possible, the shoulders should reach a position of hyperflexion, whereby the hands are positioned behind the frontal plane of the body (Figure 9.35). Stretch should be encountered in the shoulders and arms. This stretch can be assisted by a helper.

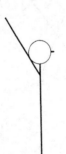

Figure 9.35

Shoulder and arm stretch 2

This is a variation of the previous stretch. The participant lies face down with their arms extended above their head. Clasping the hands together, they try to raise their hands off the floor (Figure 9.36). During the exercise the participant should attempt to raise their hands as high as possible whilst keeping their elbows extended and chin on the floor. This should produce stretch in the arms and shoulders.

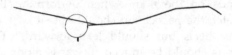

Figure 9.36

Shoulder and arm stretch 3

The participant flexes one elbow and adducts their arm across in front of their body in an attempt to touch the opposite shoulder blade (Figure 9.37). Additional stretch can be achieved by pushing up on the elbow of the stretched shoulder with the hand of the opposite arm.

Figure 9.37

Shoulder and arm stretch 4

First, the shoulder is fully flexed until the arm is in a vertical position. Then the elbow is flexed so that the lower arm extends down the back and the hand can touch the spine. The participant should attempt to reach as far down the spine as possible. This should produce some stretch in the shoulder and arm. The stretch can be enhanced by placing the hand of the opposite arm on the elbow of

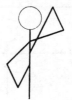

Figure 9.38

the 'stretched' arm and pushing downwards (Figure 9.38). This produces a greater amount of stretch in the arm and shoulder regions.

Shoulder and arm stretch 5

One arm is flexed at the elbow and positioned behind the back so that the back of the hand touches the opposite shoulder blade. The arm is therefore reaching up the participant's back. The participant then attempts to reach as high up their back as they can. This produces an initial amount of stretch. The hand of the opposite arm is then placed under the elbow of the stretched arm and pushed upwards, thus applying more stretch (Figure 9.39). The position should be held for the desired duration.

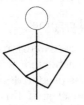

Figure 9.39

Shoulder and arm stretch 6

This is a combination of arm stretches 4 and 5. One arm performs stretch 4 so that it is reaching down the participant's back whilst the other arm performs stretch 5 and reaches up the participant's back (Figure 9.40). The participant then attempts to get their hands to touch – if they can, they should try to clasp their hands together and apply additional stretch by pulling with the appropriate arm.

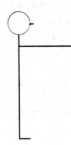

Figure 9.40

Shoulder and arm stretch 7

Both shoulders are flexed and the arms are extended in front of the body (Figure 9.41). The hands are joined by linking the fingers with the palms touching. Keeping the fingers linked, the palms are then turned outwards so that they face away from the body (in order to do this it will be necessary to flex the elbows). The hands are then pushed away from the body by extending the elbows. The arms may be raised or lowered in order to alter the stretch. This exercise produces a stretch in the arms and the shoulder region.

Figure 9.41

Shoulder, arm and chest stretch 1

The participant stands facing a wall or similar fixed object with one arm abducted so that the hand is at shoulder height and the palm touches the wall. He or she then turns away from the wall and away from the abducted arm while keeping the palm of the hand flat against the wall and the arm parallel to the wall (Figure 9.42). This will produce stretch in the shoulder of the abducted arm.

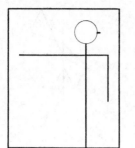

Figure 9.42

Shoulder, arm and chest stretch 2

This is a variation of the previous stretch and requires the assistance of a partner. The participant stands in the anatomical position and abducts both arms to shoulder height (Figure 9.43). From behind, the partner grasps both the participant's wrists and gently eases back the participant's arms, keeping the hands at shoulder height until an appropriate stretch is felt in the shoulders. Some individuals with very good shoulder mobility may be able to get their arms to cross behind their back; others with less shoulder mobility may only be able to get their arms just past the frontal plane.

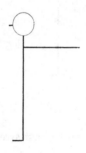

Figure 9.43

Neck lateral flexion

The neck is flexed to one side to produce stretch on the opposing side (Figure 9.44). The shoulders should be kept down and level to maximise the stretch in the neck.

Figure 9.44

Neck flexion

The participant slowly flexes their neck forwards so that their chin rests on their chest (Figure 9.45) and holds the position for a number of seconds. The neck is then slowly extended to return the head to the starting position.

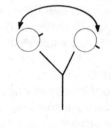

Figure 9.45

Extension of the spine

Extension or hyperextension stretching of the spine may be achieved with this exercise, which can also be used to develop the strength of the back muscles. If this exercise causes pain or excessive discomfort it should *not* be continued. The participant lies face down and places their hands behind their head or clasps them behind their back, then attempts to raise their chest from the floor by hyperextending the back (Figure 9.46). This position should be held for only a few seconds and, because of the muscle strength required, not everyone will be able to perform it.

Forward flexion of the spine

The participant sits on the floor and brings their knees up to their chest, wraps their arms

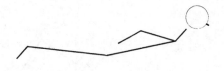

Figure 9.46

around their knees and puts their head on their knees, forming a tightly tucked position (Figure 9.47). This should be held for a number of seconds. As an advancement on the exercise the participant may then roll gently onto their back and rock forwards and backwards 6–12 times, but this should be done only on a well cushioned mat or other suitable surface. This latter variation is clearly not entirely a static stretch since movement is involved, although the spine itself is being held in a static position.

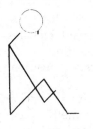

Figure 9.47

Spinal rotation

Spinal rotation is incorporated into the lower back and hip stretch and the abductor stretch

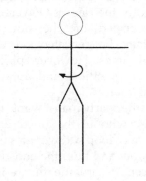

Figure 9.48

(p. 225). However, as a specific spinal rotation exercise the participant should stand with their feet about shoulder width apart and should slowly twist their upper body (rotation in the transverse plane) as far as it will go whilst keeping their feet firmly on the floor (Figure 9.48). The head should lead the rotation and greater stretch may be achieved if the arms are raised to shoulder height and are used to enhance the rotation of the spine.

General stretch

This simple stretch involves the participant lying on their back on the floor with their feet together and arms extended above their head (Figure 9.49). He or she then tries to extend their body as far as possible, making it as long as possible. This may be held for 5–10 seconds and is typical of a general stretch that someone may perform naturally first thing in the morning or after being in a constricted position for some time. It is often a useful stretch to conclude a flexibility session.

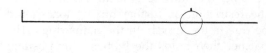

Figure 9.49

PNF

PNF is an advanced form of stretching which has the added advantage of developing the strength of some of the muscles associated with the joint being exercised. PNF works on the basis that a muscle can be stretched further if it has already undergone a maximum isometric contraction. The basis of PNF is illustrated using an example of a hamstring stretching exercise, although it can easily be applied to a number of the other static stretching exercises. PNF should be performed only after an extensive warm-up (which should elevate the muscle temperature) and a series of preliminary static stretches upon the muscles which are to be stretched using PNF. Like all forms of exercise PNF should be introduced into a programme gradually, with a systematic increase in duration, repetitions and frequency. PNF. stretching may be considered under two headings: active PNF and passive PNF.

Most PNF exercises require the assistance of a partner or assistant/therapist but in some cases the exercise may be modified to use a stretching aid, such as a rope or towel, instead. It may be unwise to use PNF stretching routines with sufferers from high blood pressure because it involves a degree of isometric muscular contraction and these individuals are generally advised to avoid isometric exercises.

ACTIVE PNF

PNF stretching for the hamstrings

The participant lies on his or her back in a relaxed position and elevates one leg as high as possible by flexing the hip joint, keeping the knee extended. At this point the restriction on further hip flexion should be due to the stretch on the hamstrings. The partner then holds the limb in this position for 10 seconds (Figure 9.50). It may be easiest for the assistant to support the limb with his or her shoulder, as this is the best position to resist the contraction of the leg that occurs during the next phase. This will almost certainly be the best position if the participant is relatively strong; although with a weaker participant the assistant may find it sufficient to resist the movement using their hands and arms. The participant then contracts the hamstrings as fully as possible, trying to push the leg down whilst the assistant holds it in position. This maximal isometric contraction is maintained for a full 10 seconds. The participant then relaxes and tries to raise the leg as high as possible (by flexing the hip joint): this should result in the leg being moved further than it was at the start of the exercise. This form of PNF is

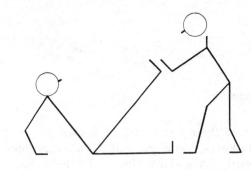

Figure 9.50

called 'active' because, at this point, it is the participant who actively moves their leg during this phase of the exercise, using the active contraction of his or her own muscles. Once the position of maximum stretch is reached, the process is repeated. An active PNF exercise may therefore include a number of cycles:

1. The participant elevates their leg to the stretched position.
2. The stretched position is held for 10 seconds.
3. The participant performs a 10-second maximal isometric contraction. The contraction is resisted by the assistant or a stretching aid.
4. The participant relaxes and then elevates the leg further to the stretched position.
5. Stages 2, 3 and 4 are repeated for the desired number of cycles.

Each cycle can be repeated three or four times before the leg is lowered and the process repeated on the other leg. The exercise may be repeated on each leg a number of times. However, progression to this level of repetitions and duration should be gradual.

Should the participant want to perform the exercise without the aid of an assistant, he or she may loop a towel or similar object over their foot and hold the ends firmly. This can be used to provide the resistive force during the contraction phase. A number of the static stretching exercises previously described can be modified to incorporate aspects of PNF.

PASSIVE PNF

Passive PNF is very similar to active PNF. However, they differ during just one phase of the process: with passive PNF it is the *assistant* who moves the limb to its point of maximum stretch rather than the participant. Passive PNF should therefore include the following stages:

1. The assistant elevates the participant's leg until an appropriate amount of stretch is felt.
2. The stretched position is held for 10 seconds.
3. The participant then performs a maximal isometric contraction for 10 seconds (as for active PNF). The contraction is resisted by the assistant or a stretching aid.
4. The participant relaxes and the assistant elevates the leg further until the participant states that an appropriate amount of stretch has been achieved.
5. Stages 2, 3 and 4 may be repeated for the desired number of cycles.

This version of PNF obviously requires good communication between the participant and the person helping them if the correct amount of stretch is to be applied. It may be more effective than active PNF but the therapist may consider active PNF preferable because it provides an opportunity for the participant to exercise other muscles (in producing the movement in active PNF). As with active PNF, the use of stretching aids such as towels make it possible for the participant to perform the exercise alone.

It should again be emphasised that PNF is a more intensive form of stretching than the simple static and loosening exercises described earlier. It should therefore be undertaken with caution and introduced gradually, paying particular attention to warm-up.

BALLISTIC STRETCHING VERSUS OTHER FORMS OF DEVELOPING JOINT MOBILITY/ FLEXIBILITY

Ballistic stretching involves a 'bouncing' action and, as such, involves a limb being moved rapidly through its full range of motion towards the full extent of the joint's permissible movement. For a number of reasons ballistic stretching is not only less effective than static stretching but also conveys a risk of injury.

1. The connective tissue within a muscle is more effectively stretched if it is held in the stretched position (as with static stretching) rather than being quickly stretched.
2. In ballistic stretching the momentum of the moving limb may force the joint beyond its normal and safe range of motion. This can overstretch and damage the muscles and associated joint structures. The slow nature of static stretching prevents the movement from exceeding the safe limits of the joint.
3. During ballistic stretching the muscle spindles, which react to both the rate and extent of a stretch, initiate a strong stretch reflex. This will cause the muscle fibres to contract and shorten. However, the momentum of the limb may force the muscle to continue to be stretched against its attempted contraction. This conflict may cause damage to the muscles or tendons.
4. During a ballistic movement the stretch reflex is likely to be initiated before the limb reaches the limits of the joint's normal range of motion. Even a gentle bouncing action may be sufficient to initiate a basic stretch reflex and cause a muscle to 'tense up'. This will prevent the connective tissue from being effectively stretched and the joint from reaching its maximum range of movement.

Therefore, in general, ballistic stretching is not advised as a means of developing joint mobility and/or increasing the length of the muscles. However, not all stretching or mobility exercises have to be static. Loosening exercises are an alternative form of stretching that may be safely used to complement static stretches. Unlike ballistic stretches which use vigorous movements, the movements used for loosening exercises are slow and controlled. In some cases it will also be performed well within the subject's range of static flexibility.

ASESSMENT OF JOINT MOBILITY AND FLEXIBILITY

Flexibility and joint mobility tests can be useful in monitoring the effectiveness of an exercise programme. Details of suggested tests are given in Chapter 6.

RECOMMENDED READING

Alter, M.J. (1996). *Science of Flexibility* (2nd ed.). Champaign, IL: Human Kinetics.

PHYSIOTHERAPY AND THE USE OF PHYSICAL ACTIVITY AND EXERCISE IN REHABILITATION

10

INTRODUCTION

For some time, sportspeople have understood the importance of following appropriate exercise programmes to both enhance performance and reduce risk of injury. This is also the case for general health, where exercise is increasingly being used to promote general physical and psychological well-being. In the words of Jerry Morris (1994), 'Physical activity may well be the country's best public health buy'. For this potential benefit to be fully realised, more well trained and qualified exercise leaders and exercise scientists are needed to work alongside health professionals.

As well as a means to promote fitness and well-being in the already 'healthy' population, exercise and physical activity are valuable rehabilitative tools, which are effective in helping those with injury, disease and disability. For example, exercise can help to promote full recovery, in the treatment of many musculoskeletal injuries (e.g. sprained ligaments). It also helps in preventing disease progression (e.g. CHD) and improves a patient's ability to cope with incurable disorders (e.g. lung disease). It is often the physiotherapist who provides the expertise to help patients achieve these outcomes. This chapter will outline how physiotherapists use exercise and physical activity as part of the rehabilitative process.

The chapter begins by explaining the role of physiotherapists within the multidisciplinary team. A broad overview of the physiotherapeutic assessment is followed by examples to show how exercise and physical activity may be applied to three categories of patient; an individual with low back pain, an injured sportsperson and a cardiac patient.

THE ROLE OF THE PHYSIOTHERAPIST

Physiotherapy is a healthcare profession which emphasises the use of physical approaches in the promotion, maintenance and restoration of an individual's physical, psychological and social well-being, encompassing variations in health status. There are 27 000 chartered physiotherapists in the UK, working as individuals or as members of health care teams. Although most work in the National Health Service, a growing number are in private practice, industry and sports clinics. All physiotherapists qualifying in recognised UK institutions are entitled to membership of the Chartered Society of Physiotherapy. This guarantees that the physiotherapist is qualified to the highest standard, governed by a code of professional conduct, covered by appropriate professional liability insurance and qualified for state registration. Once qualified, chartered physiotherapists work with people who suffer from a range of problems, in particular those associated with neuromuscular, musculoskeletal, cardiovascular and respiratory outcomes (CSP, 1997).

A physiotherapist's primary expertise is in the use of movement and exercise within the rehabilitative process, and matching these interventions to a patient's physical and psychological needs to optimise recovery. In some cases, they may use additional techniques such as electrotherapy (e.g. ultrasound), manual therapy (e.g. manipulation) and other comfort measures (e.g. cold and heat) to facilitate rehabilitation and return to normal activity.

Physiotherapists work as important members of various multidisciplinary teams. Their role within the team varies according to the needs of the patient and the other professionals involved. The physiotherapist may act as an equal team member with the general practitioner (GP) or, when dealing with an injured sports performer, the team may include a surgeon, coach, psychologist and sport scientist, all concerned with returning the sportsperson to the field. Management of the cardiac patient may include the cardiac nurse, exercise physiologist, psychologist, dietitian, cardiologist and various health and exercise specialists. In each case, the physiotherapist brings expertise in analysing abnormalities of movement and limitations in function, with the aim of negotiating appropriate rehabilitative programmes to achieve realistic goals. The physiotherapist's main aim is to help the patient achieve as much functional recovery as possible within the limits of their condition and motivational status. The ability to walk about the house independently is as important for some as it is for a sportsperson to return to full competition.

Another important role of physiotherapy is in the prevention of injury and disease, which is largely achieved through education. In the sporting environment, injury may be prevented through coach and player education about fitness conditioning, warming up, cooling down and first-aid procedures. Physiotherapists are increasingly working with exercise leaders, exercise scientists and psychologists on GP referral schemes aimed at rehabilitation and disease prevention, to promote health in society.

PHYSIOTHERAPY ASSESSMENT

Patients are usually referred to the physiotherapist by a medical practitioner, but often without a diagnosis of the problem. It is therefore important that, as well as an ability to plan and instigate a rehabilitation programme, the physiotherapist has skills in differential diagnosis. Patients amenable to physiotherapy must also be distinguished from those requiring help from a different healthcare provider. If the physiotherapist is a co-worker in a team that is lead by a specialist, who has already made a specific diagnosis and planned patient management, he or she needs to be able to determine the specifics of rehabilitation, obstacles to recovery, motivation of the patient and establish realistic and achievable goals. The physiotherapy assessment must thus be tailored according to the patient's needs.

The physiotherapy assessment, once based upon a traditional medical model, has evolved into a broader, more holistic approach, with increasing recognition of the influence that psychosocial factors can have upon the course and outcome of many illnesses. As a result, each patient is examined and treated as an individual, with consideration for the psychological and social, as well as physical, aspects of their condition.

The physiotherapy assessment can be loosely divided into two sections, the interview and the physical examination.

INTERVIEW

In the interview the physiotherapist aims to obtain an exact description of the patient's problem, including an account of how it occurred and developed. Each problem has a pattern of presentation which the patient is encouraged to describe generally, in the first instance. The physiotherapist will then use more specific questioning (e.g. Does your knee lock? Does it give way?) to clarify the picture and gain a deeper understanding of the condition. This helps to identify a specific pathology and discriminate between possible diagnoses. The patient is also asked specific screening questions to exclude possibly serious pathology and conditions not suitable for physiotherapy management. Further questioning upon general health, drugs taken and past medical problems will help to identify any obstacles to the patient's rehabilitation and recovery. Any of these factors may have an influence upon the present condition and the rehabilitation process.

Several psychosocial factors may also influence a patient's return to normal activities, and are important in shaping the appropriate level of intervention. Psychological issues include the patient's attitudes and beliefs concerning both the nature of their condition and their taking part in physical activity. The degree to which a patient takes responsibility for their condition and recovery, and any symptoms of psychological distress and depression, must also be explored in the interview. These must be addressed if they are likely to have a negative effect upon the patient's recovery.

PHYSICAL EXAMINATION

The physical examination consists of general screening, identification of factors that may point to a specific diagnosis or affect rehabilitation, and specific tests to confirm the presence of a given condition. The extent of the physical examination is determined by the pathology suspected and the activity that the patient wishes to return to.

The patient assessment principally aims to provide a diagnosis and prognosis (if this has not already been made) and to identify any obstacles to patient recovery so that an appropriate rehabilitation programme may be designed. The assessment may, however, confirm a suspicion that a presenting pathology is beyond the scope of rehabilitation at that time, and may more appropriately be seen by another team member. The relevant findings of the assessment are discussed with the patient at a level appropriate to their understanding, using jargon-free language. It is important to give the patient accurate infor-

mation in a positive manner and emphasising personal responsibility for their rehabilitation: any negative statements or descriptions of pathology that may lead to fear and a reluctance to take part in physical activity must be avoided. Once the goals of therapy have been agreed, a rehabilitation programme is negotiated. Throughout the ensuing programme, evaluation, discussion and negotiation allows continuous and appropriate modification of the rehabilitative process, as the patient progresses towards recovery.

THE ROLE OF PHYSICAL ACTIVITY AND EXERCISE IN LOW BACK PAIN

Low back pain is the most common musculoskeletal complaint in the adult population, with approximately 60% of people reporting back pain at some time in their lives. In 1993 there were about 14 million GP consultations for back pain and approximately 1.6 million people attended a hospital outpatient clinic, which represents a fivefold increase over the previous decade. Back pain is one of the most common and rapidly increasing causes of absenteeism from work, demand for health care and need for state benefit, and recently this problem has been described as a western society epidemic (Clinical Standards Advisory Group, 1994b).

Back pain may occur spontaneously with the patient unable to recall any trauma, or occasionally a strain of the back is remembered. Only a small proportion (approximately 10%) of people reporting lower back pain have underlying specific diseases which may or may not originate in the back itself. Non-spinal causes include renal, abdominal and gynaecological diseases. Causes involving the spine more directly include infections, tumours, inflammatory diseases, osteoporosis, Paget's disease and osteochondrosis, spinal stenosis and lumbar intervertebral disc herniation. However, all of these diseases are rare. It is important to differentiate individuals with these conditions as quickly as possible, so that appropriate management may follow. In the past, medicine has been relatively successful in treating and preventing many serious spinal diseases, deformities and even paralysis (Waddell, 1987).

For the remaining 90% of the population who seek help for low back trouble, the term mechanical low back pain (MLBP) is currently used to describe their symptoms (Evans and Richards, 1996). MLBP may refer pain to one or both hips or thighs, yet patients with this diagnosis show no evidence of underlying pathological or disease processes. The condition itself is benign and often self-limiting. It can be diagnosed with a reasonable degree of certainty from specific causes of low back pain from the history and signs on examination alone (Evans and Richards, 1996).

Most MLBP improves considerably in a few days, or at most a few weeks, but some symptoms persist. Von Korff (1996) has stated that 33% of people with MLBP may have symptoms for up to one year. Most patients will also have some recurrences from time to time (Coste *et al.*, 1994; Von Korff and Saunders, 1995). The majority of people cope with the problem themselves without seeking medical help (Waddell, 1987). However, approximately 10% of those with MLBP become intolerant of activity and, through a complex interaction of biological, psychological and social factors, become disabled (Waddell, 1987).

Medicine has struggled to find successful treatments for MLBP – at best these have been described as 'too little care, too late' (Waddell, 1987). Traditionally, bed rest has been the most common treatment after analgesics, yet there is now little doubt that bed rest, especially if prolonged, can be harmful and lead to weakness, chronic disability and increasing difficulty in rehabilitation (Waddell, 1987).

A recent surge of interest in MLBP has produced several comprehensive reviews of the epidemiology, existing patterns of care, assessment, diagnosis and treatment approaches used (Clinical Standards Advisory Group, 1994a,b; Evans and Richards, 1996; Waddell *et al.*, 1996). As a result of these reviews, a whole new approach to the problem has been proposed. This new 'biopsychosocial' model argues that the increase in disability due to MLBP is a consequence of changes in the way that back pain is understood in society. It suggests that changes in society's attitudes and expectations, combined with changes in medical ideas and management techniques, have appeared to promote, rather than alleviate, the disability associated with back pain (Evans and Richards, 1996). The biopsychosocial approach reinforces that, alongside the physical aspects of MLBP, management must consider a patient's psychological and social factors (which have been shown to play an important role in influencing patient response to treatment) as well as their disability (Waddell, 1992). This approach advocates an active exercise and rehabilitation approach to back pain because, contrary to popular belief, there is little evidence to suggest that activity is harmful, and it does not necessarily make the pain worse (Waddell, 1987).

Within this holistic approach to the management of MLBP, promoting physical activity as an appropriate form of intervention, the physiotherapist is in an ideal position to play a key role. The emphasis within physiotherapy is moving away from the traditional provision of symptomatic pain control in a passive patient. There is some evidence that manipulation is an effective method in providing some relief in some patients (Lewis, 1995) but it must be placed into context, used in the first six weeks to assist restoration of function through symptom reduction and confidence building. Evidence strongly favours an active approach to the patient, encouraging patient responsibility for their own recovery as the best means to manage MLBP (Clinical Standards Advisory Group, 1994a; Evans and Richards, 1996; Waddell *et al.*, 1996). The physiotherapist therefore aims to reactivate the patient and treat the whole person through physical activity and exercise. It is hoped that this will help to prevent chronicity and disability; once these are established any form of intervention is more difficult and has much lower chances of success (Burton *et al.*, 1995). The following text looks at the role of physical activity, exercise and patient education in the rehabilitation of patients with MLBP to promote return to normal activity and improved fitness.

ACTIVE REHABILITATION

It is now well recognised that the traditional treatment of rest for MLBP is not beneficial to the patient, and that the guiding principle should be to return the patient to an active lifestyle as soon as possible. There is evidence supporting activity and exercise-based rehabilitation programmes as the best means to achieve lasting relief of pain and prevent disability (Malmivaara *et al.*, 1995). Active rehabilitation uses normal physical activity and exercise to help to restore function and gain physical fitness. The particular type of exercise may be less important. This is largely based on extensive research into chronic MLBP, but theoretical principles and several controlled trials suggest that the earlier it is commenced the better (Clinical Standards Advisory Group, 1994a). Aerobic endurance exercises such as walking, cycling and swimming improve physical fitness and modify pain mechanisms (Evans and Richards, 1996). They also produce minimal mechanical stress to the back and are tolerated by most patients during the initial stages. There is little evidence to support any specific type of back exercise (Lewis, 1995). The exercise programme must be active, promoting the patient's responsibility for their rehabilitation. Exercises should start from a tolerable level and increase by planned increments, rather than progression being pain contingent. Patients treated with active exercise and early return to work have fewer recurrences, less additional time off work and less healthcare over the following two years (Clinical Standards Advisory Group, 1994a).

EDUCATION

There is increasing awareness of the need to provide patients with accurate and up-to-date information and advice, since it may have lasting effects upon their attitudes and beliefs about their condition and how it should be managed. Such information has also been shown to reduce anxiety and improve patients' satisfaction with care (AHCPR, 1994). The physiotherapist is in an influential position to gain the confidence of the patient, and therefore to begin to address any inappropriate attitudes or beliefs.

All information should be given in a positive manner to reduce apprehension and encourage participation in progressive normal activity. The patient needs reassurance as to the benign nature of their condition and the absence of any serious spinal pathology, and accurate information on the prognosis for rapid recovery. The patient must also receive practical advice on gradual return to normal activity and work, with assurance that activity is not harmful. The benefits of building their physical fitness also require reinforcement. In addition, any of the patient's concerns must be highlighted and settled in a positive manner to increase their confidence.

Such intervention should assist the patient through rehabilitation, but the patient must be aware that recovery may not mean the absence of pain, that residual symptoms may remain, or that pain may recur. Continued management therefore depends upon providing the patient with accurate information and advice, including realistic expectations and setting of goals. Again, it is important that the overall responsibility for recovery and continued management is firmly placed with the patient (Waddell *et al.*, 1996).

The level of intervention required will depend upon the individual patient. Most of the population with MLBP, and even those with some disability, cope with the problem without medical treatment (Waddell, 1987). Many of those seeking help recover well from an episode of MLBP, simply requiring reassurance and advice about a gradual return to normal activities (Waddell *et al.*, 1996). For these patients it is also important to promote the uptake of regular exercise to promote general fitness, since it has been shown that physically fit people have fewer and shorter attacks of MLBP and are more tolerant of pain (Waddell, 1987). Some patients may require encouragement and supervision through the initial stages of an exercise programme.

The management of the patient who has already become disabled by their back pain may be more complex. In these patients there appears to be a greater contribution of psychological and social factors to their chronic pain and disability (Waddell, 1992). This finding has lead to the inclusion of a wide range of psychological therapies to help to rehabilitate chronic pain patients, together with a move towards active rehabilitation and return to fitness in spite of their pain.

There is still a need for further investigation into the effectiveness of specific components of interventions used in the management of MLBP. Current evidence suggests that there must be a shift away from the negative philosophy of rest for pain reduction towards a more active restoration of function. The patient's role must correspondingly change from passive recipient of treatment to an active sharing of responsibility for his or her own recovery. It is unlikely that there will ever be a cure for MLBP (indeed, it may be a normal bodily experience) and the role of all those concerned is in helping the patient to cope with their problems.

A CASE STUDY

Karen, a 35-year-old busy mother of two young children, has had niggling back pain for years. In the past she has managed to look after her children, despite severe backache at times. However, her last bout of back trouble was so painful that she felt unable to do anything at all. She felt frightened to move and resorted to lying flat on the floor for two whole days, depending upon her husband to care for the children. Concerned that she may have seriously damaged her back, Karen visited her GP as soon as she could get herself to the surgery. Her doctor examined her and, much to Karen's relief, was able to reassure her that she had 'mechanical low back pain'. He described the condition and explained that, despite its being very painful, there was no serious spinal pathology and no need for any further investigations. He explained that she needed to gradually get herself moving again, and prescribed her some analgesia to help her return to normal activities. She was reassured that she would recover, and that a return to light activities would not be harmful; indeed it would be much more beneficial to her than rest.

The GP then referred Karen to a physiotherapist, who reinforced the GP's advice, and gave her some practical advice to help her return to activity. Through discussion with the physiotherapist, Karen realised that since the birth of her first child, she had been so occupied with her family that her own fitness had been neglected. She no longer went to regular aerobics classes with her friend. They then discussed how best she could be supported in returning to normal activities and regular exercise, enabling her to cope with her children and get back to her former physical fitness. The physiotherapist gave Karen some guidance on pacing of activities to help over the initial stages.

Karen got back to caring for her children and was keen to help herself cope with any future episodes. She felt, however, that she needed further guidance to overcome the fear of beginning any formal exercise although she knew it would help her to improve her fitness. She also felt that she lacked motivation to exercise and wasn't sure that she could do it alone. The physiotherapist invited Karen to join an 8-week programme which involved exercise and relaxation classes twice a week.

The exercise class included the following circuit of general exercises.

1. Warm-up: walking and general stretches to the whole body
2. Circuit: 2 minutes at each station
   - treadmill walking
   - step overs
   - static cycling
   - side leg raise
   - step ups
   - wall press-up
   - sit to stand
   - shoulder press with light dumbbells
   - half squats
   - standing row with spring resistance
3. Cool-down: walking and general stretches to the whole body.

Over the first few classes, advice about pacing enabled Karen to set her own exercise levels. She performed as many repetitions as she felt confident to do in the 2 minutes allowed, and then paced these over the initial classes to provide a baseline upon which to improve. At regular intervals her targets were increased under the supervision of the physiotherapist.

Alongside this programme, Karen was encouraged to take up another form of exercise that she could continue independently. She decided that walking was an activity that she could best afford and fit into her daily schedule. Eventually she hoped to return to aerobics classes, something she enjoyed and felt motivated to resume. The physiotherapist also addressed the effects of stress and tension on Karen's pain through relaxation sessions within the rehabilitation programme. Soon, Karen learnt to use these techniques independently, away from the class setting.

Despite some initial discomfort at taking part in more physical exercise, Karen gradually became more confident in her abilities and her exercise programme progressed steadily. At the end of the programme, a final consultation with the physiotherapist ensured that Karen had gained a good understanding of her condition and how it should be managed. She felt in control of her recurring MLBP and

equipped to cope with any episodes that might happen in the future.

THE ROLE OF EXERCISE IN THE REHABILITATION OF A SPORTS INJURY

As exercise and sporting activities have become more popular we have seen a considerable increase in the incidence of serious injuries to the knee (Johnson, 1988). Therefore in this section the rehabilitation of a person with an injury to the anterior cruciate ligament of the knee will be considered.

The knee joint requires two main properties that are conflicting in nature in order to withstand the stresses imposed upon it through normal activities (Johnson, 1988). *Stability* is vital to support the weight of the entire body, yet considerable *mobility* is also necessary to meet the demands of normal movement. The key to providing these two properties is a complex interplay of two pairs of ligaments, the collateral (medial and lateral) and the cruciate (anterior and posterior) ligaments, helped by other knee structures. However, if the femur and tibia (the bones comprising the knee joint) are forcefully rotated or angulated upon each other, damage to these and other joint structures may occur.

The anterior and posterior cruciate ligaments are extremely important in providing stability to the knee joint, and it is the anterior cruciate ligament (ACL) that is disrupted more often than any other ligament in the knee (Feagin and Curl, 1976; Johnson, 1988). This often occurs through participation in sporting activities such as rugby, football, netball, skiing, horse riding and gymnastics.

The ACL plays a stabilising role throughout flexion and extension of the knee. It primarily prevents the tibia from moving anteriorly relative to the femur, but it also resists internal tibial rotation and valgus forces. Damage to the ACL often occurs on suddenly side stepping, or changing direction whilst running or decelerating. Landing, perhaps awkwardly from a height, is also a common cause of injury. In contact sports, a force to the lateral side of the knee often injures the medial meniscus and medial collateral ligament as well as the ACL, an injury known as the 'unhappy triad'. It is therefore clear that, although serious knee injuries are usually associated with the high forces of contact sports, an individual may be injured with no external force involved at all.

Ligament injuries vary in extent from a partial tear, where only a few fibres may be damaged, to a rupture involving complete disruption of all ligament fibres or detachment of the ligament from the bone. Owing to a reasonable blood supply, the cruciate ligaments are capable of a certain amount of repair if only partially torn but a complete rupture will not heal spontaneously and may render the knee unstable. Instability at a joint implies that the supporting structures are no longer able to prevent abnormal movements at that joint. Such an unprotected joint may have impaired function and will be vulnerable to further injury. Typically, the patient with an ACL-deficient knee will report an inability to 'trust' the knee, together with frequent giving way and repeated swelling of the joint. However, some people with the same condition report no such instability, and are able to continue with normal activities without problems. Other knee joint structures may also be damaged (e.g. a tear to the meniscus), and such damage may also contribute to, or cause, loss of function. These concurrent injuries must be addressed and may require treatment, even if the ACL is not replaced surgically. Any suspicion of serious injury to knee joint structures justifies referral to an orthopaedic specialist.

Despite a huge volume of literature, the management of the patient with an ACL-deficient knee remains controversial. Whether the patient is carrying an acute or chronic injury, the knee must be assessed for the likelihood of further episodes of instability. Several factors, however, including sports participation and activity level, will put a patient at high risk (Johnson and Shelbourne, 1993). If instability at the knee is causing a significant loss of function, then the specialist and patient must discuss the options of preventing instability to allow an informed decision to be made. Conservative or non-surgical treatment may provide good functional recovery: some patients may return to full function with an ACL-deficient knee (Snyder-Mackler *et al.*, 1997); others, however, have difficulties with running, cutting and pivoting, and where such instability remains surgical reconstruction of the ACL may be the treatment of choice. Surgical techniques have progressed significantly, and minimally invasive methods are now widely used.

The rehabilitation of patients following surgical reconstruction of the ACL has evolved dramatically over the last decade, changing from a very slow progression to a more aggressive, active and individualised approach. Despite extensive research, however, knowledge of the biological effects of exercise upon the new graft replacement is still limited. Therefore recent protocols for rehabilitation following ACL reconstruction are largely based upon clinical experience (Irrgang and Harner, 1997). Modification to such protocols may be necessary according to factors such as the surgical technique used, the graft type, the presence of any associated pathology, and any surgery performed in conjunction with the ACL reconstruction. The patient's previous activity levels, condition before surgery, pain tolerance and motivation are also important factors to be considered in constructing the appropriate programme and environment to optimise patient recovery.

Most rehabilitation is based upon a protocol laid down by the specialist according to his or her experience. There is only a small scope for variation from the protocol – e.g. weight-bearing times, amount of flexion or extension block, how long to continue in a brace (if at all), type of exercises and prevention of complications (e.g. anterior knee pain, limited extension, over-stressing of the graft and persistent instability).

PREOPERATIVE MANAGEMENT

Up to the point of surgery, the focus of rehabilitation is on education and preparation of the patient. In the acute patient, surgery is usually delayed until the initial pain and swelling have subsided, since it is generally agreed that this reduces the likelihood of knee stiffness after surgery. Intervention may be necessary to reduce pain and swelling, regain full mobility, and encourage muscle activity and strength. There is also a strong emphasis upon maintenance and development of proprioception in order to enhance knee stability. This begins preoperatively and continues throughout all stages of rehabilitation.

Alternatively, the patient may have already completed a period of conservative treatment. This involves a progressive rehabilitation programme addressing knee mobility, strength and proprioception, aiming to bring the patient back to full function. If this aim is not achieved, then the ultimate decision may be to take the surgical route.

Preoperatively, the patient is advised upon the nature of the surgery. The postoperative rehabilitative process is also explained, which usually involves the use of a brace and crutches, as well as exercise. It is important to listen to the patient, encouraging expression of concerns and goals of rehabilitation. The patient's understanding of the responsibility that he or she must take for his or her own rehabilitation will be a significant factor. The rehabilitative process lasts months, and is indeed one which requires the patient to be well motivated in order to achieve optimal success.

POSTOPERATIVE MANAGEMENT

Working under the guidance of the surgeon and physiotherapist, the patient is actively rehabilitated after surgery with the utmost care to protect the graft.

Postsurgical goals of rehabilitation are to:

- prevent complications;
- minimise the effects of postoperative immobilisation on the knee;
- restore normal range of knee motion;
- restore normal strength to the lower limb musculature;
- restore normal proprioception to knee joint structures;
- restore patient confidence; and
- return the patient to his or her previous activity levels.

The main principles of rehabilitation are early mobilisation, early weight bearing, neuromuscular training and strengthening, whilst always protecting the healing tissues.

Research has provided an understanding of the joint forces and muscle recruitment patterns that occur during rehabilitative exercises. This knowledge, together with that available upon the physiological processes that occur following ACL reconstruction, enables the introduction of safe and effective exercises at appropriate stages in the rehabilitation programme. Much attention is placed upon the appropriate use of open and closed-chain exercises. The nature of muscle contractions during exercises (isometric versus isotonic, concentric versus eccentric), and resulting forces upon the joint and graft are all important considerations. The physiotherapist is challenged to balance general body-maintenance work with more specific knee-rehabilitative exercises. Full restoration of flexibility, power, co-ordination, balance and skill must be achieved by means which preserve the integrity of the graft. Careful patient monitoring, with vigilance for potential complications, allow for appropriate modification of the rehabilitation programme to promote a smooth and full recovery.

The rehabilitative procedure is therefore of utmost importance and may dictate the success or failure of ACL reconstructive surgery. Damage to the graft may be caused by several means:

- repetition at the extreme ends of joint range can create fatigue and failure of the graft at points of high stress;
- movements causing overelongation of the graft may lead to excessive anterior movement of the tibia and thus reduce the ability of the graft to perform its intended role;
- excessive loading associated with abnormal joint displacement, which may occur during a twist or fall, may also damage the graft.

This stresses the necessity for a carefully planned, monitored and progressed rehabilitative programme. Failure to improve occurs in approximately two out of ten cases, with ongoing instability present, with or without further joint problems.

Rehabilitation is a gradual and progressive procedure which is dictated by the surgeon, together with the physiotherapist. Initially the patient is monitored closely; as he or she recovers, the patient may be seen less frequently to monitor progress and adjust the programme. Over the later stages, the sportsperson may be seen more frequently by the sport scientist who will be working closely with the rehabilitative team. The final stages of rehabilitation will depend on the goals of the patient. Return to normal activities will progress gradually, to allow development of motor control to dynamically stabilise the knee and to allow the body time to adapt to the new stresses imposed upon it. Final rehabilitation of the sportsperson will require sports-specific training to ensure that all demands for the sport are met in terms of general fitness, as well as knee stability. The decision as to whether the patient can cope with both the mental and physical demands of the sport will be lead by the specialist but will involve the whole team, which may include the physiotherapist, sport scientist, psychologist and coach. Return to sports usually occurs 6–9 months following surgery (Irrgang and Harner, 1997).

CASE STUDY

George is a 24-year-old builder and promising sportsman, who was carried from the rugby pitch following an injury to his right knee during a tackle. He received first-aid treatment on the side line and went home limping on a swollen knee. Concerned that the swelling had failed to go down over the weekend, George then visited his GP, who referred him to an orthopaedic specialist and for physiotherapy.

The specialist determined that George had completely ruptured his ACL. Fortunately, there was no other damage to the joint structures, and it was decided that conservative treatment would follow. This required George to regularly attend for physiotherapy. The physiotherapist and George agreed upon an exercise programme which was progressed gradually, and may have eventually included any of the exercises in the list entitled 'rehabilitative knee exercises' (below). As George made progress, he attempted to return to work, but his knee gave way beneath him on the building site. George's knee became painful and swollen again, setting his exercise programme back considerably. George felt he had little confidence in his knee and was concerned for his job as well as for his sporting future.

The knee continued to give way, making further rehabilitation impossible and risking further injury and increased degenerative changes. It was then decided that his ACL should be surgically reconstructed. Twelve months after the initial injury, George underwent surgery using a microsurgical technique that took a graft from his patellar tendon to replace the ruptured ligament. There were no complications and George was encouraged to commence exercises soon after the operation. These included:

- knee bending to 60° initially, then increasing to 90°;
- full passive (involving no muscle work) knee extension;

- isometric quadriceps exercises (45° or more flexion) and isometric hamstring co-contractions. No straight leg raises for 6 weeks;
- muscle pump exercises;
- simple closed kinetic chain exercises (e.g. heel raises, mini-squats);
- proprioceptive exercises (e.g. weight transference).

George was fitted with a knee brace on the second day and began to take some weight through his foot, using crutches. He was discharged on the fourth day and referred to physiotherapy for rehabilitation. Over the next 12 weeks, George had regular checks with the specialist who, together with the physiotherapist, guided the progression of his exercise programme. George was weaned from his crutches and was allowed to progress his exercise programme to gain greater mobility (determined by his brace until 6 weeks postoperatively), strength and proprioception. George's recovery, although requiring much motivation and determination, ran smoothly as he began gentle running. At this stage, his physiotherapy programme had progressed considerably and may have included any of the exercises in the list below. Eventually the specialist allowed non-competitive sporting activities, and George began to work on more sport-specific training, anticipating his return to rugby. Here George focused upon general conditioning to meet the fitness demands of rugby, as well as ensuring that his knee could withstand the stresses imposed upon it by the game. Here, the physiotherapist worked closely with the sport scientist to construct an appropriate programme addressing all components of fitness to allow George to safely join in the non-contact aspects of the fitness training sessions at the club. Final consultation with the specialist gave George permission to resume full sporting activity. Again negotiation between George, his physiotherapist, coach and sport scientist ensured gradual progression of his programme to ensure return to full contact rugby competition with optimal recovery and preparation, and minimal risk of re-injury. George played his first rugby match one year after his surgery.

Rehabilitative knee exercises

- Prone knee bend
- Knee flexion/extension in sitting
- Hip abduction in side lying
- Hip adduction in side lying
- Squats:
  (a) double leg
  (b) single leg
- Bridging
  (a) both legs
  (b) single leg
- Wobbleboard
  (a) both legs
  (b) single leg
- Trampet
  (a) walk
  (b) jog
  (c) hop on spot
  (d) hop, varying directions
- Hamstring curl with other leg resisting
- Wall slide squats
- Balance exercises in standing
- Static bike
- Sit to stand
  (a) double leg
  (b) single leg
- Balance exercises on gym ball
- Step ups
  (a) strong leg first
  (b) weak leg first
- Step downs, single leg lowering
- Calf raises on step
  (a) double leg
  (b) single leg
- Lunges
  (a) over weak leg
  (b) over strong leg
- Running
  (a) circling
  (b) shuttling
  (c) zig zag

(d) sideways zig zag
- Jumping
  (a) on spot
  (b) all directions
  double leg then single leg
- Controlled running against resistance of elastic in all directions.

THE ROLE OF EXERCISE IN CARDIAC REHABILITATION PROGRAMMES

In CHD there is a gradual narrowing of the coronary arteries and the coronary blood flow (supplying the heart muscle itself) becomes insufficient for the needs of the heart. Many affected people may be unaware of any abnormality until a narrowing blocks an artery completely, leading to irreversible damage. Such an event is termed a myocardial infarction (MI), commonly known as a heart attack. It is one of the leading causes of death in affluent populations.

Recent decades have seen radical changes in the rehabilitation of the cardiac patient. In the 1940s, the patient faced as much as 8 weeks of bed rest for recovery from an MI. It was soon found, however, that a patient's guarded return to normal activity within a few days after an MI produced no adverse effects: early activity was indeed shown to reduce some of the harmful effects of bed rest and to have significant beneficial psychological effects (Levine and Lown, 1952). Now, the patient with stable MI or one who has undergone low-risk coronary artery bypass (CABG) surgery requires as little as a day of complete bed rest and as few as three or four days in hospital, with a much more rapid return to normal activities and work (Greenland and Chu, 1988). The emphasis upon early ambulation and exercise-based rehabilitation after MI and other cardiac illnesses or procedures has increased significantly.

Cardiac rehabilitation is best defined as 'the sum of activity required to ensure cardiac patients the best possible physical, mental and social conditions, so that they may by their own efforts regain as normal as possible a place in the community, and lead an active and productive life' (World Health Organization, 1964). It is now well accepted that CHD has physiological, psychological and social impacts upon the individual, all of which need to be addressed through rehabilitation. Therefore a holistic approach to managing the cardiac patient is developing which may provide exercise therapy, patient education and psychological counselling, risk-factor modification, vocational counselling and group support meetings. Ideally, the multidisciplinary team should involve a cardiac nurse, physiotherapist, exercise physiologist, psychologist, dietitian, cardiologist and various exercise and health educators. Most often, however, the overlap in educational backgrounds of these professions allows fewer personnel to provide high-quality programming in many areas of specialisation (Hall, 1993). In all rehabilitation programmes the final responsibility for recovery must remain with the patient.

Cardiac rehabilitation services were originally designed for patients recovering from an acute MI. They have since, however, been expanded by modifying some of the procedures and therapeutic exercises to other cardiac patients, including those recovering from CABG surgery, angioplasty and heart transplantation, those with stable angina or silent ischaemia and those with chronic arrhythmias, congestive heart failure, valvular heart disease or other heart disorders. Cardiac rehabilitation may also be offered as part of a primary prevention programme for patients with a high risk factor profile for a future CHD event. The incorporation of physical activity (now a core component of cardiac rehabilitation programmes) into the patient's lifestyle has been shown to have an inverse association with the incidence of heart disease (Powell *et al.*, 1987).

In Britain, cardiac rehabilitation is routine at most hospitals following uncomplicated MI or CABG surgery. The patient may go through three main phases of rehabilitation: inpatient, outpatient and community-based programmes. The inpatient programme begins once a patient is medically stable and all contraindications are excluded. Outpatient exercise training usually begins within a few weeks of discharge, and a patient may then progress to a medically unsupervised, less intensely monitored community programme. During this period efforts are made to gradually reduce supervision and to promote self-regulated programmes, hopefully for life (Leon *et al.*, 1990).

Exercise therapy now forms the core of the majority of cardiac rehabilitation programmes because it has many potential physiological, psychological and social benefits for the cardiac patient. Indeed, it has been suggested that, together with the commonly known physiological effects of CHD, it is the emotional, behavioural and social impacts of the disease that may be most debilitating to the patient.

Since cardiac disease affects both a patient's psychology and their coronary blood supply, standard prescriptive methods to determine exercise levels cannot be applied directly to these patients. Particular care must be taken to negotiate individualised programmes, in accordance with the psychological and physiological limitations imposed by CHD. As with any patients undertaking an exercise programme, exercise recommendations must take into account the patient's stage of recovery, any limitations due to medication, and other orthopaedic or neuromuscular problems.

The initial challenge to the therapist is to make the patient feel confident in their ability to resume and progress activity. Initially, the uncertainties that a patient experiences during recovery from an MI may be overwhelming, since they may be unsure of what to do and how to do it. It is widely reported that giving information and involving patients in their therapy is beneficial in both reducing patient anxiety and increasing their sense of control over the condition (Kincey *et al.*, 1975;

Ley, 1988). Advice about gradual pacing, progression of activity and recognition of signs and symptoms that may occur through exercise will increase the patient's feelings of control, and allow them to progress their exercise programmes appropriately. Patients must also be encouraged to express their concerns and beliefs about their condition, which, together with their attitude, motivation and goals, will all influence the planning and progress made through rehabilitation. A confident and reassuring attitude shown by the therapist will also help to promote and progress physical activity.

Inpatient activities, such as simple self-care procedures, will eventually progress to walking. Outpatient and community rehabilitation programmes usually introduce exercise, principally as a means to increase patient confidence in their ability to perform physical activities. Patients are encouraged to include a variety of exercise modes into their programmes, perhaps using cycle and arm ergometers, bench stepping and treadmills. Circuit-type training has been recommended in the early phases because rest periods can be taken as required; this may be particularly important in the initial stages of recovery (Hall *et al.*, 1984). Continuous conditioning training such as walking, swimming and cycling may be more appropriate to promote improved work capacity at later stages. However, use of a single mode of exercise may indeed become boring and lead to poor adherence (American College of Sports Medicine, 1991; Bethell, 1992), so the exercise mode must be chosen to suit the patient. Weightlifting (particularly isometric strengthening work) and dynamic sports such as squash and contact sports are not recommended for cardiac patients due to the sudden rise in blood pressure that accompanies such effort.

Outpatient and community programmes usually offer a group setting which may have several advantages in achieving the goals of rehabilitation. The social aspects in themselves are often sufficient to divert a patient's attention from their disease and improve morale by providing enjoyable companionship. All encounters are social events and as such have the potential to be highly therapeutic. Considerable patient surveillance and extensive therapist attention to guide and monitor exercise aims to provide support and promote confidence as well as safety. These factors may be particularly important in activating patients during the initial stages of rehabilitation.

Although there have been few quantitative studies, the psychological benefits of exercise programmes have been noted anecdotally (Fletcher and Cantwell, 1974). It is intended that improved confidence and sense of wellbeing will provide sound foundations upon which further benefits may be gained. It is hoped that patients will gradually progress their levels of exercise, initially under supervision, and will eventually incorporate more unsupervised activity into their lifestyle. Only when a patient has gained sufficient confidence can exercise progress to levels that promote increases in work capacity. It is generally accepted that cardiac rehabilitation services limit the physiological effects of cardiovascular disease and do improve a person's functional status, while increasing the threshold for the onset of chest pain in patients with angina (Greenland and Chu, 1988; Oldridge *et al.*, 1988; O'Conner *et al.*, 1989; Leon *et al.*, 1990). Exercise has also been shown to have a positive effect upon risk factors for CHD (e.g. by contributing to weight reduction, increasing high-density lipoprotein levels, lessening the adrenergic response to stress; Oberman, 1988).

It must be remembered that, as in most chronic diseases, the rehabilitation of patients with cardiac disorders does not effect a cure. It aims to improve a patient's quality of life by enabling them to resume active and productive lives, within the limitations imposed by their disease process, for as long as possible, with a balanced, healthy and optimistic attitude.

A COMMUNITY CARDIAC REHABILITATION PROGRAMME

Kerland Sports and Lifestyle Clinic and Taunton and District Cardiac Support Group, supported by the Somerset Physical Activity Group, arranged for the provision of a community cardiac rehabilitation service. Sessions are held in a community centre under the direct supervision of a nurse and qualified exercise leaders. Participants attend a 75-minute session once per week, and the intervention consists of an exercise conditioning and education programme in which patients are invited to participate, with their spouses if they so wish. Each session begins with a revision of exercise safety and self-monitoring issues. A 'buddy' system is employed, in which patients are allocated a partner (if not accompanied by their spouse), and patterns of communication and recognition of warning signs are reinforced. Patients are also encouraged to express any concerns they may have felt over the preceding week.

A 10-minute warm-up is followed by a 20-minute cardiovascular circuit of exercises (see below), in which patients are encouraged to exercise within their levels of confidence. A 10-minute cool-down concludes the exercise component. Patients are encouraged to progress their programmes independently and, if confidence and exercise intensities increase sufficiently, the Borg scale (Borg, 1982; Figure 5.1, p. 104) is employed to provide further guidance to encourage a training effect, if appropriate. Under the recommendations of the American College of Sports Medicine (1991) cardiac patients are encouraged to exercise between the levels of 12 and 14 on the Borg scale for effective training and safety. However, actual levels of exercise are secondary to building a patient's confidence in increasing their activity levels above those to which they are accustomed, whatever the level.

Each exercise session is concluded with a discussion of one of several health issues relevant to the patient population. All components of the session are directed towards building confidence, stamina and long-term compliance to an active lifestyle for both patient and spouse.

Basic cardiovascular circuit included in the exercise component of the intervention

- High knee stepping on the spot
- Arm circles (various)
- Spot steps/step-ups (small)
- Push aways from wall
- Half squats
- Stretch (various)
- Chest press with ball
- Side steps/split squats
- Lateral arm raises with ball
- Shuttle walking

REFERENCES

AHCPR (1994). *Management Guidelines for Acute Low Back Pain*. Rockville, MD: Agency for Health Care Policy and Research, US Department of Health and Human Services.

American College of Sports Medicine (1991). *Guidelines for Exercise Testing and Prescription*. Philadelphia: Lea and Feibiger.

Bethell, H.J.N. (1992). Exercise in post infarct rehabilitation. *British Journal of Clinical Practice*, **46**, 116–122.

Borg, G.V. (1982). Psychophysiological basis for perceived exertion. *Medicine and Science in Sports and Exercise*, **14**, 377–387.

Burton, A.K., Tillotson, K.M., Main, C.J. and Hollis, S. (1995). Psychological predictors of outcome in acute and subchronic low back trouble. *Spine*, **20**, 722–728.

CSP (1997). *The Case for Physiotherapy, Delivering Effective Patient Care*. London: Chartered Society of Physiotherapy.

Coste, J., Delecoeuillerie, G., Cohen de Lara, A., Le Parc, J.M. and Paolaggi, J.B. (1994). Clinical course and prognostic factors in acute low back pain: An inception cohort study in primary care. *British Medical Journal*, **308**, 577–580.

Clinical Standards Advisory Group (1994a). *Report on Low Back Pain*. London: HMSO.

Clinical Standards Advisory Group (1994b). *Epidemiology Review: The Epidemiology and Cost of Low Back Pain. Annex to the CSAG report on Back Pain*. London: HMSO.

Evans, G. and Richards, S. (1996). *Low Back Pain: An Evaluation of Therapeutic Evaluations*. Bristol: Bristol Health Care Evaluation Unit, University of Bristol.

Feagin, J. and Curl, W. (1976). Isolated tear of the anterior cruciate ligament: 5 year follow-up study. *American Journal of Sports Medicine*, **4**, 95–100.

Fletcher, G.F. and Cantwell, J.D. (1974). Outpatient gym exercise program for patients with recent myocardial infarction; a preliminary report. *Archives of Internal Medicine*, **134**, 63–68.

Greenland, P. and Chu, J.S. (1988). Efficacy of cardiac rehabilitation services. *Annals of Internal Medicine*, **109**, 650–663.

Hall, L.K. (1993). *Developing and Managing Cardiac Rehabilitation Programs*. Pittsburgh: Human Kinetics.

Hall, L.K., Meyer, G.C. and Hellerstein, H.K. (eds) (1984). *Cardiac Rehabilitation: Exercise Testing and Prescription*. La Crosse Exercise and Health Series. Illinois: Life Enhancement Publications.

Irrgang, J.J. and Harner, C. D. (1997). Recent advances in ACL rehabilitation: clinical factors that influence the programme. *Journal of Sport Rehabilitation*, **6**, 111–124.

Johnson, R. (1988). Prevention of cruciate ligament injuries. In *The Crucial Ligaments: Diagnosis and Treatment of Ligamentous Injuries about the Knee*, Feagin, J. (ed.). New York: Churchill Livingstone.

Johnson, G.E. and Shelbourne, K.D. (1993). Patient selection for anterior cruciate ligament reconstruction. *Operative Techniques in Sports Medicine*, **1**, 16–21.

Kincey, J., Bradshaw, P. and Ley, P. (1975). Patient satisfaction and reported acceptance of advice in general practice. *Journal of the Royal College of General Practitioners*, **25**, 558–562.

Leon, A.S., Certo, C., Cosmoss, P. and Franklin, B.A. (1990). Scientific evidence of the value of cardiac rehabilitation services with emphasis on patients following myocardial infarction: exercise conditioning component. *Guidelines for Cardiac Rehabilitation Programs*. Champaign, IL: Human Kinetics.

Levine, S.A. and Lown, B. (1952). 'Armchair' treatment of acute coronary thrombosis. *Journal of the American Medical Association*, **148**, 1356–1369.

Lewis, M. (1995) MEDLINE Reviews from January 1992 to September, 1995 of RCTs of Exercise and Manipulation for Acute Low Back Pain. Available on request from Royal College of General Practitioners.

Ley, P. (1988). *Communicating with Patients*. London: Croom Helm.

Malmivaara, A., Hakkinen, U., Aro Heinrichs, M.L., Koskenneimi, L., Kuosma, E., Lappi, S., Paloheimo, R., Servo, C., Vaaranen, V. and Hernberg, S. (1995). The treatment of acute low back pain – bed rest, exercises or normal activity? *New England Journal of Medicine*, **332**, 351–355.

Morris, J.N. (1994). Exercise in the prevention of coronary heart disease: today's best buy in public health. *Medicine and Science in Sports and Exercise*, **26**, 807–814.

Oberman, A. (1988). Rehabilitation of patients with coronary heart disease. In *Heart Disease: A Textbook of Cardiovascular Medicine*, Braunwald, E. (ed.). Philadelphia: WB Saunders Company.

O'Conner, G.T., Buring, J.E., Yusuf, S. and Paffenburger, R.W. (1989). An overview of randomised trials of rehabilitation with exercise after myocardial infarction. *Circulation*, **80**, 234–244.

Oldridge, N.B., Guyatt, G.H., Fischer, M.E., Rimm, A.A. (1988). Cardiac rehabilitation after myocardial infarction. *Journal of the American Medical Association*, **260**, 945–950.

Powell, K.E., Thompson, P.D., Caspersen, C.J. and Kendricks, J.S. (1987). Physical activity and the incidence of heart disease. *Annual Review of Public Health*, **8**, 253–287.

Snyder-Mackler, L., Fitzgerald, G.K., Bartolozzi, A.R. and Ciccotti, M.G. (1997). The relationship between passive joint laxity and functional outcome after anterior cruciate ligament injury. *American Journal of Sports Medicine*, **25**, 191–195.

Von Korff, M. (1996). Studying the natural history of back pain. *Spine*, **21**, 2059–2063.

Von Korff, M. and Saunders, K. (1995). The course of back pain in primary care. *Spine*, **21**, 2833–2837.

Waddell, G. (1987). A new clinical model for the treatment of low back pain. *Spine*, **12**, 632–644.

Waddell, G. (1992). Biopsychosocial analysis of low back pain. *Clinical Rheumatology*, **6**, 523–557.

Waddell, G., Feder, G., McIntosh, A., Lewis, M., Hutchinson, A. (1996). *Low Back Pain Evidence Review*. London: Royal College of General Practitioners.

World Health Organization (1964) *Report of a WHO Expert Committee: Rehabilitation of Patients with Cardiovascular Diseases*. Technical Report # 270. Geneva: World Health Organization.

EXERCISE BENEFITS AND PRESCRIPTION FOR SPECIFIC CONDITIONS

11

INTRODUCTION

According to the Health of the Nation report (1993), 80% of all-cause mortality can be attributed to CHD (45%), cancer (25%) and respiratory disease (10%). On a global scale this accounts for millions of deaths each year. A lack of physical activity has been linked with the incidence of many of these disorders, some of which can have fatal consequences. In this chapter we will explore the underlying mechanisms of these and other diseases and explain the preventive and rehabilitative roles exercise can play. In addition, and when appropriate, we will also make reference to the insights that exercise psychology can provide.

Whilst there is evidence of a dose–response relationship, with increasing amounts of exercise producing further reductions in the risk of these diseases, considerable benefits (indeed, the largest health benefits) have been shown to be associated with the change from no exercise to some exercise. A major reduction in the risk of many of these diseases can be achieved by persuading individuals to incorporate a moderate amount of activity into their lifestyle (Åstrand, 1992; Blair 1994, 1995; Shephard, 1997). For example, moderate bouts of regular walking several times a week are sufficient to induce substantial improvements in health status (Hardman 1996; Woolf-May et al., 1997). Such beliefs were expressed by the Greek physician Hippocrates over 2000 years ago, when he wrote 'All parts of the body which have a function, if used in moderation and exercised in labour in which each is accustomed, become thereby healthy, well developed and age more slowly, but if unused and left idle they become liable to disease, defective in growth and age quickly' (Hollmann, 1991).

Given the research evidence, inactivity itself is considered to be a health risk by many authorities (Blair 1994), which causes them to recommend participation in appropriate forms of exercise as a means of promoting or maintaining health. Morris (1994) concludes that exercise is 'the best health buy'. For additional information a number of key texts, review and research articles are listed at the end of this chapter (Åstrand and Grimby, 1986; Fentem et al., 1988; Bouchard et al., 1994; Morris 1994; Blair, 1995; 1990; Hardman, 1996; Shephard, 1997). In particular, the work of Blair and colleagues at the Cooper Institute in Dallas has demonstrated that, even when individuals exhibit other health risk factors such as high blood pressure, smoking and high cholesterol, if they are fit their risk of premature death is less than that of unfit individuals who exhibit none of the other risk factors (Blair et al., 1996). Likewise the health risks associated with high body mass index (BMI >30) values and/or high body fat (>25%) and/or large abdominal girth (>100 cm) in men appear to disappear if the individual is physically fit. In their research (Blair, 1997) the risk of premature death in the fit group was half that of the unfit group regardless of the factors related to obesity and body composition.

Unfortunately, despite the evidence to support the benefits of exercise upon health, many people still participate in relatively little physical exercise. Butler (1987) presented figures which suggested that over 75% of adults in Britain exercised less than twice a week, despite the fact that about half of those interviewed believed that they did not take enough exercise. More recently, the results of the Allied Dunbar National Fitness Survey (Sports Council/Health Education Authority, 1992) indicated the scale of this national problem, with inactivity increasing with age and being more prevalent in women. Similar conclusions have been drawn from numerous studies world-wide, and show that, while there is a general belief in the population that 'exercise is good for you', people do not exercise because of lack of time or incentive. Despite an apparent awareness of the health-promoting benefits of exercise, relatively few people are willing to make a commitment to exercise on a regular basis. It may therefore be the role of the exercise adviser to provide the opportunity, advice, motivation, incentive and expertise required to encourage a person to undertake appropriate forms of health-promoting exercise.

Some of the key questions which research has only partially resolved are how much exercise, and of what type, duration and intensity, have which health benefits? Linked to this is the appreciation that not all exercise programmes convey the same benefits or have the same magnitude of effect. Even the same programme may have different impacts upon different individuals

This chapter will review the evidence for the benefits of exercise for the population in general and will particularly consider specific conditions. Recommendations for exercise prescription will be made in each of these groups. In all cases it should be remembered that a reduced risk of developing certain diseases is only one beneficial aspect of exercise. Other very important gains include improving physical capacity (which may or may not be linked to the maintenance of independence and quality of life), social and mental benefits.

EXERCISE FOR THE PROMOTION AND MAINTENANCE OF GENERAL HEALTH IN ADULTS

For the adult, the reported health-related benefits of exercise are diverse and often interrelated. However, for convenience they may be considered under the following broad headings:

1. Promotion of physical capacity to enhance a person's ability to cope with the physical demands of his or her lifestyle.
2. Promotion of mental health.
3. Provision of a social environment.
4. Reduction in the risk of certain hypokinetic diseases.
5. Enhancement of recovery from, or minimising the adverse effects of, an accident, illness or other trauma.

The remainder of this chapter will centre upon a number of specific conditions for which exercise can be prescribed. An extensive amount of research suggests an important role for exercise at all ages. Where appropriate, these findings will be discussed within each section.

EXERCISE FOR THE ASYMPTOMATIC ADULT

If a sedentary or 'low-active' adult wishes to commence an exercise programme it is recommended that they undergo a full health check. The results of this check will either reassure the exercise adviser that the participant is unlikely to suffer any harm from the exercise or will identify health problems of which the participant may have been previously unaware, and which should be taken into consideration in the exercise prescription.

A general 'needs assessment' of the client will usually reveal a number of desired outcomes from their exercise programme, typically a combination of wishing to lose weight, wanting to tone-up their muscles and generally hoping to feel fitter. Some individuals may have specific goals such as getting fit for a sporting event like running a marathon. The reality of such intentions and/or their desirability will depend on the current condition of the individual and their capacity to achieve it.

For most adults a programme involving aerobic exercise (walking, jogging, swimming, cycling, rowing and exercise classes) coupled with general toning exercises and flexibility work, undertaken three times a week, should be recommended. This programme could also incorporate lifestyle changes such as walking or cycling to work and/or some activity during any lunch-break they may have.

Unless indicated to the contrary, the intensity of the aerobic exercise should be within the 'heart rate training zone' and performed for a minimum of 20–30 minutes. However, some benefits can be attained from repetitive bouts of exercise of a shorter duration. Research has also indicated that exercise of an intensity below the heart rate training zone does convey some health benefits. The toning exercises should work all the major muscle groups and should be performed in sets of 12–20 repetitions. Loosening and stretching exercises should be included as part of a general warm-up and cool-down. At the start of the programme light resistances and gentle aerobic exercise should be used before progressing gradually over a period of weeks: this is because it is in the early stages of an exercise programme that a previously sedentary individual is most vulnerable to injury and a possible cardiovascular incident.

EXERCISE AND THE OLDER ADULT

Elderly people show beneficial adaptations to exercise similar to those seen in younger adults, although generally more slowly.

Therefore, when devising a programme for an elderly client the starting point may need to be at a very easy level and subsequent progression should be applied very gradually. Furthermore, since the maximum physical potential of the participant is likely to be lower due to the effects of ageing, the goals of the programme will also need to be set accordingly. However, the general content and type of exercises included can be very similar to those for younger adults, including walking, swimming, cycling, flexibility and strengthening exercises (MacHeath, 1984; Rikkers, 1986).

In western society it is becoming more acceptable for older people to be physically active and to pursue physically demanding hobbies. With these trends, the physically active older person is becoming more common, as are some middle-aged individuals who (through continued participation in exercise programmes) find themselves as physically fit as they were 10 years ago. Unfortunately, such individuals are still in the minority and the population as a whole still tend towards inactivity. Strauzenberg (1981), in a review of the literature, concluded that the ageing process was slowed down by regular participation in exercise and that older people who had regularly participated in vigorous physical activity since their youth were biologically younger than their sedentary counterparts. Such research is always open to criticism, since participants in long-term studies are almost inevitably volunteers and therefore self-selected. It can thus always be argued that it is only the 'biologically younger' individuals who are capable or willing to participate in vigorous exercise. Hence, although there is a clear link between exercise participation and biological age the exact cause and effect is still not proven (Kasch, 1976; Holloszy, 1983; Thornton, 1984).

Findings from investigations such as the Allied Dunbar National Fitness Survey (Sports Council/Health Education Authority, 1992) indicate that a significant proportion of older adults have fitness levels below or close to levels which can affect their independence as well as their quality of life. The implications of training for older woman have been reviewed by Taunton *et al.* (1997), who suggest that strength training may be the most important form of exercise for elderly people because it will help to 'maintain strength, physical function, bone health and psychosocial health'. When considering exercise training for elderly people particular emphasis should thus be placed on the implications of loss of muscular strength, which severely impedes the completion of everyday activities, such as lifting objects, opening jars and general mobility. Declines in strength of 15% per decade after the age of 60 have been reported in the literature (Vanderport and McComas, 1986). Owing to the slower adaptation of older individuals, strength training programmes need to be of a more prolonged duration (16–18 weeks) before substantial improvements can be detected, although some gains may be seen within a few months. Programmes of weight training and 1RM exercises both improve strength. An additional benefit of strength gains is the improved balance and co-ordination, which can prevent injurious falls.

Swimming, walking, cycling and flexibility exercises are likely to be considered as the most appropriate forms of activity although, for those who have the capacity and inclination, weight training may also convey considerable benefits in preventing the reduction in lean tissue mass (and hence strength) which tends to accompany ageing. For individuals with specific problems such as arthritis, activities such as swimming may be ideal although they should not be pursued if the exercise causes pain. Swimming is often recommended for a number of disorders because of its beneficial effects on joint mobility, muscular strength and cardiovascular fitness. The activity requires relatively slow and controlled movements through a wide range of motion, which helps to maintain flexibility. In addition, working against the resistance of the water helps to maintain muscular strength and, if performed at a moderate intensity, swimming will have positive aerobic effects. Swimming is often preferable over other forms of activity because the buoyancy of the water supports the body and thereby reduces pressure on the joints, which may be an important consideration for patients for whom land-based exercises are problematic – such as those with joint problems, lower limb dysfunction or who are excessively overweight. If possible, weight-bearing exercises should be included within a programme to help reduce the risk of osteoporosis, although the first stage for people already suffering from the disease may be simply walking in the water. Osteoporosis is discussed further later in this chapter.

An exercise programme for elderly patients should commence at a very low intensity and progress very gradually. This is especially important with older individuals, where there is a possibility of asymptomatic cardiovascular disease.

EXERCISE, ATHEROMA AND CORONARY DISEASE

The heart is made up of specialised muscular tissue (cardiac muscle) which, like other muscles in the body, requires a constant supply of blood to provide it with the oxygen it needs to contract. Whereas skeletal muscle can resort to anaerobic metabolism for short periods during intensive exercise, cardiac muscle cannot work anaerobically. The coronary arteries supply the cardiac muscle with all the blood and oxygen it needs, even during intensive forms of exercise. These blood vessels form an extensive network in and around the heart muscle itself (Figure 11.1).

In the case of what is usually referred to as coronary heart disease (CHD) the coronary arteries become constricted by a build-up of fatty deposits (atheroma) on the inside of the artery wall (Figure 11.2). This is the condition referred to as *atherosclerosis*. The exact details of the processes leading to atherosclerosis are

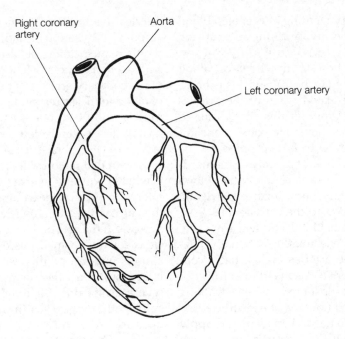

Figure 11.1   The coronary arteries

not clearly understood; however, factors such as high concentrations of fats in the blood (hyperlipidaemia), high total blood cholesterol (hypercholesterolaemia), high blood pressure (hypertension), damage to the walls of the arteries, blood platelet aggregation, high carbon monoxide levels in the blood, cigarette smoking and a relatively low ratio of high-density (HDL) to low-density lipoproteins (LDL) in the blood are all thought to increase the risk of atherosclerosis. The two main theories of atheroma formation are therefore generally referred to as: (1) the hypercholesterolaemia and cholesterol metabolism theory and (2) the cell injury theory. The former centres on the issue of cholesterol, the latter on injury to the endothelial layer of the arteries, which (when damaged) promotes platelet adherence and aggregation, thereby promoting the formation of an atheromatic lesion. For a more detailed review of the current hypotheses see Moore (1994). The overall effect of atheroma is to reduce the diameter of the blood vessels, restricting the flow of blood to the area of muscle they supply. The formation of fatty streaks (atheromatous thrombi) on the walls of the arteries conveys additional risks because these could rupture or become dislodged. A dislodged thrombus can block a

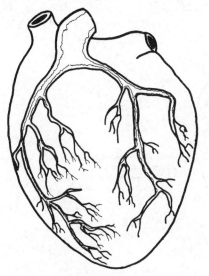

Figure 11.2   Build-up of atheroma

coronary artery, preventing oxygenated blood from reaching the myocardium and causing ischaemia.

Further restriction to the flow of blood through arteries may be caused by a hardening of the elasticated walls of the arteries (*arteriosclerosis*). Although this may occur to some extent as an inevitable consequence of ageing it is believed to be worsened by the presence of atheroma. The walls of the hardened arteries fail to stretch fully when blood is pumped through them, further restricting the supply of blood to the cardiac muscle.

At rest the flow of blood, and hence oxygen, reaching the cardiac muscle is usually adequate even if the arteries are partially constricted. However, if the heart has to work harder (as, for instance, when walking upstairs) the blood flow may be insufficient to supply the oxygen needed. Inadequate supply of blood is known as *ischaemia*. Inadequate supply of oxygen to a region of the heart may result in chest pains and the conditions known as angina pectoris or angina decubitus.

Angina symptoms tend to appear when atherosclerosis is already somewhat advanced, with the diameter of the coronary artery (or arteries) having been reduced by about 75%. Angina is a serious condition which often requires medication; it also predisposes the sufferer to a greater risk of complete blockage of the coronary arteries. If this occurs, the flow of blood to the corresponding region of cardiac muscle will be stopped, and that part of the heart will be severely deprived of oxygen. If the lack of oxygen persists then an area of cardiac muscle in that region will die (Figure 11.3); this is what is typically referred to as a myocardial infarction (MI) or 'heart attack'. The death of the cardiac muscle cells is also referred to as necrosis. If the area of damage to the heart muscle is relatively small this occurrence may go almost unnoticed (this is termed a 'silent' infarction). On other occasions it can cause severe chest pains and, if the area of damage is sufficiently large, it can have fatal consequences.

According to figures published by the British Heart Foundation (1986), heart and circulatory diseases account for 44% of all premature deaths in the UK. In the USA the American Heart Association (1984, 1995) has estimated that about 51% of all American deaths were caused by cardiovascular disease

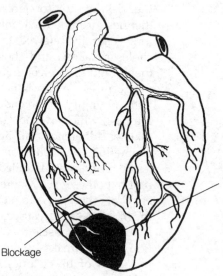

Area of cardiac muscle damaged, due to a lack of oxygen

Blockage

Figure 11.3   A myocardial infarction

and that nearly half of these occur in individuals under the age of 65 years (American Heart Association, 1997). Similar figures are reported by Hutchinson (1985) and Kannel *et al.* (1985), who also report that in addition to the premature fatalities over 8 million people in the USA suffer from some form of disability as a result of CHD. Additional reports on the scale of the problem have been presented by the British Cardiac Society (1987), who stated that by the age of 40–44 one in six men in the UK will have clinical evidence of CHD; by the age of 55–59 one in three is affected.

It is widely known that cardiovascular disease is far more common in men than in women. The reason for this observed inequality is believed to be due to hormonal differences between the sexes. The key difference seems to be the significantly higher levels of oestrogens in women. These hormones appear to convey a form of protection to premenopausal women but after the menopause, when the hormonal differences are greatly reduced, women appear to be as much at risk from CHD as their male counterparts. Further support for the suggestion that oestrogens convey protection against CHD comes from clinical investigations in which oestrogens were administered to men recovering from MI. Oestrogens effectively reduced the risk of further attacks.

A major and increasing concern over the incidence of CHD is its frequency in the relatively young. Autopsy studies indicated that over 77% of American soldiers killed in the Korean War had signs of coronary artery disease despite the fact that their average age was only 22 (Enos *et al.*, 1953). Similar findings were found in later studies conducted on American soldiers killed in Vietnam (McNamara *et al.*, 1971). CHD is not just a disease associated with old age, it is a major killer of men between 35 and 44 years and there is also an apparent increase in CHD in women of this age group. Some investigations have shown that the early stages of cardiovascular disease can be observed in young children, including some

younger than 5 years of age (Kannel and Dawber, 1972).

It is thus clear that CHD is a major health problem for a large proportion of the population: it is not a disease that just affects elderly people. Any preventive measures that can be taken to reduce the magnitude of the problem are of great importance. One of the major difficulties in trying to persuade people to take preventive measures such as exercises is that, although CHD is a gradual process which may begin in childhood or even infancy, the symptoms and debilitating effects of the disease do not become apparent until it is fairly advanced.

Some individuals are inherently more likely to suffer from CHD than others. This may be due to factors such as age, sex, race and genetic traits over which the individual has no control. However, a number of risk factors which increase the chances of a person suffering from CHD can be influenced by the individual:

- hypertension
- smoking
- obesity
- high total blood cholesterol levels
- a relatively low ratio of high-density lipoprotein cholesterol to low-density lipoprotein cholesterol
- stressed emotional state
- lack of physical exercise
- poor haemostatic profile of fibrinolytic activity, thrombus formation and platelet aggregation.

All of these factors can by influenced by the individual, and thus a person is able to exert some influence over their chances of developing CHD. Exercise in particular can have a positive effect on these factors, either through the direct physiological changes brought on by physical activity or by psychosocial changes, including behavioural modifications such as stopping smoking.

These 'optional' risk factors are often interrelated, and altering one factor (such as taking up exercise) can have beneficial effects upon the others. For example, exercise may reduce body fat levels, lower blood pressure, reduce blood cholesterol levels, produce a more favourable ratio of HDL to LDL-cholesterol, increase insulin sensitivity, promote fibrinolytic activity, decrease blood clotting and alleviate stress. These changes will all contribute towards decreasing an individual's chances of suffering from CHD. Evidence comes from a large number of investigations which are reviewed by Astrand and Grimby (1986), the Coronary Prevention Group (1987), Morris *et al.* (1987), Powell *et al.*, (1987), Fentem *et al.* (1988, 1990), Blair (1994) and Bouchard *et al.* (1994). Overall, research suggests that death due to ischaemic heart disease is twice as common in the physically inactive as in the physically active. Some of the discrepancy between research findings may be due to methodological deficiencies, and Blair (1994) suggests that 'if physical activity is carefully assessed, CHD accurately measured, and appropriate epidemiological methods are used, it is virtually certain that a significant inverse association will be found between activity and CHD'.

There is also general agreement that, in order to effectively reduce the risk of CHD, the exercise needs to be 'aerobic', undertaken regularly and be of sufficient duration. Thus, many authorities recommend activities such as swimming, cycling, jogging and brisk walking. Most authorities would recommend a frequency of three times a week, with each session lasting a minimum of 20–30 minutes (American College of Sports Medicine, 1991). However, whilst there is an association between physical activity and reduced risk of CHD, the exact physiological processes that reduce the risk remain unclear. In general, it is widely accepted that exercise produces its effects by improving the overall condition of the cardiovascular system and by exerting numerous effects upon the various risk factors associated with CHD. Suggested effects of exercise include:

- improvement of blood lipid profiles
- reduction of arterial blood pressure
- improvement of overall body composition by reducing the percentage of body fat
- reduction of sympathoadrenal activity
- reduction or inhibition of atheroma
- improvement of the efficiency of the heart
- control of stress
- promoting fibrinolysis, reducing platelet aggregability and preventing unwanted blood coagulation, although considerably more research is needed to elucidate the exact mechanisms by which these factors work
- growth of collateral coronary blood vessels.

Thus there is much evidence to support the role of exercise in reduction of CHD risk factors which, even without the implications of CHD, are considered in themselves to be detrimental to the overall health and well-being of the individual.

In summary, exercise has an important role to play in reducing the risk of CHD, and may therefore be prescribed as a form of preventive medicine. It would also appear that significant benefits may be obtained from relatively modest doses of exercise such as walking for 30–40 minutes a day, and that it may not be necessary to complete this duration of activity within a single session (DeBusk *et al.*, 1990). The issue of 'accumulating' exercise during a day still requires much research. Individuals who currently do not pursue an active lifestyle need to be reassured that to gain health benefits they do not need to undertake very strenuous exercise (Duncan *et al.*, 1991). Indeed, the link between exercise and benefit appears to be curvilinear, with the greatest decline in risk occurring with the change from doing no exercise to doing some regular activity of a relatively moderate intensity.

In addition to its reported preventative effects exercise is used very extensively in the rehabilitation programmes of people with MI and in the treatment of coronary artery disease (Cox, 1997), both to help restore physical capacity and to try to reduce the risk of a further attack (for details see Chapter 10).

If evidence from research studies does support the notion that exercise can reduce the risk of CHD, the following question may be asked: 'Can the participation in very large amounts of exercise provide complete immunity against CHD?' This question was investigated by Noakes *et al.* (1984), who studied the incidence of CHD in marathon runners. They concluded that, while exercise did indeed reduce the incidence of CHD, very large doses of exercise did not provide complete immunity, especially when other risk factors such as smoking and poor blood fat profiles were involved. Thus, most authorities recommend a basic level of exercise with appropriate levels of intensity, duration and frequency; few would advocate excessive amounts of exercise as a means of substantially reducing the risks further. In summary, there is much evidence to support the belief that exercise can reduce the risk of CHD but any health-promotion programme must also consider the other risk factors associated with CHD and advise patients accordingly.

With much of the research evidence it is difficult to entirely exclude the influence of subject self-selection. It could be argued by sceptics that only those who are predisposed to good health feel inclined to exercise. It is virtually impossible to exclude this hypothesis entirely, but many of the intervention studies clearly demonstrate favourable changes due to exercise in previously sedentary subjects, and therefore strongly support the causal link between exercise and good health. However, for the exercise scientist the question 'how much exercise?' remains to be resolved. Issues of modality, intensity, frequency and duration must all be addressed for different population groups with a variety of ages, pre-intervention health status and gender. It is possible that different risk factors require different exercise criteria. For each risk factor it is still not known whether the important criteria are the total amount of exercise completed per week and/or the amount performed above a set threshold intensity and/or the amount completed beyond a certain duration in each session. When we have answers to these questions we will be able to prescribe exercise programmes in a far more specific way.

EXERCISE, BLOOD PRESSURE, HYPERTENSION AND CHD

Blood pressure is a measure of the pressure exerted by the blood on the walls of the arteries. The pumping action of the heart moves the blood through the arteries in surges rather than in a steady flow. This causes the pressure exerted on the walls of the arteries to vary. The greatest pressure occurs as the heart contracts; this surge of blood can be felt as the pulse in arteries close to the surface of the body. The pressure during these surges is known as the *systolic* pressure. Between the surges, whilst the heart is refilling with blood, the pressure in the arteries is at its lowest. This is known as the *diastolic* pressure.

Blood pressure is usually measured at the left brachial artery whilst the subject is seated (or, occasionally, lying down) using a sphygmomanometer which is strapped to the upper arm over the artery. When measuring 'blood pressure' both the systolic and diastolic pressures are taken. The blood pressure is then expressed as the systolic pressure over the diastolic pressure (e.g. 125/75). Although they appear to be expressed as a fraction they are always expressed as two figures, with the difference between the two being the 'pulse pressure'. There are a range of accepted values for both systolic and diastolic pressures: typical adult systolic values are 120–145 mmHg; typical diastolic pressures 60–85 mmHg. Owing to the stiffening of the arteries there is a slight rise in blood pressure with age, and some authorities suggest a much wider range of acceptable values.

If a pressure exceeds the 'normal' range it is said to be high; if it is below, it is said to be low. Blood pressure is expressed in millimetres of mercury (mmHg). Most traditional sphygmomanometers measure blood pressure using a column of mercury. Digital sphygmomanometers, whilst not using mercury, express blood pressure in the same units.

An individual's blood pressure is influenced by a number of factors, including their emotional state, posture, recent exercise, smoking and recently ingested food or drink. A persistently high resting blood pressure (e.g. 175/100) is known as *hypertension*. High blood pressure is due to a greater than normal pressure within the arteries. This may be caused by the arteries being constricted, possibly as the result of tension or fatty deposits (atheroma), or by the arteries losing their elasticity and hence their capacity to stretch as the blood passes through them.

High blood pressure is not only undesirable in terms of overall health, it is also a major risk factor in many diseases including CHD (Horan and Lenfant, 1990; Horan and Mockrin 1990). The incidence of high blood pressure (160/90 mmHg) is in the region of 10% in European countries, and in the USA over 58 million people have elevated blood pressure (Fagard and Tipton, 1994). The actual mechanisms which cause hypertension are complex and not fully understood but contributing factors include stress, diet, smoking, age body mass, large sodium intakes, substantial alcohol consumption, an inherited tendency towards high blood pressure and lack of exercise. Therefore changes in diet, medication, lifestyle and exercise participation have been employed to reduce hypertension.

During exercise the increase in stroke volume and cardiac output have the potential to cause an increase in blood pressure. However, this is largely counteracted by dilation of the blood vessels, which decreases the peripheral resistance and thus gives a small increase in systolic blood pressure and little change in diastolic. However, in some normotensive subjects a more dramatic increase in blood pressure has been observed – which, it is

suggested, could be predictive of a tendency towards hypertension (Benbassat and Froom, 1986; Tipton 1991).

Studies such as that of Choquette and Ferguson (1973) have shown that appropriate exercise programmes are effective in reducing blood pressure, at rest and during exercise. Reports and reviews investigating the value of exercise in reducing resting blood pressure include those of Boyer and Kasch (1970), Kukkonen *et al.* (1982), Kiyonaga *et al.* (1984), Roman *et al.* (1984), Seals and Hagberg (1984), Tipton (1984, 1991) and Duncan *et al.* (1985). Overall it is suggested that prolonged aerobic activity is most effective in reducing high blood pressure, while resistance training has a minimal effect. An inverse relationship between physical activity and/or fitness with hypertension has been demonstrated (Folsom *et al.*, 1985; Reaven *et al.*, 1991). Other investigations (Goldberg *et al.*, 1980) have also shown that exercise reduces the amount of medication required to control hypertension, and thus exercise has gained much support in the control of hypertension, especially in patients where the condition is considered to be relatively slight. The underlying causes of this hypotensive change are not clear, although Fagard and Tipton (1994) suggest that reduced sympathetic activity is a strong candidate. Work by Hagberg *et al.* (1989) demonstrated a decline in both systolic and diastolic blood pressure after 9 months of relatively low to moderate-intensity exercise. Meta-analysis suggests average reductions of 6–7 mmHg in well controlled studies.

The arteries have a tendency to lose their elasticity as part of the ageing process and there is a slight increase in blood pressure with age. However, the investigations of Blair *et al.* (1984) and Kasch and Wallace (1976) indicate that this loss of elasticity may be largely prevented by continued participation in endurance exercise throughout life.

Exercise also has acute effects on blood pressure. For example, following an acute bout of exercise resting blood pressure falls to below that of its pre-exercise levels (Tipton, 1991). This post-exercise hypotension is believed to have important long-term consequences and to be of significant benefit if exercise is repeated frequently (Pescatello *et al.*, 1991). Such responses are even seen in exercise programmes which prescribe short repetitive bouts of exercise (3 × 10 minutes per day) (Davis *et al.*, 1998).

In summary, research would suggest that exercise can be used to reduce the risks of hypertension, to reduce blood pressure in hypertensive subjects and to reduce the amount of medication needed to control hypertension. It should be remembered that high blood pressure can occur in children (Blumenthal *et al.*, 1977) and therefore appropriate forms of exercise may also be recommended for this age group as a means of controlling blood pressure (and hence promoting good health).

Isometric exercises should not be recommended for those with high blood pressure. Any exercise programme devised for those with hypertension should include exercises that are of a dynamic nature, such as walking, swimming or cycling. The reason for avoiding isometric exercises is that holding a muscle in a strong static contraction will restrict the blood flow through it, causing a build-up of metabolic waste products which can then stimulate an unwanted rise in blood pressure as the cardiovascular system attempts to send more blood to the muscle. Dynamic exercises tend to avoid this problem due to the cyclic contractions and relaxation of the muscles which facilitate the venous flow of the blood out of the muscle and back towards the heart.

EXERCISE, STRESS AND CHD

Various pieces of research have indicated that a person's emotional state, or the amount of 'stress' they experience, is another significant factor affecting risk of CHD. This is of course in addition to its contribution to many debilitating stress-related disorders (Friedman and Rosenman, 1959, 1974; Friedman, 1969). A major problem encountered when trying to assess the significance of stress on a person's health is that stress is difficult to measure quantitatively. It is also difficult to separate the potential effects of stress from other factors and its precise relationship with certain disorders. Thus the significance of stress as a risk factor for CHD remains largely unknown. However, some authorities consider it as a major determinant both directly and indirectly because of its influence upon other risk factors such as blood pressure.

Individuals most at risk from stress are those exhibiting 'type A' behaviour – those with a strong competitive drive at work and/or in their leisure time. These people also tend to work in a tense state with some degree of urgency. Exercise can reduce the amount of stress a person experiences and may therefore be an effective means of controlling it, thereby reducing the risk of CHD and other disorders (Folkins and Amsterdam, 1977; Blumenthal *et al.*, 1980; Ledwidge, 1980; Seals and Hagberg, 1984). Work by Long (1983) suggests that the psychological aspects of exercise programmes are important in reducing stress (and may indeed be more significant than the more easily measured physiological effects). Thus exercise may be used to control this increasing problem in modern society which affects both children and adults. However, exercise advisers will need to ensure that any exercise programme does not become too competitive as this could increase the amount of stress experienced by the individual rather than reduce it.

EXERCISE, BLOOD LIPIDS, ATHEROMA AND CHD

Abnormally high levels of fat in the blood (hyperlipidaemia) are associated with cardiovascular disease. In particular there is a link between high levels of serum cholesterol (hypercholesterolaemia) and risk of CHD (Grundy, 1986). Cholesterol values above 200 mg dl^{-1} are a significant CHD risk factor, with a fourfold increase in risk if the level exceeds 300 mg dl^{-1} (Goodman, 1988).

It is therefore clearly desirable to have blood cholesterol well below these levels (less than 180 mg dl^{-1} is recommended) in order to reduce the risk of CHD. The value of exercise in reducing blood cholesterol levels has been demonstrated in various studies (Hartung, 1984; Haskell, 1984a): thus, by implication, this research provides support for the notion that physical activity can reduce the risk of CHD.

The most common types of fat found in the blood are triglycerides (triacylglycerols) and cholesterol, which circulates in the blood in association with protein carriers to form what are known as lipoproteins. Several types of lipoproteins are found in the blood: according to structure they are designated high-density lipoproteins (HDL), low-density lipoproteins (LDL) and very-low-density lipoproteins (VLDL). The relative abundance of these different types of lipoproteins has a significant effect upon the probability of the formation of atheroma in the blood vessels and hence the incidence of CHD. Thus, not only the absolute concentration of fat within the blood but also the relative abundance of these lipoproteins can influence risk of CHD. In particular the ratio of HDL cholesterol to LDL cholesterol affects CHD: an increased risk is associated with HDL cholesterol levels below 35 mg dl^{-1} and LDL cholesterol levels above 130 mg dl^{-1} (National Institutes of Health, 1985). A ratio of LDL cholesterol to HDL cholesterol greater than 4.5 is associated with increased risk and a ratio of 3.5 or less is desirable (Manninen et al., 1988).

HDL appears to reduce the incidence of atheroma formation by transporting cholesterol to the liver, where it is metabolised and removed from the body in the bile. Relatively high levels of LDL appear to cause the formation of atheroma on the walls of the arteries. Numerous studies have shown that exercise increases the HDL/LDL ratio in the blood (Huttunen et al., 1979; Wood and Haskell, 1979; Rotkis et al., 1981; Thorland and Gilliam,

1981; Cowan, 1983; Gordon et al., 1983; Roberts, 1984; Goldberg and Elliot, 1985; Castelli et al., 1986; Chandrashekar and Anand, 1991; Thompson et al., 1991; Wood et al., 1991), thereby reducing the rate of deposition of atheroma on the walls of the arteries and increasing the rate of removal of cholesterol from the blood (Haskell, 1984a,b). It may even facilitate the regression of atheroma (Kramsch, 1981).

Training and cross-sectional studies also suggest that the metabolic adaptations to exercise include an enhanced capacity to use triacylglycerols via enhanced lipoprotein lipase activity. However, detraining studies also suggest that these benefits begin to decline within 2–3 days of the last exercise bout, although the rate at which they decline and the level to which they fall in trained athletes remains to be determined (Hardman et al. 1998).

Further interest in the effects of exercise upon blood lipid profiles comes from studies on children (Gilliam and Burke, 1978; Widhalm et al., 1978; Nizankowska-Blaz and Abramowicz, 1983) in which higher levels of HDL-cholesterol were seen in children who were more physically active than those who were relatively sedentary. Other studies of the relationship between physical activity level and blood lipid profiles in children have been less conclusive (Valimaki et al., 1980; Linder and DuRant, 1982) but this may be due to the fact that the children tended to have 'normal' blood lipid profiles even before the exercise programme commenced and, hence, little or no change would be expected. Other factors such as the type, intensity and duration of the exercises undertaken in the different programmes may also go some way to explain the inconsistencies of the findings.

EXERCISE, FIBRINOLYSIS, BLOOD CLOTS, PLATELET AGGREGATION AND CHD

A further factor which needs to be considered when discussing the effects of exercise upon the incidence of CHD is the formation of blood clots which can cause blockages in arteries that are already partially closed by atherosclerosis. A blood clot can block a coronary artery and cause an MI. A clot that blocks the artery in which it was formed is called a thrombus; if it becomes detached and is then transported in the blood causing a blockage elsewhere it is an embolus. Work by Elwood *et al.* (1991) has shown a relationship between high platelet counts and their tendency to aggregate, which increases the risk of death due to ischaemic heart disease. In some groups high levels of fibrinogen are considered more of a risk factor in CHD than high cholesterol levels (Wilhelmsen *et al.* 1984; Stone and Thorpe, 1985; Meade *et al.* 1986). Platelet aggregation has been proposed as a possible cause of thrombosis and MI in individuals who exhibit few other risk factors (Burgess-Wilson *et al.*, 1984; Trip *et al.*, 1990). Blood platelets appear to be involved in the atherosclerotic process via an interaction with LDL cholesterol, although the exact mechanisms remain unclear (Davis and Thomas, 1984; Schneider *et al.*, 1988).

The formation of blood clots is a complex process requiring a series of reactions between clotting factors in the blood (Furie and Furie, 1992). The clotting process is initiated by factors released by damaged tissues and cells. In the case of a small cut or graze on the skin blood will coagulate in the vicinity of the damaged tissue and the wound will close. Clots (thrombi) can also form internally, damage to the artery walls being a prime initiator. The reverse process, whereby blood clots are dissolved and removed, is called fibrinolysis (thrombolysis).

It has been suggested that atherosclerotic arteries are similar to other damaged tissue in that they stimulate the formation of thrombi. At present, although there is a clear link between thrombi, atherosclerosis and cardiovascular disease, the exact mechanisms of cause and effect are unclear. An increase in the incidence of thrombi would increase the chances of one of them causing a blockage in an artery – and, hence, the probability of a MI and/or stroke.

Even within an individual differences occur in atherosclerotic arteries and those which are free of atheroma. A key difference is the level of fibrinolytic activity, which is higher in the atheroma-free arteries (Ljungner and Bergqvist, 1984).

It has been proposed by some authorities that if exercise were to promote fibrinolysis it could reduce the incidence of blood clots and hence the risk of heart attack (Fentem and Turnbull, 1987). However, current research is not conclusive and evidence is contradictory. Some work indicates that exercise increases the rates of both clot formation and fibrinolysis. If the effects on both processes were of equal magnitude they would offset each other, perhaps resulting in no overall benefit. However, despite this there is generally a view that moderate exercise can be antithrombotic (Astrup, 1973; Davis *et al.*, 1976; Joye *et al.*, 1978; Meade *et al.*, 1979; Vogt and Straub, 1979; Hyers *et al.*, 1980; Andrew *et al.*, 1986; Eichner, 1987). It is postulated that exercise could cause relative changes in plasminogen activator and its inhibitor. However, Rauramaa and Salonen (1994) suggest that the elevated fibrinolytic effect of exercise is transient and declines within a few minutes of exercise ceasing. Therefore sustained high levels of fibrinolytic activity may not be detected in many studies and the real benefits of this anti-thrombotic effect are seen only in frequent repetitive bouts of exercise.

Additional work by Stratton *et al.* (1991) indicates that, particularly in older men, sustained exercise can favourably affect the balance between thrombosis and thrombolysis. This could have further significance given that fibrinolytic activity tends to decline with age (Takada and Takada, 1988).

However, it must be remembered that if exercise has a beneficial effect upon the condition of the atherosclerotic arteries themselves it could indirectly reduce the formation of blood clots. In some studies has been shown to reduce platelet aggregation (Rauramaa *et al.*, 1986). In addition to the reduction in the amount of atheroma (and, hence, constriction within the arteries) this will reduce the chances of a blood clot becoming stuck in a constricted artery and the risk of a complete blockage. This is clearly an area in which further research may yield valuable information.

EXERCISE, CARDIAC FUNCTION AND THE PROMOTION OF COLLATERAL CORONARY BLOOD VESSELS

Support for the role of exercise in benefiting cardiac function comes from the work of Tharp and Wagner (1982), who suggest that one of the major benefits is the training effect, which causes a reduction in the heart rate at a given sub-maximal exercise intensity. The slower heart rate will result in a longer diastolic period in the cardiac cycle. This will increase perfusion of blood into the heart muscle itself and thereby enhance the supply of oxygen to the cardiac muscle.

Research by Woolf-May *et al.* (1997) demonstrated an enhanced rate of ventricular relaxation with even moderate doses of exercise (walking) in previously sedentary and low-active adults.

Support for the effects of exercise in promoting the growth of additional coronary blood vessels comes from the work of Eckstein (1957), Schaible *et al.* (1981) and Wyatt and Mitchell (1978), who suggested that exercise may promote alternative coronary arteries to perform the function of blocked ones and hence reduce the impact of atherosclerosis or even MI. The review by Laughlin *et al.* (1994) suggests that such structural changes occur in striated (skeletal and cardiac) muscle, with increases in arterial length and cross-sectional area and in the number of capillaries (angiogenesis).

In summary, exercise can promote the development of additional blood vessels within the cardiac muscle ('vascularisation'), which has been extensively observed in skeletal muscle following a programme of aerobic exercise. Similar effects are believed to occur in cardiac muscle; however, research into the subject is difficult and most studies supporting the idea have involved the use of other animals or are based on indirect evidence (Blumgart *et al.*, 1940; Stevenson *et al.*, 1964; Ferguson *et al.*, 1974; Barnard, 1975; Connor *et al.*, 1976; Scheuer 1982; Bloor *et al.*, 1984) and may not be applicable to heart disease in the human. Therefore, whilst this suggested benefit promotes much interest it is still subject to speculation and debate.

The results of such research are complicated by indications that the deprivation of oxygen to part of the heart muscle, caused by a blockage within a coronary artery, also appears to be a stimulus for initiating the development of collateral arteries within the myocardium. These bypass the blockage, forming what is known as a collateral circulation, and hence the heart muscle in this area can be supplied with the blood it requires via an alternative set of blood vessels (Schiesinger, 1938; Zoll *et al.*, 1951; Ferguson *et al.*, 1974). Therefore, in studies where exercise has been used and coronary collateralisation has been observed, the extent to which the exercise itself was responsible for the changes is not entirely clear.

Aerobic exercise has also been shown to increase the size of blood vessels in skeletal muscle, thus enhancing blood flow to the muscles. Studies on rats indicate that a similar process may also occur in cardiac muscle (Tepperman and Pearlman, 1961; Stevenson *et al.*, 1964; Bloor and Leon 1970; Tharp and Wagner, 1982). This would again enhance the delivery of blood to the myocardium. The larger diameter of the coronary arteries would reduce the risk of a complete blockage and, hence, MI. Studies on this aspect in humans are complicated by possible genetic and other lifestyle factors, but some indirect evidence does support these suggestions (Currens and White, 1961; Qu Xia, 1990).

EXERCISE PSYCHOLOGY INSIGHTS INTO CHD

Psychological as well as physiological risk factors are apparently associated with CHD. Stress and an inappropriate emotional response to it, along with 'type A behaviour', are commonly recognised as increasing an individual's vulnerability. Psychological variables such as attitudes and social norms also help to determine those individuals who are more likely to adhere to health-promoting behaviours such as physical activity. Health-promotion interventions aimed at reducing the incidence of CHD need to recognise these psychological factors and address issues related to stress management and the behavioural skills needed to live a healthy lifestyle.

Exercise and health psychology can also help us to understand the challenges and difficulties faced by patients who are undergoing rehabilitation following MI. Whilst evidence shows that physical activity should play an important role in the process this may appear counterintuitive to the patient and their family. The concept of complete bed rest following a heart attack may long ago have been rejected by the medical community but its legacy still lingers in the minds of some patients! For them a heart attack may be a signal to 'take things easy' and for their partners to ensure that they do not do 'too much'. Although these phrases contain an element of truth, if they are inappropriately turned into reasons to be sedentary they may hinder the rehabilitative process, causing the patient either to drop out of the programme or not to start it. These issues and the importance of ensuring that any exercise programme is set at an appropriate rating of perceived exertion are explored in more detail in Chapter 10.

EXERCISE, OBESITY AND CHD

An obese individual has an excessively high amount of fat stored in their body. It is gener-ally agreed that for health a man's body mass should be approximately 15% fat and that of a woman approximately 23%, although some authorities recommend values slightly below this. Fat stores in excess of these values are generally considered to be detrimental to health. Definitions of what constitutes moderate and severe obesity vary between authorities. In part this may be related to the difficulties associated with accurately assessing body composition and the problems inherent in the use of the body mass index (BMI = weight (in kilograms)/height (in metres)^2), which does not distinguish between fat and lean tissues. Abdominal girth has also been used as a defining measurement in some studies. Given these difficulties, suggested values for moderate obesity in men include 25–30% body fat and/or a BMI of 26–34, and for women 35–40% body fat and/or a BMI of 25–33. Values in excess of these would be classified as severe obesity. At the other end of the spectrum, exceptionally lean individuals (such as male and female endurance runners) may have body fat values as low as 6% and 12% respectively. These low values are not generally considered to be 'unhealthy' but below this there may be health implications, especially for women, who may become more prone to osteoporosis if they lose too much fat.

A certain amount of fat is essential for the body as it fulfils certain vital functions: it forms a major component in the structure of cell membranes, provides insulation, provides physical protection, acts as an energy store, is essential for the manufacture of biochemicals such as steroid hormones, and is required in numerous metabolic processes.

In addition to its social implications, obesity reduces a person's physical capacity and is considered to be a major risk factor in a number of diseases and disorders, such as:

- CHD, possibly through the association between obesity and other CHD risk factors such as hypertension, inactivity and blood lipid profiles;

- impaired cardiac function;
- hypertension;
- diabetes (about 80% of people with adult-onset diabetes are overweight)
- renal disorders;
- pulmonary disease and impairment of lung function;
- osteoarthritis;
- cancer;
- gallbladder disorders;
- abnormal plasma lipid and lipoprotein profiles.

Obesity is a complex phenomenon which may be caused by a number of factors, including inactivity, overeating, hormonal disturbances, genetic and socioeconomic factors. The amount of fat stored in the body depends on the number of fat cells a person has and the size of those fat cells. Fat cells have the capacity to increase or decrease in size as a person stores or uses fat. Studies have suggested that there are two basic types of obesity: in *hyperplasia obesity* the individual has an increased number of fat cells, in *hypertrophy obesity* the individual has a normal number of fat cells but they are larger and contain more fat.

Problems of excessive fatness may originate before birth. Research by Udall (1978) showed that mothers who put on too much fat during pregnancy produced fatter babies, who appeared to possess a greater number of fat cells (adipocytes) than less fat babies whose mothers had not put on excess fat during pregnancy. This hyperplasia is believed to make the overfat babies more prone to obesity throughout their lives (Charney, 1976). A second period of vulnerability to obesity may occur during infancy: according to Brook (1972), if infants are overfed in their first year they may become overfat, with a resulting increase in the number of fat cells. This hyperplasia again has implications for obesity throughout life. A third period of potential hyperplasia may then occur between the ages of 9 and 13, just before the adolescent growth spurt (Hirsch, 1972; Salans *et al.*, 1973). It may

therefore be suggested that fatness in childhood can make the individual more prone to obesity in adulthood, although some authorities would dispute these reported changes in the number of fat cells.

Studies on obese adults suggest that if they were not overfat as children then their obesity is more likely to be of the hypertrophy-obesity type than hyperplasia. Such conclusions are reached because these individuals appear to have a normal number of fat cells, but the cells are larger than in non-obese individuals (Sims, 1974; Hirsch and Batchelor, 1976). It is also interesting to note that when the amount of fat stored within the body is reduced the fat cells shrink, but there appears to be no reduction in the actual number. Rognum *et al.* (1982) and Vinten and Galbo (1983) showed that, whilst exercise reduced the fat stores of the body, the effects were on the size of the fat cells and the amount of fat stored within them rather than on the actual number of fat cells. Such findings may indicate why many obese individuals find that having lost fat they are very prone to putting it back on. Bjorntorp (1974) suggested that individuals suffering from hyperplasia obesity have more difficulty in reducing their body fat levels and do not respond as well as those with hypertrophy obesity to normal diet and exercise regimens. Therefore, in the case of obesity, as with any disorder, preventive measures should be initiated early in life.

Although obesity is linked with CHD, the exact relationship is unclear due to the association of obesity with other risk factors. For example, many obese individuals have high blood pressure, consume too much fat in their diet and take very little vigorous exercise. It is also apparent that obesity limits an individual's physical capacity and puts more strain upon their cardiovascular system, muscles and joints, even during relatively low-intensity activities such as climbing stairs. Therefore an individual's body composition is an important consideration in terms of both physical capacity and general health.

The amount of fat stored in a person's body basically depends upon their calorific balance, the relationship between the number of calories consumed in the diet and the number of calories used up by basal and general metabolism, growth processes and the energy requirements of physical activity. If the number of calories taken in greatly exceeds the number used up then substantial amounts of fat may accumulate in the body, much of this fat being stored in fat cells under the skin (subcutaneous fat). If more calories are consistently used up than are taken in then the fat stores of the body are reduced. If an individual wishes to maintain his or her body composition, it is necessary to ensure that the calorific intake and expenditure are balanced but if the individual wishes to reduce their fat stores, then more calories must be used than are consumed. This calorific balance, and the tendency to store fat, therefore depends on a number of factors, including diet, the level of physical activity, general metabolism, and certain inherited characteristics. Of these factors the amount of exercise undertaken by a person is one which can be altered. By increasing calorific expenditure – by undertaking more exercise – it is possible for an individual to reduce their fat stores.

Aerobic exercise has long been advocated as a means of losing weight and to produce significant reductions in body fat levels in both obese and non-obese individuals, even without being undertaken in conjunction with a calorie-restricted diet (Boileau *et al.*, 1971; Bjorntorp, 1978; Leon *et al.*, 1979; Wilmore, 1983). Various authors (Mayer and Thomas, 1967; Chirico and Stunfard, 1976; Mayer, 1980) present evidence to suggest that obesity is very often due to inactivity rather than overeating, even in children (Corbin and Pletcher, 1968). These suggestions are supported by research indicating that many obese individuals do not have a higher than average calorific intake (Fry, 1953; Peckos, 1953; Johnson *et al.*, 1956). It is therefore not surprising that many investigators recommend a combination of exercise

and a calorie-controlled diet as the optimal means of controlling and/or reducing body fat – see the reviews by Bjorntorp (1983), Pace *et al.* (1986) and Segal and Pi-Sunyer (1989).

To reduce body fat levels many authorities recommend a calorific deficiency of about 500 kilocalories (kcal) per day. This amounts to a deficiency of 3500 kcal per week, which is equivalent to approximately 0.5 kg (1 lb) of fat. Such a deficit may be achieved through exercise, dietary modifications or both. Whilst a fat loss of 0.5 kg per week may not appear to be spectacular it should be remembered that people do not become obese overnight and that the more rapid weight losses that are observed under certain regimens have drawbacks: these are discussed more fully later. Aerobic forms of exercise appear the most effective means of burning up excess calories and will, of course, convey other health benefits. However, the exercise undertaken needs to be of a sufficient duration, intensity and frequency (see Chapter 7 for details). Authorities such as the American College of Sports Medicine and the Health Education Authority (UK) recommend participating in some form of exercise at least three times a week if the exercise is to be effective in reducing fat levels. It is also recommended that the exercise sessions should be of at least 20–30 minutes duration; during each session the participant should thus use up a minimum of 300 kcal.

To lose 0.5 kg of fat it is necessary to burn up about 3500 kcal, approximately equivalent to 12 30-minute exercise sessions, 35 miles of jogging or walking, 20 hours of golf or 12 hours of cycling. Such figures are often quoted by sceptics to illustrate, as they would put it, the 'futility' of exercise in a weight-control programme. However, to put these values into perspective, to walk 3 miles five times a week represents an expenditure of 75 000 kcal per year – the equivalent of 10 kg (about 20 lb) of fat. In addition to this significant contribution to weight control, the walker would gain numerous other health benefits from the exercise.

There is very little difference in calorific expenditure of jogging 3 miles in 24 minutes and walking the same 3 miles in an hour. It is the *duration* of the exercise completed which dictates the calorific cost, not the speed at which it is completed. If two individuals were to perform a 45-minute exercise class and one completed more exercises than the other within that period, he or she would have used more calories, in the same way that a runner running 8 miles in an hour will use more calories than a person walking 3 miles in an hour.

A major problem encountered by the exercise adviser or therapist is that many people wish to lose considerable amounts of fat very quickly without much effort, despite the fact that they probably put on the fat over many months and years through an inappropriate lifestyle. Those wishing to lose weight are also subjected to much commercial advertising which leads them to believe it can be done without effort or changing their lifestyle. However, many advertised methods cause weight loss due to fluid imbalance and/or loss of important energy stores such as muscle glycogen, whilst being relatively ineffective in losing fat: they can also convey other health implications for some individuals. In weight-reduction programmes that do not include exercise there is a tendency for the subject's metabolic rate to fall as the programme progresses. This means that the individual actually needs fewer calories each day – and further fat reduction becomes more difficult. The inclusion of exercise into a fat-reduction programme helps to prevent this unwanted fall in resting metabolic rate (Donahoe *et al.*, 1984; Mole *et al.*, 1989) and also helps to prevent the undesirable loss of important lean tissue, which may occur if dieting is the sole means of reducing body fat (Zuti and Golding, 1976). Research has also suggested that regular participation in exercise can elevate the metabolic rate for some time after the exercise session has finished, thereby further enhancing a reduction in fat stores.

It is also important to note that exercise will be really effective in reducing the fat stores only if the calorific content of the diet does not exceed the overall calorific expenditure of the individual. Therefore the level of physical activity and the diet both need to be considered. Depending upon the individual's circumstances, current dietary habits and the amount of fat which needs to be lost, a calorie-restrictive diet may not be essential to produce the desired reduction (Leon *et al.*, 1979). However, it is often argued that exercise alone will not reduce body fat levels, since it stimulates an increase in appetite which more than compensates for the calorific expenditure of the exercise. This appears to be an area of some controversy, a number of investigations indicating that there is little or no increase in calorific intake as a result of exercise (Katch, 1969) whilst others suggest that there is (Woo *et al.*, 1982a,b; Woo and Pi-Sunyer, 1985). A further consideration on this matter is that in some investigations it has been shown that, although non-obese individuals may tend to increase their calorific intake to compensate for the additional exercise, obese individuals do not. This would illustrate a very effective homeostatic control of calorific balance, which should result in an appropriate body composition. In addition, some authorities believe that exercise can enable obese individuals to become more 'sensitive' to their calorific needs and hence reduce their calorific intake (Allen and Quigley, 1977).

Another area of controversy and misconception concerns the topic of 'spot reduction': the idea that specific exercises can promote the reduction of body fat at specific sites around the body. One example is that of recommending sit-ups to reduce subcutaneous fat in the abdominal region. However, there is no conclusive evidence to support such ideas. During exercise the fat stores of the body may be used as an energy source. They are mobilised from the fat cells by the action of various hormones secreted from endocrine glands. These hormones travel around the body in the blood and hence can promote the utilisation of any fat stores that the blood passes through. Thus, fat stores that are some distance from the exercising muscle groups may be mobilised in the same way as those close to the exercising muscles. Therefore any exercise is likely to reduce the fat stores at numerous sites around the body, and not just close to the exercising muscles. However, whereas specific exercises may not reduce the fat stores around specific muscles they may well be effective in improving the general muscle tone of the muscles concerned and hence make an area of the body appear less 'flabby'. In summary, current research suggests that exercise has a *general* effect in reducing the fat stores of the body rather than specifically reducing the fat stores around the exercising muscles (Schade *et al.*, 1962; Noland and Kearney, 1978). This is supported by the work of Katch (1984) on the effects of sit-ups on fat reduction. To further dispel the misconceptions over spot reduction, Gwinap (1971) compared the dominant and non-dominant arms of high-level tennis players. Whilst the muscles of the dominant arm were significantly larger, as may be expected considering the additional work they perform, there was no significant difference in the skin fold thickness. Gwinap concluded that there was no difference in the amounts of fat stored in the highly exercised and less exercised arms.

A further factor to consider when discussing the topic of obesity is the difference between body composition and body weight. Body composition, or more specifically the percentage of the body that is fat, is the key issue rather than body weight. However, because it is easier to measure body weight than body composition this tends to be the measurement that concerns most individuals. Thus complications can occur when individuals, who may be extremely muscular with a very low percentage body fat, are classified as being 'overweight' according to height/weight charts. Conversely, and somewhat more commonly, a person may be of the correct weight, but in reality too much of that weight may be fat rather than lean tissue. For the exercise adviser the use of BMI has the same inherent problems.

Additional complications can occur when an individual diets. During some forms of excessive dieting much of the initial weight loss is due to reduction in muscle glycogen and water. This is not a healthy situation – and, indeed, most authorities would recommend that for most people a gradual reduction in weight (fat) of 0.5–1.0 kg (1–2 lb) per week is optimal. Therefore, whilst a reduction in weight may indicate a reduction in body fat levels it may not be a good indicator of the *actual* amount of fat lost. For this reason alternative means of estimating body composition may be employed. These include the use of hydrostatic weighing, body densitometry, anthropometric measurements (including skin fold thickness), radiography and various forms of technological instrumentation which use conductance, impedance and/or absorbance. By using these methods, monitoring of fat levels can be more precise and specific, helping to ensure healthy reduction in fat levels rather than inappropriate loss of lean tissue.

For those attempting to lose weight via diet only, while the initial loss in weight may be encouraging it may not significantly reduce the fat stores. It also has the undesirable effect of making them feel physically tired (owing to a lack of muscle glycogen) – and it is also temporary, since the water and muscle glycogen will be replenished once normal eating habits are resumed. Exercise promotes a reduction in the fat stores by increasing calorific expenditure, prevents reduction in metabolic rate (thereby aiding further fat loss) and conveys numerous other health benefits.

However, some additional care should be taken when prescribing exercise to excessively obese people because of their physical condition. Apart from their health-related problems, such as an increased risk of CHD, their lack of physical fitness may mean that they are not fit enough to exercise at an intensity and duration that is sufficient to use up a significant number of calories and hence reduce their fat stores. Exercise may still be included because of its health-promoting benefits and as a means of initiating long-term lifestyle changes, or it may be left out of the programme until some fat reduction has occurred because weight-bearing activities such as jogging could put an excessive strain on the joints. Non-weight-bearing activities such as swimming and/or cycling may be preferable. Work by Blair (1997) has demonstrated that, in terms of all-cause mortality risk, fitness and activity have an overriding effect over body composition. They discovered that the effects of a high BMI (>30), high body fat percentage (>25% in males) and large abdominal girth (>100 cm in males) are insignificant compared with the effects of fitness. These somewhat controversial findings showed that the risks in the high-fat group (high BMI, high percentage of body fat, large girth) were similar to those in the low-fat group (low BMI, low percentage of body fat, narrow girth) in similarly fit people but that low fitness doubled the risk of all-cause mortality in both groups.

It has been demonstrated that exercise adherence and compliance with recommended exercise programmes are much higher in supervised than in unsupervised programmes (MacKeen *et al.*, 1983). Therefore, for an exercise programme to be effective it should be carefully designed, monitored and supervised, with the exercise adviser being in regular contact with the participant.

Reviews of the research on the role of exercise in the prevention and treatment of moderate and severe obesity have been produced by Hill *et al.* (1994) and Atkinson and Walberg-Rankin (1994) respectively. Despite the controversies, the recent epidemiological work by Blair (1997) has clearly demonstrated that fitness reduces risk of CHD in obese individuals to below that of non-obese but unfit individuals.

INSIGHTS INTO OBESITY FROM EXERCISE PSYCHOLOGY

Whilst obesity is undoubtedly a health issue it should also be recognised that a 'desirable' body shape and size are culturally determined. In societies in which food is scarce and famine not unknown being overweight can be a sign of high social status and a sound insurance against future catastrophe. To appreciate how our concept of what constitutes a 'beautiful body' has changed over time visit a local art gallery and look at portraits painted in the seventeenth and eighteenth centuries. These clearly indicate that the wealthy 'supermodels' of the day were rather plump, and possibly obese. Whilst most sections of our society would appear to endorse the idea of weight control it is interesting to speculate whether these attitudes will change in the future and once again associate fat with beauty, wealth and health.

On a more practical note we would suggest that health professionals who work on obesity programmes may like to reflect and discuss with their colleagues the following questions.

What would it feel like to be diagnosed as obese?

If you reflect upon this question for even a short period of time it is not difficult to empathise with the emotional response of many patients when this word is applied to them. Obesity is one of those diagnoses that can have a 'social stigma' and may, quite wrongly, carry an assumption that the patient is lazy or slow. Health professionals who work on weight-control programmes must ensure that these stereotypes are challenged and should empower their patients to help build self-esteem and confidence.

Does exercise feel harder the heavier you are?

A simple practical experiment involving walking up a set of stairs carrying a 10 kg weight is usually enough to help most students answer this question and develop some empathy with those who suffer from obesity! This problem is not just related to carrying extra weight but also to thermoregulation (fat is a great insulator) and the chaffing of skin surfaces which rub together during movement. Many of these problems can be overcome through the prescription of non-weight-bearing activities, the use of the rating of perceived exertion and feeling scales, and advice on clothing and the use of lubricants such as Vaseline.

Have most people who suffer from obesity tried to lose weight before?

The answer to this question is almost invariably yes, but they have usually either failed to lose weight on these previous attempts or (more likely) have failed to maintain that weight loss. This may cause the client to attribute being overweight to factors over which they have no control ('all my family are fat – it is just the way we are') and to lose perceived behavioural control ('every time I try to do more exercise I end up dropping out – so what's the point in trying again?'). To tackle these issues health professionals need to focus on process goals (e.g. walking 10 minutes extra every day) rather than outcome goals (losing weight). This may mean that the programme moves away from measuring weight and body composition to rewarding distance walked and new activities.

EXERCISE AND STROKE

Stroke is one of the major causes of death and disability in Europe and the USA. Its causes are cerebral infarctions or cerebral haemorrhages. Typically a *cerebral infarction* is caused by a thrombus in the cerebral microcirculation, extracranial carotid system or within an intracranial artery. An embolus originating from the heart or extracranial carotid system can also cause the blockage (Wolf and Kanel, 1986). With this form of stroke the blood, and

hence oxygen supply, to the brain becomes restricted and if the deprivation of oxygen to the brain cells is prolonged the cells will die and brain functions will be interfered with, resulting in disability. Cerebral infarction is therefore also known as an *ischaemic stroke*. Other terms for this type of event include cerebrovascular accident or brain infarction. The fundamental causes of ischaemic stroke are therefore the formation of thrombi and atheroma and, by implication, the risk factors associated with their development.

A stroke may also be caused by the bursting of an artery supplying the brain (a *cerebral haemorrhage*). As a consequence of this haemorrhage the cells normally supplied by the artery are deprived of oxygen and may die. Hypertension is believed to be a key risk factor for this type of stroke. Some people may have an increased risk of haemorrhagic stroke if they have weak areas in their cranial arteries (aneurysms).

A stroke can have a number of effects. These may be temporary or permanent, with the degree of severity varying with the area of brain damaged. The effects can include paralysis of one side of the body (hemiparesis), loss of memory and a reduction in the ability to communicate.

In general, the risk factors associated with a stroke are the same as those for CHD (high blood pressure, smoking, age, poor blood lipid profile) and therefore behavioural factors that can reduce the risk of CHD, such as physical activity, are also likely to reduce the risk of stroke. Paffenbarger *et al.* (1984) and Salonen *et al.* (1982) presented evidence to this effect, with the major benefits being reduction of blood pressure and improvement in blood cholesterol profiles. However, the number of published studies which specifically investigate the link between physical activity and the incidence of stroke is limited.

The effects of a stroke may be partially or fully reversible. As with many disorders, the level of activity of stroke victims is commonly reduced. Some sufferers may not be able to participate in exercise because of the severity of their disorder. However, for those who do it reduces the risk of a further attack, improves physical capacity (affecting quality of life and independence), reduces risk of other hypokinetic diseases and improves mental state. Exercise programmes should be designed in consultation with the individual's medical team. General exercise prescription guidelines will be influenced by the individual's overall condition. Clinical sessions concentrating upon redevelopment of movement patterns and co-ordination will be necessary and low to moderate-intensity aerobic activities are generally recommended along with stretching and strengthening exercises.

INSIGHTS FOR EXERCISE PSYCHOLOGY INTO STROKE

It should be recognised that exercise psychology is a relatively new area of study and that most of the published work related to specific conditions clusters around CHD, obesity and mental illness. It is thus difficult to make any definite recommendations on how best to use exercise as part of the rehabilitation process for stroke patients. However, it is possible to make some general comments, which may encourage readers to watch for developments in this area of work or even to contribute through their own research and professional practise. A useful starting point is the following quote from the charity Different Strokes: 'many of us [stroke patients] have had no previous experience of serious illness, making the serious after effects of a stroke even more difficult to deal with. We find it very hard to relate to ourselves as "ill" people, let alone disabled in some way' (Different Strokes. The Invisible Side of Strokes). Implicit within this statement is the knowledge that strokes do not just happen to 'old people' but to individuals across the age range. Sport and physical recreation may have been an important part of the social life and sense of identity of some stroke sufferers, for whom exercise may be important

in the management and rehabilitation of their condition and may provide them with important social contact and an opportunity to continue the leisure pursuits they enjoyed before their stroke. Wake (1998) reported on innovative work by exercise leaders at the YMCA (London) with stroke patients; it would appear that exercise can help to develop confidence and a sense of general well-being.

EXERCISE AND DIABETES MELLITUS

Diabetes mellitus is found in both adults and children. It is a complex disease with many side-effects. The primary effects of the disease include failure to control blood sugar levels and inability to store glucose in the form of muscle or liver glycogen. Further problems include increased risk of atherosclerosis, hypertension, stroke, kidney dysfunction, neuropathies (autonomic and peripheral) and retinopathies due to microvascular disease. Diabetes therefore has implications for both the quality of life and longevity.

Glucose circulates in the blood, via which it is delivered to actively metabolising tissues. The brain and all parts of the nervous system require a constant supply of glucose (and at rest they account for approximately 80% of the body's glucose requirements). During exercise, although the brain and nervous system continue to require glucose, an even greater requirement occurs in the skeletal muscles. Glucose enters the body in the form of dietary carbohydrate, which, given the sporadic nature of meals, is an irregular supply. Despite the erratic supply and utilisation of blood glucose its concentration must be regulated within fairly narrow limits. Levels are kept stable after a meal by storing excess as glycogen, mainly in the skeletal muscles. This prevents blood glucose levels from becoming too high (hyperglycaemia). During fasting, to prevent blood glucose levels declining to below permissible levels the liver releases glucose back into the blood, thereby preventing the levels becoming too low (hypoglycaemia).

Glucose storage and use is primarily under the control of the hormone insulin. Failure to produce appropriate amounts of insulin and/or failure of the tissues to respond to its presence (insulin resistance or reduced insulin sensitivity) are the defining characteristics of diabetes mellitus.

There are two basic types of diabetes mellitus. The first is caused by the destruction of the β cells of the pancreas, which normally produce insulin. As a result the sufferer is unable to produce this hormone in sufficient amounts. Such an individual is dependent upon regular injections of insulin, usually a combination of short-acting and sustained-release insulin injected subcutaneously twice a day, the exact dose depending on the individual. This form of diabetes is referred to as insulin-dependent diabetes mellitus (IDDM). It most commonly appears during childhood and is therefore sometimes referred to as juvenile, primary or type 1 diabetes.

The second form of diabetes mellitus is known as non-insulin-dependent diabetes mellitus (NIDDM). Individuals with this condition are capable of producing insulin, but it is less effective than it should be. Insulin secretion from the β cells of the pancreas may be affected to a greater or lesser degree, resulting in elevated, reduced or normal levels of insulin. However, a key characteristic of the disorder is reduced sensitivity of the liver and skeletal muscles to insulin, which affects their responses to it and hence their ability to store glucose. Individuals with NIDDM also have a tendency for an increased basal production of glucose from the liver, which results in higher fasting levels of blood glucose (fasting hyperglycaemia). So, whilst the NIDDM individual's muscles have a reduced capacity to store glucose and subsequently to utilise glycogen, they may have fasting blood glucose levels of >7.7 mmol l^{-1} (140 mg per 100 ml blood). They will also have elevated plasma glucose levels during an oral glucose tolerance test. In a glucose tolerance test an individual consumes a prescribed amount of glucose (usually

50–100 g) and their blood glucose concentration is monitored over several hours. In normal individuals blood glucose concentrations will be maintained within acceptable limits, reaching a peak of about 7 mmol l^{-1} (125 mg per 100 ml) 30 minutes after ingestion of 50 g of glucose and falling to about 4 mmol l^{-1} (75 mg per 100 ml) at the 2 hour point. This indicates that the pancreas has secreted adequate insulin and that the peripheral tissues have responded by promoting the uptake of the additional glucose. In individuals with an impaired response the glucose is not stored at the required rate and so accumulates within the blood, causing hyperglycaemia. In an oral glucose tolerance test a diabetic's blood glucose level may exceed 11 mmol l^{-1} (200 mg per 100 ml) within 30 minutes of ingesting the glucose and remains high for several hours. This type of diabetes more commonly occurs later in life and is therefore also known as secondary, maturity-onset, or type 2 diabetes.

An intermediate condition, called 'impaired glucose tolerance', exists. In this condition there is a partial failure in glucose regulation due to a partial loss of insulin sensitivity within the skeletal muscles, but this is not of a level to be classified as diabetes mellitus. It is characterised by high fasting blood glucose levels (6.4–7.7 mmol l^{-1}) and higher than normal levels of circulating insulin (hyperinsulinaemia). Individuals with impaired glucose tolerance appear to have an increased risk of NIDDM and it is therefore a condition which should be monitored.

A diabetic's inability to store glucose following consumption of a meal containing large amounts of carbohydrate causes the level of glucose in their blood to rise rapidly. At very high blood glucose concentrations the kidneys are unable to reabsorb all the glucose from the blood that passes through them, and the glucose is excreted in the urine. The failure to store glycogen also means that the individual has a very limited supply of glucose available between meals. In patients with IDDM the lack of stored glycogen means that glucose cannot be released back into the blood as the blood glucose levels fall, which can result in a state of hypoglycaemia and certain metabolic disturbances (of key importance is the supply of glucose to the brain and nervous system). A severe hypoglycaemic condition stimulates the incomplete breakdown of certain fats into ketones to provide energy. This production of ketones alters the acidic balance of the body, which in extreme cases can induce a diabetic coma that can be fatal.

Diabetes mellitus is linked with additional health complications. The incidence of CHD in diabetics is 2–3 times higher than in the non-diabetic population. NIDDM is associated with an increased incidence of other CHD risk factors such as obesity, hypertension and lipid abnormalities. Other problems include neuropathies (autonomic and peripheral) and effects upon the blood vessels within the eye, causing proliferative retinopathy. Insulin resistance co-exists with several other metabolic risk factors, which as a cluster may be referred to as metabolic syndrome, Syndrome X or Reaven syndrome (Maheux *et al.*, 1994; Reaven 1994; Reaven and Laws 1994). These risk factors include compensatory hyperinsulaemia, glucose intolerance, high triacylglycerol levels, low levels of HDL cholesterol and hypertension; all of which are linked to atheroma formation. Consequently the overall benefits of exercise for the diabetic are enhanced insulin sensitivity, which improves lipid and glucose metabolism; this, coupled with increased HDL cholesterol levels and generally improved blood lipid profiles, results in reduced atherogenic tendencies.

A more recently identified effect of insulin is its role in acutely vasodilating skeletal muscle: the blood flow to the muscles is impaired in patients lacking insulin (Laakso *et al.* 1990, 1992). However, the exact implications of this have yet to be elucidated.

BENEFITS OF EXERCISE FOR IDDM

IDDM is treated by careful control of diet and regular injections of insulin. In addition, exercise can improve an individual's sensitivity to insulin (Rodnick *et al.*, 1987): this can help in the control of the disorder and enable the insulin-dependent diabetic to substantially reduce the daily amount of insulin they require. However, the long-term implications remain uncertain, although the benefits of reducing the incidence of CHD are supported by strong research evidence (Giacca *et al.*, 1994). Exercise-induced improvements in insulin sensitivity or reduced insulin resistance are believed to be linked to changes in the skeletal muscles. Skeletal muscle adaptations to chronic exercise programmes include increased muscular capillarisation and blood flow, enhanced glucose transport systems across the muscle fibre membrane, and increases in the enzymes associated with glucose storage. All of these will enhance glucose uptake by the skeletal muscles.

For the patient with IDDM who has no additional complications, exercise has numerous benefits. Planned exercise programmes are usually desirable as they enable careful adjustments in insulin injections and timing, along with control over exercise type, duration and intensity (American Diabetes Association, 1990). Owing to individual variations it is not possible to produce definitive exercise prescriptions here, but programmes should be based upon general recommendations concerning diet and insulin therapy. Overall the American Diabetic Association's Position Statement states 'A uniform recommendation for preventing hypoglycemia and improving metabolic response to exercise cannot be made. Rather, self monitoring of blood glucose should be incorporated into the exercise program to provide the glycemic information necessary to adjust the patient's diet or insulin dosage.'

For several hours after exercise there is a tendency for diabetics with IDDM to experience hypoglycaemia. This is believed to be caused by increased sensitivity to insulin and the increase in muscle uptake of glucose for glycogen synthesis following its depletion during the exercise (Vranic *et al.*, 1990; Giacca *et al.*, 1991).

EXERCISE IN PREVENTION AND AMELIORATION OF NIDDM

The incidence of NIDDM is estimated to be 3–7% of the adult population and primarily affects older individuals. World-wide it accounts for hundreds of thousands of deaths annually and causes disability in millions. Factors contributing to its incidence include genetic and environmental influences. The disorder varies in severity and exact expression of symptoms but generally it appears to progress from an impaired glucose tolerance, which may not have been diagnosed, to impaired β cell function and/or insulin resistance, which may reach sufficient severity to be classified as NIDDM (Wallberg-Henriksson *et al.*, 1998). Inactivity, obesity and stress all appear to be influential risk factors that can be modified by behavioural changes to prevent and treat NIDDM. Whilst there is an increase in the incidence of NIDDM with age it is unclear whether this is due to age in itself or to the other risk factors such as obesity and inactivity that become more prevalent with age (Zavaroni *et al.*, 1986). Current treatment of the disease focuses on management of the diet, use of sulphonylurea drugs to lower fasting plasma glucose levels and (in some cases) administration of insulin to promote β-cell responses to glucose. Treatment may be supported by an exercise programme that increases the insulin sensitivity of skeletal muscles and reduces associated health problems. Evidence is now accumulating for the role of exercise in preventing the incidence of insulin resistance, impaired glucose tolerance and NIDDM (Ivy 1997); a growing body of evidence supports the benefits of exercise in alleviating these conditions.

Aerobic exercise can play an important role in preventing and/or controlling NIDDM by reducing an individual's weight – or, more specifically, their percentage of body fat. This is believed to be important because obese individuals appear to be more at risk of developing NIDDM (over 80% of type 2 diabetics are obese; National Diabetes Data Group, 1979). Exercise also helps to reduce blood pressure and normalise dyslipoproteinaemia as well as increasing insulin sensitivity, thereby ameliorating some of the problems. Research has demonstrated improved insulin sensitivity through training (Ruderman *et al.*, 1979); however, this response starts to be lost within 5–7 days of the last bout of exercise, which emphasises the importance of regular frequent exercise (Dela *et al.*, 1995). Strengthening exercises are also believed to be important in reducing the risk of NIDDM in people over 50 years of age because the maintenance of muscle mass is thought to help prevent the impairment of glucose tolerance.

Exercise greatly reduces the risk of developing NIDDM (Helmrich *et al.*, 1991; Manson *et al.*, 1991), both in high-risk groups (where the subjects exhibit a combination of obesity and a family history of diabetes) and in low-risk groups (non-obese and with no family history of diabetes). In these studies a good level of fitness has been linked to very substantial decreases in the risk of NIDDM.

The acute responses to exercise of a diabetic are generally a more pronounced decline in blood glucose levels than that observed in non-diabetics (where little change is seen). Conversely, a hyperglycaemic state is observed in some individuals following exercise; this is believed to be due to an exaggerated compensatory response. The long-term benefits of exercise to the individual with NIDDM include improved metabolic control of the condition (Zierath and Wallberg-Henriksson, 1992; Friedman *et al.*, 1992). This may be linked to reductions in body fat and associated improvements in peripheral insulin sensitivity which may be attributable to an increase in the number of insulin receptors (Olefsky and Reaven 1974; Olefsky 1976). Further benefits include improvements in blood lipid profiles (reducing VLDL-cholesterol and increasing

HDL-cholesterol) and reductions in blood pressure, which will reduce the risk of CHD. Since high levels of circulating free fatty acids stimulates hepatic glucose production, exercise-induced improvements in their regulation may also contribute to the lowering of basal hepatic glucose production and hence reducing fasting hyperglycaemia (Ivy 1997).

SPECIFIC CONSIDERATIONS FOR PREVENTION AND TREATMENT OF DIABETES MELLITUS

The increased incidence of CHD amongst people with IDDM prompted some authorities to recommend that an exercise ECG is taken before commencing an exercise programme, especially in older adults. The severity of the disorder and complicating factors may preclude some diabetics from exercising. However, many should be encouraged to exercise because of its diverse benefits upon general health and its specific implications for their condition. The general recommendations for a health-based exercise prescription are similar to those for general health, with additional implications for obese individuals with NIDDM who are trying to lose weight: exercise frequency of 5–7 times per week, with aerobic activities being performed at 50–70% VO_{2max} and resistance training with light weights (Braun *et al.*, 1995; Howley and Franks 1997). Diabetics participating in sport will adjust their training regimes in accordance with the demands of the sport and their capabilities.

A key issue whilst exercising is the prevention of hypoglycaemia and exercise advisers as well as patients need to be aware of the symptoms (sweating, feeling weak, difficulty in concentrating, dizziness, trembling, visual disturbances, and feeling drunk). Many of these symptoms occur in non-diabetics who are approaching a hypoglycaemic state and/or glycogen depletion. The remedy is the ingestion of rapidly assimilated carbohydrate, preferably preceded by a blood glucose check if this does not involve a prohibitive delay.

Although exercise may benefit the diabetic, the nature of the disorder requires that specific precautions are taken. The American College of Sports Medicine, (1991) recommend that before undertaking an exercise programme an individual with NIDDM should be screened for ischaemic heart disease, hypertension, proliferative retinopathy, microalbuminuria and peripheral and/or autonomic neuropathies. When exercising the following points should be considered:

1. The blood sugar level should be normal before commencing an exercise session. Exercise should be postponed and insulin taken if blood glucose levels exceed 16.5 mmol l^{-1} and food should be taken if blood glucose levels are below 4 mmol l^{-1} (Giacca *et al.*, 1994).

2. A supply of sugar should be available during exercise. This is especially important during prolonged forms of exercise when blood sugar levels are most likely to become depleted.

3. A diabetic should try to ensure that they do not exercise alone, in case they become hypoglycaemic.

4. When exercising, the person accompanying a diabetic should be aware of the condition and know what to do in the event of collapse.

5. Carbohydrate may be consumed 20–30 minutes before exercise (1 g per minute of vigorous exercise) and intake should be repeated every 30–60 minutes during prolonged exercise (approximately 40 g per hour). A further 15–30 g should be taken after exercise to prevent post-exercise hypoglycaemia (Lefèbvre *et al.*, 1986).

6. Exercising 1–3 hours after a meal is generally recommended. Insulin intake may be reduced by 30–50% if a post-meal bout of prolonged exercise is planned (Sonnenberg *et al.*, 1990).

7. Patients using an insulin regimen of one or

two injections daily should not exercise at the peak time of insulin action.

8. Exercising earlier in the day is recommended to avoid hypoglycaemia at night (Giacca *et al.*, 1994).

If a diabetic does feel hypoglycaemic (or collapses) during exercise, sugar should be taken (or given) immediately in order to restore the blood glucose levels. Most diabetics are fully aware of their condition and the symptoms they should look out for. Therefore, provided that they adhere to these additional safety aspects, diabetics should be able to exercise in the same manner as non-diabetics and gain all the desired health-related benefits.

For individuals with diabetic complications there are specific considerations, which include the following (Giacca *et al.*, 1994; Gudart *et al.*, 1994):

1. Patients with proliferative retinopathy should not perform isometric weightlifting, exercises which involve the Valsalva manoeuvre, exercises which require a head-down position or head-jarring exercises.

2. Patients with peripheral neuropathy should not perform exercise which involves jarring impact to the lower extremities, such as jogging. The lack of sensitivity of the foot may allow injury to occur due to the lack of neurological afferent feedback. Such people should always use well cushioned footwear when exercising and check for abrasions, blisters and pressure marks on their feet.

3. Patients with autonomic neuropathy should exercise in a comfortable environment which minimises the risk of dehydration and homeostatic imbalances. Other problems include bouts of hypotension and a reduced maximal heart rate. Activities such as swimming are feasible for such individuals because it promotes venous return.

In summary, exercise may reduce the incidence of NIDDM (Helmrich *et al.*, 1991; Manson *et al.*, 1991) by its effects upon insulin sensitivity and weight control (Heath *et al.*, 1987). It can help with regulation of the condition and (as per the non-diabetic population) can reduce the risk of CHD, which has a higher prevalence in diabetics. General recommendations are for moderate-intensity exercise which can be incorporated as a regular component of the lifestyle (Wallberg-Henriksson *et al.*, 1998), although the review by Ivy (1997) indicates that prolonged, vigorous aerobic exercise training protocols have more favourable physiological results. The benefits of resistance training, which prevents muscle atrophy and stimulates muscle growth, thereby improving glucose tolerance, are also strongly advocated by Ivy (1997) and Miller *et al.* (1984). Further recommendations include adjusting food intake and insulin doses in accordance with the exercise demands, avoiding dehydration, wearing the correct footwear and daily foot inspections (Wallberg-Henriksson *et al.*, 1998).

EXERCISE AND OSTEOPOROSIS

Osteoporosis is 'a disease characterised by low bone mass and microarchitectural deterioration of bone tissue leading to enhanced bone fragility and a consequent increase in fracture risk' (Drinkwater, 1994). It occurs in men, women and children, but is most common in women, particularly following the menopause (Smith *et al.*, 1990). According to the National Osteoporosis Society it can affect one in three women and surveys by Looker *et al.* (1995) and Melton (1995) suggest that it can affect one in five women over the age of 50 years.

Osteoporosis occurs when minerals such as calcium are gradually lost from the bone, making it weak, brittle and vulnerable to fracture. It is a major health problem and is thought to contribute to over a million fractures a year, commonly wrist, spine and hip fractures. Some of these fractures can cause serious permanent disability; hip fractures are estimated to result in fatality in 20% of cases (Ray *et al.*, 1990). Other effects of osteoporosis include loss of height, curvature of the spine and chronic back pain.

Contributing factors are a diet deficient in vitamin D and/or calcium, inactivity and (in women) low levels of the oestrogen hormones, which may be due to the menopause or amenorrhoea. The reduced oestrogen levels increase the risk of calcium loss from the bone. Much of the initial concern about osteoporosis has focused upon older, post-menopausal women; however, younger amenorrhoeic women are also at considerable risk, particularly if they have not attained a high bone mineral density, which means that they could be vulnerable throughout their lives (Erikson and Sevier 1997).

EXERCISE FOR PREVENTION OF OSTEOPOROSIS

In healthy individuals on a diet containing adequate calcium and vitamin D who are undertaking appropriate levels of exercise, bone density should increase to a peak in the late twenties and early thirties. Following this, bone density declines by about 7% in the lumbar spine and 16% at the neck of the femur by the age of 50 years (Drinkwater, 1993).

Bone, like other tissues of the body, is capable of adapting to the physical stresses placed upon it and, conversely, is liable to regress and become weak if unused. Active individuals exhibit greater skeletal mass than inactive people of the same stature. Significant losses in bone density are observed in those who are bedridden for some time, and are also experienced by astronauts in zero gravity.

The role of exercise in preventing osteoporosis has received considerable attention and is one of the advertised benefits of exercise for all adults – particularly women, for whom it is advocated as a means of maximising bone density before age-related losses occur, thereby minimising the risk of it falling to undesirably low levels later in life. However, if an individual is already suffering from osteoporosis exercise prescription becomes more problematic, as it needs to promote mineral retention without subjecting the weakened bones to a level of stress that will cause them to fracture.

In healthy non-osteoporotic individuals exercise promotes favourable adaptations to the pressure on the bone in weight-bearing forms of activity and the stresses placed upon the bone when the muscles attached to it contract. Some researchers also suggest that the electrical activity generated by the exercise is beneficial.

The effects of exercise on the strength of the skeleton begin in childhood, and it is generally considered that skeletal strength peaks between the late teens and early thirties. Appropriate exercise during adult life should help to maintain this strength, enhance it if the skeleton is already weak, or at least attenuate the usually observed decline associated with ageing. However, as with other adaptations to exercise, the observed effects are related to the principles of training, including that of specificity, such that non-weight-bearing activities such as swimming appear to have little effect on bone density. Therefore, young adults should be encouraged to participate in weight-bearing activities such as walking and related exercise which involves a moderate amount of impact. It is important to recall the specificity of adaptations: leg exercises are unlikely to improve the density of the bones in the upper limbs (Brewer, *et al.*, 1983) and should be supplemented with additional resistance work which, research suggests, provides some positive benefits (Heffron *et al.*, 1997). However, the research in this area is equivocal; some report benefits upon bone mineral density (Dalsky *et al.*, 1988), others do not (Gleeson *et al.*, 1990). Howley and Franks (1997) suggest performing a variety of upper body exercises with a regime of 3–6 sets of 10 repetitions, although sets of higher intensity and lower repetitions could also be tried. Whether this will improve bone mineral density or whether the benefits will be confined to improved muscular strength remain to be resolved.

Further benefits of exercise on the musculo-skeletal system include the strengthening of tendons, ligaments and their points of attachment to bones, all of which help to ensure an overall healthy physical condition. Exercises that improve muscular strength, flexibility and co-ordination can help to prevent falls, which is particularly important in the incidence of osteoporotic fractures in elderly people. The American College of Sports Medicine position statement on osteoporosis and exercise (1995) concludes that exercise is beneficial to bone health as well as general health. However, they also state that much research evidence is cross-sectional (active people exhibit better bone health than sedentary people) rather than longitudinal (demonstrating clinically and functionally significant improvements in bone health and a reduction in osteoporotic fractures via the commencement of exercise programmes) and at present there is no conclusive evidence to suggest that exercise can be used as an alternative to hormone replacement therapy in postmenopausal women.

In summary, exercise throughout life is believed to be important in reducing the risk of osteoporosis, although, according to Drinkwater (1994), further research is required to clarify the exact role.

EXERCISE IN THE TREATMENT OF OSTEOPOROSIS

Exercise is not a cure for osteoporosis, but it may be used in conjunction with other treatments such as hormone replacement therapy. For middle-aged and older adults whose bones are already weak, it is important for the prescribed exercise programme to progress gradually: increasing the volume of exercise too rapidly can increase the risk of osteoporotic fractures, especially to the metatarsals (Shephard, 1994). Walking, moderate-impact activities and resistance training can prevent further calcium loss (American College of Sports Medicine, 1993) and may improve bone mass, although some authorities question whether increases in bone mineral density are possible (American College of Sports Medicine, 1995; Brooks *et al.*, 1996).

EXERCISE, OSTEOPOROSIS AND THE ACTIVE/ATHLETIC WOMAN

The link between exercise, low body fat and amenorrhoea has specific osteoporotic implications for the woman involved in hard training, particularly activities associated with a restricted diet such as gymnastics, dancing or endurance running. This is sometimes known as the 'female athlete's triad' of hard training, restricted diet and low body fat, which reduces oestrogen levels and causes amenorrhoea. This combination may weaken the skeleton to the extent that the impact of hard training is more than can be tolerated by the bones and instead of promoting bone strength it will contribute to fractures.

It is it is ironic that, although exercise has positive benefits upon bone health, the extreme levels of training undertaken by some athletes may actually contribute towards osteoporosis. The coach, exercise adviser, therapist and medical practitioner should be aware of this possibility amongst this group of individuals. In some cases oestrogens may be prescribed to combat the potential effects of hard exercise upon bone density and, hence, the risk of osteoporosis in later life.

GENERAL RECOMMENDATIONS

The American College of Sports Medicine's (1995) position statement on exercise and osteoporosis makes five key points:

1. weight-bearing exercise is essential for the development and maintenance of a healthy skeleton;
2. strength training may be beneficial for non-weight-bearing bones;
3. for the sedentary, an increase in activity may prevent further loss of bone minerals

and may even cause some increase in bone density;

4. exercise is not a substitute for post-menopausal hormone replacement therapy; and

5. an exercise programme for the older woman should include exercises for strength, flexibility and co-ordination as these will reduce the risk of falls and consequently lessen the risk of fractures (Erickson and Sevier, 1997).

EXERCISE AND ARTHRITIS

The term 'arthritis' means joint inflammation. The many types of arthritis can be grouped into two general categories: *osteoarthritis* and *rheumatoid arthritis*. Osteoarthritis is characterised by a physical degeneration of the articular cartilage which is linked to ageing and physical trauma. Rheumatoid arthritis is an autoimmune disease characterised by inflammation of the synovial membrane, swelling of the joint and deterioration of the articular cartilage. In severe cases it can also affect the underlying bone.

EXERCISE AND RHEUMATOID ARTHRITIS

Rheumatoid arthritis is a chronic inflammatory disease which can affect the cardiovascular system, lungs, peripheral nerves, tendons and muscles as well as the joints (Shephard, 1994). Typically, the sufferer will experience phases of inflammation and general deterioration that may be separated by bouts of remission during which the symptoms are greatly reduced. During severe phases of inflammation exercise is not recommended as it can lead to a more severe inflammatory response and joint damage. However, during remission exercise should be encouraged (Ike *et al.*, 1989). In a longitudinal study, Nordemar *et al.* (1981) demonstrated that exercise minimised the degenerative changes and reduced the risk of the hypokinetic problems that were observed in sufferers who did not

participate in an exercise regimen. Indeed, immobility appears to worsen the condition (Spector 1990) and prolonged bedrest can result in muscular atrophy, loss of strength and contracture of soft tissues and tendons. Therefore, when their condition permits, sufferers should be encouraged to participate in exercises which help to retain their joint range of motion. They should also participate in aerobic activities such as swimming and, if possible, moderate-impact activities such as walking to help retain bone density. Light resistance training which does not aggravate the affected joints is also recommended.

For the rheumatic arthritic participation in exercise will convey various other benefits: enhancement of mental state, provision of a social activity, an increased tolerance to pain, increased ability to maintain independence and general improvement in quality of life.

EXERCISE AND OSTEOARTHRITIS

Osteoarthritis affects 30–40% of adults aged over 60 years (Hadler, 1985). Its causes may be primary (age-related and more common in diabetics and the obese) or secondary (related to a previous joint injury) (Eriksson *et al.*, 1990). Whilst there is some epidemiological data to indicate that a previous joint injury, such as damage to the knee, may increase the risk of later osteoarthritis, the belief that exercise in itself increases the risk of osteoarthritis is refuted by epidemiological evidence (Lane *et al.*, 1986; Panush and Brown 1987). The persistence of this misconception may be perpetuated by reports in the media of former athletes suffering from osteoarthritis – no attention is given to former athletes who never suffer from the disease, or to the many sedentary individuals who do.

The joints most commonly affected by osteoarthritis are the hip and knee. Therefore general exercise regimens, fitness training and sporting activities which do not increase the risk of traumatic joint injuries are not associated with an increased incidence of osteoarthritis (Bouchard *et al.*, 1993; Fries *et al.*, 1994; Kujala *et al.*, 1995; Newton *et al.*, 1997). The development of osteoarthritis after a joint injury is believed to be linked to the limited repair capacity of the articular cartilage. This can result in the formation of fibrocartilage, bony spurs and adhesions in the surrounding membranes and ligaments which can reduce joint mobility (Howley and Franks, 1997). If the joint is not used fully additional adhesions can develop, reducing the ease of movement still further. Flexibility and general joint-loosening exercises which utilise a full range of movement are advocated for osteoporotic individuals (Brooks *et al.* 1996).

It is common for patients with arthritis to be encouraged to assume a less active lifestyle, and their painful joints will often reinforce this tendency. Consequently they become more susceptible to the deleterious effects: loss of strength, joint mobility, cardiovascular fitness, weight gain and an increased risk of numerous hypokinetic diseases (DiNubile, 1997a). These adverse changes will all affect the individual's independence and quality of life. A particular effect of reduced activity in osteoarthritic patients is reduced production of proteoglycans within the joint. It is suggested that this decline may cause a more rapid degeneration of the joint (Howell and Manicourt, 1988). The osteoarthritic individual may become trapped in the downward spiral of osteoarthritis, inactivity, loss of mobility and independence, leading to further reductions in activity, etc. and the exercise adviser may need to reverse this trend by applying the physiological and psychological principles of exercise prescription.

Given the nature of arthritis it is prudent for the exercise adviser to confirm the client's capacity to exercise with their medical practitioner. Passive mobility exercises can be utilised with (if appropriate) resistance exercises and water-based activities. Land-based activities such as cycling and walking are possible, depending upon the individual, but exercises involving significant amounts of jar-

ring and impact should be avoided. When prescribing exercise for people with arthritis, it is essential to ensure that the activity does not aggravate the condition and cause additional pain. Therefore it is important to carefully monitor the patient's sensations during particular exercises and adjust the programmes as necessary. This is particularly important during phases of the condition when the inflammation may be more aggressive than usual. The general maxim 'appropriate exercise is beneficial to health, whereas inappropriate exercise can be detrimental to health' can be applied whilst reinforcing the importance of individualising an exercise regimen to each person's condition.

Exercise has been shown to improve the condition of osteoarthritic joints. This is believed to be because it enhances the supply of nutrients to the joint and stimulates its general maintenance. It will also help to maintain the strength of the stabilising structures around the joint, thereby enhancing its resilience and reducing the risk of further injury. Exercise will have more general additional benefits, such as helping to minimise weight gain and retaining physical capacity by maintenance of muscle strength and aerobic fitness. It may also reduce the sensation of pain (Kovar *et al.*, 1992).

Choosing a mode of exercise that does not irritate the condition should be possible for most individuals. For example swimming, cycling, walking and/or upper-body ergometry should all convey aerobic and cardiovascular health benefits. One of the specific problems associated with arthritis is the development of contractures, which are a result of a shortening of the muscles, tendons and other joint structures. Stretching and loosening exercises may help to prevent these and/or reduce their severity.

The American College of Rheumatology recommends exercises similar to those given to most individuals. They identify the need to include aerobic/cardiovascular exercise, resistance/muscular strengthening exercises and flexibility/joint mobility work, and recommend that some exercises should focus on specific joints (DiNubile, 1997b). The recommendations for duration, frequency, intensity and recovery are similar to those for non-arthritic people, but additionally suggest avoidance of high-impact exercises if the weight-bearing joints are severely damaged.

EXERCISE AND CHRONIC OBSTRUCTIVE PULMONARY DISEASES

The term chronic obstructive pulmonary disease (COPD) includes a range of conditions from asthma and simple bronchitis to chronic obstructive bronchitis and emphysema. All are characterised by an obstruction to the airways which restricts the flow of air in and out of the lungs. This will manifest with a combination of the following factors, the values for which will depend upon the severity of the disorder: reduced vital capacity (VC), forced expiratory volume in one second ($FEV_{1.0}$) and forced expiratory flow rates (FEF) at 25% and 75% of the FEV (American College of Sports Medicine, 1993). More extensive lung function tests which assess pressures and diffusion capacities are used to classify the disorders and quantify the condition. Given its common occurrence, a separate section will be devoted to the discussion of asthma.

For most individuals the capacity of the lungs to take in oxygen is not a limiting factor in the ability to perform physical activities. However, individuals with COPD may be unable to ventilate sufficient air, which may indeed be the constraining limitation on physical capacity.

CHRONIC OBSTRUCTIVE BRONCHITIS AND EMPHYSEMA

Chronic asthmatic bronchitis, chronic obstructive bronchitis and emphysema are all debilitating diseases and some can be fatal, especially emphysema, in which gas exchange is impaired due to destruction of the alveolar capillary membranes (over 50% of sufferers are likely to die within 10 years). Chronic bronchitis is almost always associated with tobacco smoking. It is characterised by an inflammation of the small airways and increased sputum production, reduced ciliary function and consequently coughing and wheezing. The breathing difficulties in chronic bronchitis result in inadequate ventilation of the alveoli (hypoventilation) and perfusion of blood through the lungs, causing a reduced partial pressure of oxygen in the blood. Persistent chronic obstructive bronchitis may deteriorate into emphysema.

Emphysema is usually linked with heavy smoking or similar environmental conditions, although it is occasionally caused by a genetic defect. The disease is characterised by progressive destruction of the alveoli, which reduces the surface area for gas exchange. As the disease progresses it causes increased pressure in the pulmonary arteries (pulmonary hypertension). This, coupled with fibrosis and atherosclerosis, results in right heart failure (Brooks *et al.*, 1996). Individuals with this condition therefore experience severe breathing difficulties. To assist with their breathing they use accessory muscles; consequently they develop chest deformities.

The abnormal condition of the lungs of many individuals with COPD results in a greater 'dead space' than normal. Consequently, a greater minute ventilation is required to achieve normal aeration of the alveoli. Sufferers also tend to breathe rapidly and shallowly in response to reduced inspiratory and expiratory flow rates.

Individuals with COPD will almost inevitably have a low physical capacity and experience dyspnoea (shortness of breath) even at rest. The dyspnoea associated with these disorders makes exercise prescription a sensitive issue and pre-exercise programme clearance should be obtained from the client's medical consultant. It is also possible that the exercise specialist will need to work in combination with other health professionals such as physiotherapists and occupational therapists, and may often operate in a clinical setting.

There are a number of 'triggers' which can make a COPD sufferer's breathing even more difficult. These include cigarette smoke, respiratory infections and air pollutants. Therefore the exercise adviser should endeavour to ensure that their client is not exposed to these triggers. The aims of an exercise programme will be to alleviate the condition as well as convey the usual health benefits of exercise to the participant. Cardiovascular health and fitness will improve through the adaptations previously described for this form of exercise; in addition exercise capacity will be increased, ventilation for a given oxygen consumption reduced (improved $\dot{V}O_2/\dot{V}E$ ratio), dyspnoea reduced and maximal oxygen consumption increased. The general increase in exercise capacity is also likely to be related to improvements in confidence, motivation and the previously mentioned factors (Mink, 1997). However, since the lungs are not 'trainable' and these are destructive diseases, actual improvements in lung condition may be minimal in severe cases.

The limited physical capacity of individuals with COPD must be reflected in any exercise prescription. Moderate levels of cycle ergometry and walking are appropriate and can be linked to breathing exercises. The general benefits of aerobic exercise training are to improve the respiratory muscles and facilitate the removal of mucus. When following a prescribed exercise programme, although the changes achieved in lung function tests may be minimal, improvements in other factors can reduce the severity of the symptoms, most notably the degree of breathlessness when performing specific tasks. This will obviously improve functional capacity, is likely to improve their quality of life and help to maintain independence. These improvements in exercise capacity are thought to be linked to an increased tolerance of dyspnoea and/or improved muscular movement effi-

ciency (American College of Sports Medicine, 1993).

Many patients with COPD will commence an exercise programme from a very low level of fitness, due to the sedentary lifestyle their condition has imposed upon them. Consequently there is also a high incidence of CHD in this group. The onset of COPD is usually gradual and the wish to avoid breathlessness tends to reinforce the individual's sedentary lifestyle. This may have resulted in a vicious cycle, in which they become less active as their condition worsens. If it is prescribed appropriately, aerobic exercise can produce functional improvements (Shephard, 1976), but to achieve this the exercise adviser will need to overcome the individual's fear of dyspnoea.

A general exercise recommendation for this group would be similar to that for older sedentary adults, but may be of lower intensity. It should include stretching, strengthening and aerobic/activity-based exercises of moderate intensity. An initial intensity below the usual training zone of 60% of maximum heart rate may be appropriate, with the total bout of aerobic activity being divided into repetitive sets (for example, 2–5 minutes walking, repeated with a short rest interval, for up to six sets). A normal response to exercise is an accelerated rate of breathing due to the increased demand for oxygen and need to exhale carbon dioxide. In patients with COPD this can lead to very rapid but shallow breathing which reduces breathing efficiency. This is because with shallow breaths a significant proportion of the fresh inhaled air does not reach the alveoli (where gas exchange occurs), but remains in the airways. A slower and deeper breathing pattern should be encouraged in these individuals. Exercise prescriptions from the American College of Sports Medicine (1993) include the suggestions of 'walking to an end point of dyspnoea' and working at '80% of maximum tolerated workload for 15–20 minutes, twice daily, 5 times a week'. Mink (1997) suggests that, whilst high-intensity programmes have produced aerobic benefits, other less structured programmes of a lower intensity have also produced improvements. He also supports the use of resistance training to offset the causes of muscular fatigue, which is a common limitation to physical capacity in individuals with COPD. Shepard (1994) suggests that under clinical conditions a COPD sufferer may be encouraged to commence an exercise programme by walking on a treadmill whilst breathing oxygen.

Key safety aspects for exercise prescription with COPD patients include:

- clearance from an appropriate medical practitioner;
- consultation with other health professionals who may be involved with the treatment;
- the use of appropriate medication and an awareness of its potential effects upon exercise responses, such as heart rate;
- awareness of the symptoms of cardiorespiratory complications.

For a more detailed consideration of the physiology of respiratory diseases and the issues of exercise prescription see the review by Cooper (1995).

CYSTIC FIBROSIS

Cystic fibrosis is an autosomal recessive genetic disorder. This means that both parents can be carriers but appear normal, showing no signs of the disease. It occurs in approximately 1/2500 Caucasians and 1/17 000 African Americans (Klinger, 1985). A characteristic of cystic fibrosis is the production of mucus which is thick and viscous, causing an obstruction in the airways and adversely affecting ventilation due to enlargement of the respiratory dead space. The alveolar ventilation and oxygenation of the blood is therefore the limiting factor in the aerobic capacity of most sufferers. The disease also makes the sufferer more susceptible to respiratory infections. The benefits of exercise to

individuals with cystic fibrosis have been recognised for many years. They include increased endurance of the respiratory muscles and facilitation of the removal of mucus, as well as the established health benefits that are common to all individuals. The level of physical fitness that can be achieved will depend upon the individual and the severity of their condition. Aerobic exercise is particularly helpful and some sufferers have achieved notable athletic successes, such as completing marathons and participating in relatively high standards of other sporting endeavours. For a review see Boas (1997). The sweat of people with cystic fibrosis has a high concentration of salt, and in conditions which promote copious sweating patients should increase their electrolyte intake (Shephard, 1994).

EXERCISE AND ASTHMA

Asthma is characterised by a reversible airway narrowing which restricts the flow of air through the airways. There are two basic kinds of asthma; bronchial asthma and exercise-induced asthma.

Bronchial asthma

Bronchial asthma is caused by contraction of the bronchial smooth muscles, which constricts the bronchial airways (bronchospasm), and/or inflammation, mucosal oedema and increased production of mucus. This is due to a hyperreactivity of the 'mast cells' that line the bronchial airways. When stimulated, these cells produce chemical mediators (such as histamine) which cause inflammation and constriction of the bronchial airways (bronchospasm). This restricts airflow in and out of the lungs, particularly exhalation, causing a build-up of pressure in the lungs which inhibits the action of the diaphragm. Consequently the individual has further difficulty in breathing (dyspnoea).

The stimuli for an asthmatic attack include allergies, infection, environmental irritants and emotions. Bronchial asthma may be classified as chronic, intermittent or seasonal (Anderson and Hall, 1995). Chronic asthma is persistent, sufferers experiencing symptoms on a daily basis without remission. Intermittent asthmatics will suffer on a much less frequent basis and may go for many days without symptoms. Seasonal asthma occurs when the condition is caused by a specific allergen, such as a particular pollen which is produced at a certain time of the year.

Bronchial asthma can be treated using oral medication and inhalants which inhibit bronchospasm and mucosal inflammatory responses.

EXERCISE-INDUCED ASTHMA

Exercise-induced asthma (EIA) is a condition in which exercise is responsible for initiating an 'asthma attack, ' typically 6–15 minutes into a bout of exercise. The symptoms of dyspnoea tend to be most severe 8–15 minutes after exercise has ceased but breathing returns to normal within 60 minutes (Tan and Spector, 1998). According to Gong (1992) approximately 80% of asthmatics suffer from EIA, but it is also experienced by 3–4% of the population who are otherwise not 'asthmatic' (Voy, 1986). An EIA 'asthma attack' is characterized by constriction of the bronchi and production of excess fluid by the associated membranes. The constriction of the airways and excess fluid or mucus makes breathing more difficult and a characteristic 'wheezing' often occurs. The causes of EIA are believed to be the increased volume of air being ventilated through the bronchioles during exercise, which increases evaporation of water from the bronchial mucosa and has a cooling effect (Whipp and Casaburi, 1994). The loss of bronchiolar heat and water affects the osmolarity of the cells lining the airways and stimulates the release of chemical mediators, such as histamine, which then cause bronchospasm (Tan and Spector, 1998). An alternative theory (which is still subject to some debate) is that post-exercise EIA bronchospasm, which can occur 4–6 hours after exercise (late phase), is caused by rewarming of the airways, increasing blood flow and resulting in oedema.

In accordance with these theories exercise-induced asthma appears to be most common when the exercise is performed in a cold dry environment, which would have the greatest evaporative and cooling effect and it occurs relatively infrequently in environments where the air is warm and moist. Consequently, activities such as swimming are far less likely to induce EIA than, for example, jogging on a cold winter's morning. However, if advocating swimming, an exercise adviser should be aware that very cold water can induce an attack. Whatever the exercise, to prevent EIA the asthmatic may be advised to use bronchodilators before a bout of exercise.

A feature of EIA is the observation that any exercise taken within 30 minutes to 3 hours after an attack is less likely to reproduce the symptoms. This is referred to as a 'refractory period' and has implications for those involved in vigorous exercise: a warm-up before the main exercise will minimise the chances of a further attack during the exercise session. Furthermore, a cool-down can reduce the incidence of the post-exercise attack (McFadden, 1995). The reason for this could be that a cool-down ensures that airway rewarming occurs gradually. Generally prescribed prophylactic medication for EIA includes β-adrenoceptor agonists such as salbutamol (which should be inhaled 15–60 minutes before exercise), sodium cromoglycate, antihistamines and nedocromil, which reduces mast cell reactivity.

SPECIFIC EXERCISE CONSIDERATIONS FOR ASTHMA SUFFERERS

Asthma varies considerably in its severity. Chronic asthmatics may be restricted in the type of exercise in which they can participate, others who are less severely affected can achieve a high level of physical performance, as illustrated by the number of asthmatics who reach an elite level in sport (Anderson *et al.,* 1989; Huftel *et al.,* 1991). The administration of bronchodilator drugs (as oral medications or inhalants) can often be used to control the problem. The exact type of medication prescribed will depend on the severity of the condition, steroidal preparations being used for more persistent conditions.

As the effects of an asthmatic attack may be prevented or minimised by appropriate medication, most asthmatics should be encouraged to participate in appropriate forms of exercise which will provide all the previously discussed health benefits. Careful management of the condition with medication will help to ensure that all except the most severe asthmatics will be able to participate in full exercise regimens, for which the principles of exercise prescription for the non-asthmatic can be applied. Exercise appears to improve lung function and can reduce dependence upon medication.

The basic guidelines for health-related exercise prescription for an asthmatic do not differ from those generally applied to non-asthmatics: aerobic exercise for 20–30 minutes five times a week, along with strength and flexibility components as required. There are, however, a few additional points which the exercise adviser should consider in their exercise prescription.

- Use prescribed medication 10–15 minutes before commencing a planned bout of exercise. Have the participant's medication readily available throughout the bout of exercise.
- Consider the environmental conditions: cold dry environments are more likely to induce EIA. Where possible, avoid specific allergens, dust and other irritants. If exercising outside in cold dry conditions, and the exercise permits, breathe through a mask or scarf as this will warm and moisten the air.
- Warm up with gentle exercise for 10–15 minutes, and cool down with a

similar set of exercises after the main exercise session.
- Where possible, breathe through the nose as this will warm and moisten the inhaled air.
- Avoid exercising alone.
- Drink plenty of fluids; this reduces the thickness of mucosal secretions and thereby reduces associated breathing difficulties.

EXERCISE AND PREGNANCY

Whilst individual opinions vary on the subject, much research indicates that a properly designed exercise programme can help to maintain the fitness of already active women without adversely affecting their pregnancy (Wolfe *et al.,* 1989; Freyder, 1989; Sternfeld *et al.,* 1995). Although specific considerations are needed during the first trimester and the final trimester (when the increase in body mass will affect what the mother can realistically achieve), research indicates that previously sedentary women can commence a gentle exercise programme in the second trimester without jeopardising themselves or their child. General guidelines for exercise during pregnancy and after birth developed by the American College of Obstetricians and Gynecologists (1985) are listed in Table 11.1. Most of the recommendations are simply extensions of the general safety considerations for all exercise programmes. Some authorities would also view them as very stringent for the already active and healthy woman who exhibits no complications.

Pregnancy results in many changes (haematological, morphological, endocrinological, cardiorespiratory and metabolic) to the mother's body. The issues associated with exercise and pregnancy centre around whether, in combination with these changes, an exercise programme can be of benefit or represents a risk to either the mother or the fetus.

When reviewing the issues of exercise and pregnancy many factors need to be considered:

Table 11.1 General guidelines for exercise during pregnancy and after birth

During the pregnancy and following birth:

1. Regular exercise (at least three times per week) is preferable to intermittent activity. Competitive activities should be discouraged
2. Vigorous exercise should not be performed in hot, humid weather or during a period of febrile illness
3. Ballistic movements (jerky bouncy motions) should be avoided. Exercise should be done on a wooden floor or a tightly carpeted surface to reduce shock and provide a sure footing
4. Deep flexion or extension of joints should be avoided because of connective tissue laxity. Activities that require jumping, jarring motions or rapid changes in direction should be avoided because of joint instability
5. Vigorous exercise should be preceded by a 5–minute period of muscle warm-up. This can be accomplished by slow walking or stationary cycling with low resistance
6. Vigorous exercise should be followed by a period of gradually declining activity that includes gentle stationary stretching. Because connective tissue laxity increases the risk of joint injury, stretches should not be taken to the point of maximum resistance
7. Heart rate should be measured at times of peak activity. Target heart rates and limits established in consultation with the physician should not be exceeded
8. Care should be taken to gradually rise from the floor to avoid orthostatic hypotension. Some form of activity involving the legs should be continued for a brief period
9. Liquids should be taken liberally before and after exercise to prevent dehydration. If necessary, activity should be interrupted to replenish fluids
10. Women who have led sedentary lifestyles should begin with physical activity of very low intensity and increase to moderate levels very gradually
11. Activity should be stopped and a physician consulted if any unusual symptoms appear

During pregnancy only:

1. Maternal heart rate should not exceed 140 beats per minute
2. Strenuous activities should not exceed 15 minutes duration
3. No exercise should be performed in the supine position after the fourth month of gestation
4. Exercise that employs the Valsalva maneuver should be avoided
5. Calorific intake should be adequate to meet not only the extra needs of pregnancy but also the exercise performed
6. Maternal core temperature should not exceed 38°C.

American College of Obstetricians and Gynecologists, 1985.

- The potential health benefits and/or risks to the mother.
- The potential health benefits and/or risks to the fetus.
- The type, duration and intensity of the exercise.
- The stage of the pregnancy.
- Whether the mother exercised regularly before her pregnancy, and if she did what exercise regime she followed.
- Any additional complicating factors.

GENERAL CHANGES ASSOCIATED WITH PREGNANCY

Pregnancy results in a variety of structural, metabolic, cardiovascular and endocrinological changes to the mother's body (reviewed by Carpenter, 1994, based on the work of Rose *et al.*, 1956; Hytten and Paintin, 1963; Walters *et al.*, 1966; Lees *et al.*, 1967; Lund and Donovan, 1967; Ueland *et al.*, 1969; Rubler *et al.*, 1977; Laiard-Meeter *et al.*, 1979; Wilson *et al.*, 1980; Longo, 1983; Clapp *et al.*, 1992). In summary, they include increases in blood volume, cardiac output, metabolic rate and body mass, calcium accretion, lordosis, generalised ligamentous relaxation and an increase in insulin resistance. Research has shown that within 6–8 weeks of becoming pregnant the mother's plasma volume increases, and continues to rise, reaching up to 45% more in week 34. Red cell volume, stroke volume, resting heart rate, resting cardiac output and ventricular wall thickness also increase.

On average the mother will experience a 10–25% increase in weight due to the fetus, placenta, amniotic fluid, additional body fluids (intra and extracellular) and tissue deposition. She will also experience insulin resistance resulting in a higher insulin:glucose ratio. All of these factors will influence her capacity to exercise to a greater or lesser extent at various stages of her pregnancy. During the final trimester the increase in body mass will reduce her exercise capacity (Carpenter *et al.*, 1990). If this becomes problematic activities such as cycling and swimming may be recommended because they provide an element of support, unlike running or jogging.

It should be remembered that, due to the mother's increased metabolic rate and increased body weight, her oxygen demand during pregnancy increases. This may make exercise more difficult for the previously active woman, and even more so for the inactive woman who may rapidly become breathless.

FACTORS AFFECTING THE MOTHER'S
HEALTH AND EXERCISE CAPACITY

In theory a fitter woman should be more able to cope with the physical demands of pregnancy (Sternfeld *et al.*, 1995). Stronger muscles should help her to deal with the additional body weight and change in centre of gravity, which could reduce the likelihood of lower back pain as well as helping with the actual birth. Any reduction in physical capacity associated with the pregnancy will have less of an effect on a fit woman than it would on an unfit woman, who may find even basic activities physically demanding. There are also suggestions that physically fit women experience easier labour and have a lower perception of pain during labour: this could be linked to the production of beta-endorphins and perhaps a higher pain threshold (Varassi *et al.*, 1989; McMurray *et al.*, 1990). However, actual length of labour does not appear to be affected by fitness (Lokey *et al.*, 1991).

The risks to the mother associated with exercise are linked to her increased body mass, change in centre of gravity and increased ligament laxity, which could increase the risk of soft tissue injury (Work, 1989; Artal *et al*, 1991; Clapp and Little, 1992). Weight training may give some cause for concern if heavy resistances are used, although those of low intensity, if used properly, should not cause any problems. The strengthening effects of exercise upon the abdominal muscles, the pelvic floor and perineum do not appear to adversely affect the labour and may make childbirth easier.

Exercise is reported to reduce the amount of weight gain associated with pregnancy and helps to maintain the woman's physical condition, thereby facilitating a more rapid recovery to pre-pregnancy fitness levels after the birth (Clapp *et al.*, 1995). The prevention of excessive fat deposition is not only important for the athletic female wishing to return to competition but also has implications for all women, given the association between excessive body fat and certain diseases. Furthermore, the general health benefits of remaining active, for example blood lipid profiles, with their implication upon cardiovascular disease, continue to affect a pregnant woman.

An additional implication is the observed increase in insulin resistance which occurs in pregnancy; for some individuals this may be sufficient to initiate gestational diabetes. This is similar to NIDDM (see p. 271), with a reduced sensitivity to insulin resulting in higher blood glucose levels. Exercise is extremely beneficial in such women. Even modest exercise programmes of 20 minutes of arm cranking at

140 beats min^{-1} (approximately 50% $\dot{V}O_{2max}$) three times a week can increase insulin sensitivity for up to 48 hours (Milkines *et al.*, 1988; Jovanovic-Peterson *et al.*, 1989; Clapp and Little, 1995). This is supported by Young and Treadway (1992), whose work indicated that glucose tolerance and insulin response are aided by exercise during pregnancy.

Swimming is often advocated for the pregnant woman, especially during the later stages of pregnancy. Pool temperatures of around 30°C are recommended for active swimmers because cooler temperatures may cause discomfort due to heat loss. Whilst swimming can help to strengthen the back and reduce the risk of lower back pain caused by lordosis resulting from the change in body mass, care should be taken with stroke technique so as not to exacerbate the problem (butterfly or breast stroke with a hyperextended back). Aquanatal classes can be useful as the buoyancy helps to support the extra weight and change in centre of gravity, whilst the water provides additional resistance for muscle toning (Gill, 1994).

CONSIDERATIONS FOR FETAL HEALTH

During physical exercise the mother experiences changes in cardiac output, ventilation and oxygen use. Concerns over the implications of these changes on the health of the fetus include the possible decrease in placental blood flow (resulting in a risk of hypoxia), substrate deprivation (causing hypoglycaemia), elevated core temperature (producing hyperthermia), biomechanical stress (causing physical damage), metabolic acidosis, developmental problems and low birthweight.

Wolfe *et al.* (1989) suggest that during prolonged strenuous exercise by the mother the fetus may suffer from hypoxia due to the competing demands of the skeletal muscles, which could affect fetal growth and development. Hypoxic damage can occur if the oxygen supply is inadequate: uterine blood supply may decrease by as much as 59%

during strenuous exercise due to the normal vasoconstrictive response to exercise (Wells, 1991). However, many authorities consider that a number of other physiological mechanisms actually prevent hypoxia in the fetus. For example, fetal haemoglobin has a strong affinity for oxygen, facilitating greater extraction of oxygen from the available blood supply. It is also suggested that uterine blood flow is re-distributed to favour the placenta (and hence the fetus), ensuring a favourable supply of oxygen. During pregnancy there is a haemoconcentration of the maternal blood, which augments its oxygen content, therefore oxygen availability may only marginally be affected despite a reduction in blood volume flowing through the uterus (Morris *et al.*, 1956; Lotgering *et al.*, 1984). Since the uterus of a pregnant woman exhibits an enhanced oxygen extraction the fetus's supply of oxygen is not thought to differ greatly between rest and exercise (Chandler *et al.*, 1985; Clapp *et al.*, 1987; Artal *et al.*, 1991).

Some concern has been expressed that the demands of exercise may deprive the fetus of nutrients such as glucose. However, Artal *et al.* (1986) showed that during exercise pregnant women obtain a greater proportion of their energy from fat and less from carbohydrate, resulting in a lower respiratory exchange ratio. It is hypothesised that this, coupled with the increased insulin resistance (Boren *et al.*, 1992), could reduce the risk of hypoglycaemia and ensure that the fetus is not deprived of glucose (Fioretti *et al.*, 1970; Holness *et al.*, 1991).

If excessive, an increase in temperature with exercise could adversely affect the development of the fetus. Temperature increases will be related to exercise intensity and duration, as well as ambient temperature and the woman's capacity to dissipate heat. Exercise normally elevates the core temperature, which could present a teratogenic risk to the developing fetus, particularly during the early stages of pregnancy when the neural tube is developing. However, Clapp (1991) and Clapp *et al.* (1987) suggest that heat dissipation is enhanced during pregnancy; coupled with an earlier onset of sweating and a reduced exercise capacity this means that core temperature (measured as rectal temperature) is not elevated to harmful levels. Caution should still be used when exercising in hot and humid conditions.

The risk of physical trauma to the fetus during exercise will depend greatly upon the activity being undertaken. Contact sports should be avoided. Some authorities have cautioned against jogging or running because of the jolting action (Synder and Caruth, 1984), although many other studies have demonstrated no ill-effect and it is suggested that the amniotic fluid provides ample cushioning.

Studies on the effects of chronic exercise upon fetal birthweight are inconclusive and contradictory. Dale *et al.* (1982), Clapp and Dickstein (1984) and Mezzapelli *et al.* (1991) suggest an increase in risk of a low birthweight baby through exercise, whereas Hatch *et al.* (1993) recorded an increase in birthweight in mothers who exercised most intensely and Pomerance *et al.* (1974), Gorski (1985), Wong and McKenzie (1989) and Lokey *et al.* (1991) in meta-analyses suggest no effect. Therefore it appears that exercise has a minimal, if any, effect on the birthweight of the infant.

Clapp and Little (1995) discovered an association between obesity in the mother and high fetal body weight. Since there is a link between fetal body weight and childhood obesity, which often leads to adult obesity, the body composition of the pregnant woman has significant implications for the future life of the unborn child. Because exercise can help to combat the excess fat deposition experienced by some women it could have long-term effects on the child.

GENERAL ISSUES

A woman who was very active before pregnancy and who wishes to remain so does not apparently risk the health of either herself or her unborn child. However, the onset of pregnancy is not a good time for a previously sedentary woman to commence a vigorous exercise programme. Common sense should prevail, and if there are any concerns a physician should be consulted. For the previous non-exerciser there may be problems if they are unable to distinguish between the common feelings associated with exercise, those of the pregnancy and those which might suggest complications. Cohen *et al.* (1989) reported the case of two competitive runners who, unaware that they were pregnant, continued to run 40–50 miles per week and raced until 20 weeks of pregnancy. Both women continued to jog 12–13 miles a week even in the third trimester and both delivered normal infants.

The effects of exercise upon the pregnancy should be considered separately for each trimester. General recommendations include:

- work at a moderate exercise intensity for a shorter duration;
- avoid ballistic exercises and/or those involving the Valsalva manoeuvre;
- take additional care in hot and humid environments;
- avoid activities which include the risk of falls and collisions.

These recommendations are generally considered by the well conditioned low-risk woman as very stringent (Clapp, 1991; Hatch *et al.*, 1993). The meta-analysis of Lokey *et al.* (1991) suggests that exercise programmes of an intensity of around 144 beats min^{-1} performed for 43 minutes, three times a week do not result in any adverse effects on either the mother or fetus. Most fit women appear able to continue with their established exercise programme almost unmodified during their first and second trimesters. In the third trimester the increase in body mass will become a limitation. Conversely, those who are unfamiliar with exercise should commence with a programme of low intensity and comparatively short duration. Activities such as swimming and walking are recommended.

For the already fit woman most forms of exercise will be possible during the early stages of pregnancy. However, as the pregnancy progresses, high-impact weight-bearing activities will become less suitable and may need to be replaced by walking and swimming. Whilst the 'athletic' woman may be worried about maintaining her fitness, these desires should not be allowed to jeopardise the fetus and serious training will become prohibitive beyond the twentieth week, if not before. Regardless of the activity the mother's calorific intake must be sufficient for her own needs, those of the developing fetus and the calorific cost of the exercise.

Opinions on the topic of weight training are extremely varied, and very little research is available to support or refute its use (Work, 1989). However, it is generally considered that maximal lifts should be avoided, and the Valsalva manoeuvre can reduce oxygen supply to the fetus during heavy lifting. The onset of pregnancy is not the best time to commence a new exercise programme (Hall and Kaufmann 1987), and even a woman who trains regularly should modify her programme as the health of the fetus must take priority. General recommendations for regular exercisers are to train all the major muscle groups, using about 15 exercises (each being performed for about a minute), with an appropriate resistance that does not cause excessive strain (Shangold, 1994).

In conclusion, the concerns about exercise participation appear to be unwarranted for a healthy asymptomatic woman and her fetus. The benefits of an appropriate exercise programme seem well-founded. If a previously active mother wishes to continue to exercise she should be encouraged to do so, with some sensible modifications at the appropriate stages of her pregnancy.

EXERCISE, CORONARY REHABILITATION AND THE TREATMENT OF CORONARY ARTERY DISEASE

Over the past two decades the inclusion of appropriately supervised exercises into coronary rehabilitation programmes has become widely accepted and previously advocated extended bedrest is now considered inadvisable for most individuals. Haskell (1994) describes physical activity for patients with coronary heart disease as 'a double-edged sword'. His comments come in a review from which he concludes that regular exercise may reduce the risk of future cardiac events, but the additional demands made on the heart during exercise increases the risk of sudden cardiac death. When comparing the benefits and risks he suggests that, overall, an exercise programme can reduce the risk of all-cause mortality and that the risk of a coronary event during exercise is only 1 per 60 000 participant-hours. However, the actual benefits of exercise extend beyond the relatively simple measure of morbidity and include improvements in physical capacity, advantages to general physical and mental health and a lessening of symptoms such as angina pectoris and shortness of breath.

Therefore, with a number of exceptions, exercises are recommended for most individuals who are rehabilitating after MI or coronary bypass surgery. Details of recommendations and guidelines have been published by several American bodies, including the American Association of Cardiopulmonary Rehabilitation (1991), the American College of Sports Medicine (1986), the American Heart Association (1991) and the American Medical Association Council on Scientific Affairs (1981). A full review of the topic was produced by Oldridge *et al.* (1988). Similar reports, with recommendations for patients who are recovering from heart transplants were produced by Squires (1983) and Badenhop (1995). The rehabilitation process must be supervised and guided by a team of individuals which may include cardiac specialists, physiotherapists, occupational therapists, nurses and specialist exercise advisers. The functions of such programmes are to restore a patient's confidence in their capabilities, restore their physical capacity to its full potential and to minimise the chances of further complications or another coronary event. For the post-MI patient, controlled exercise programmes bring no increase in risk of further complications or death, whereas a number of adverse effects are associated with prolonged bed rest: decreased aerobic capacity, increased risk of venous thrombosis and orthostatic hypotension (caused by reduction in blood and plasma volume), loss of calcium, muscle atrophy and increased risk of pneumonia.

Guidelines for the design and implementation of post-MI exercise programmes were produced by the American College of Sports Medicine (1991). Appropriately designed exercise programmes are essential in rehabilitating patients and developing their physical capacity to a level at which they can cope with the physical demands of their lifestyle. Numerous studies have demonstrated that after MI many individuals can attain good levels of fitness (and, indeed, the prescribed exercise programme can result in them becoming fitter than they were before the coronary event or operation). A number of individuals have gone on to complete marathons after a heart attack and, whilst this extreme form of physical activity is not advocated by all authorities or recommended for all individuals, it does illustrate the potential capabilities of the heart attack victim if given the correct exercises.

Following a heart attack or cardiac surgery the initial stages of the rehabilitation process will be guided by the cardiac specialist and multidisciplinary team. Rehabilitation is likely to include considerations of the four main risk factors (elevated lipids, smoking, hypertension and inactivity). In the case of a minor uncomplicated MI the programme may include gentle walking within a week of the event, although slightly more vigorous forms of exercise are unlikely to be recommended until 3–6 weeks later. Any rehabilitation programme will also include advice on lifestyle habits such as diet, smoking, drinking, stress and relaxation, as well as exercise. Before commencing any exercise programme the patient should undergo a graded exercise test, during which the responses of their heart to exercise will be monitored. The results of such tests will give the specialist information on exercise-induced arrhythmias and the extent of angina. From this information he or she will be able to make recommendations concerning the type, duration and intensity of exercise the patient should undertake. The specialist may also specify a heart rate training zone to attain during exercise sessions. This is usually the stage at which the exercise adviser becomes involved with the exercise programme.

An exercise programme for coronary rehabilitation should be conducted with the same basic principles as any other programme. Sessions should include warm-up and cool-down phases, and gradual progression should be evident. A cardiac rehabilitation programme is likely to emphasise the aerobic component of exercise. In the early stages of a programme many authorities advise that the patient's cardiovascular responses should be monitored using ECG telemetry and that a defibrillation unit should be available. The basic components of the programme should be based upon exercises which involve large rhythmic contractions and should avoid isometric work or exercises which primarily involve small muscle groups. The activity should also be non-competitive and, in the early stages, an increase in the heart rate of 30 beats min^{-1} is often recommended (although this may be modified in accordance with any medication being taken). Exercises are therefore likely to include loosening exercises, such as arm and leg swings, and activities such as walking and cycling on an ergometer. Exercise sessions should progress with the objectives of reaching a level at which the aerobic component of the session lasts for 20 minutes and the participant exercises at least three times a week. Where possible, as the programme progresses it should take on the form of a basic aerobically oriented programme (as described in Chapter 7), although modifications may be advised by the specialist according to the specific circumstances of the individual. Circuit weight-training using light to moderate intensities is effective in improving fitness without increasing risk to the patient. Research studying different exercise modes and protocols includes the work of Kelemen *et al.* (1981), DeBusk *et al.* (1985), Goble *et al.* (1991) and Sparling *et al.* (1990).

Whilst the risk of a cardiac event is slightly higher in post-MI subjects than in asymptomatic individuals it remains relatively low. Thompson and Fahrenbach (1994) report surveys by Haskell (1978) and Van Camp and Peterson (1986), who showed that in rehabilitation centres there was one cardiac arrest every 33 000–112 000, participation-hours, one MI every 233 000–294 000 participation-hours and one death every 116 000–784 000 participation-hours.

For individuals with identified coronary artery disease exercise may reverse the atherosclerotic process. This includes a possible widening of the arteries, increased stroke volume and improved contractility. For further information and a review on exercise prescription for the cardiac patient see Cox (1997) and Chapter 10.

REFERENCES

Allen, D.W. and Quigley, B.M. (1977). The role of physical activity in the control of obesity. *Medical Journal of Australia*, 2, 434–438.

American Association of Cardiopulmonary Rehabilitation (1991). *Guidelines for Cardiac Rehabilitation Programs*. Champaign, IL: Human Kinetics.

American College of Obstetricians and Gynecologists (1985). *Guidelines for Exercise During Pregnancy and Postpartum* in *ACOG Home Exercise Programs: Exercise During Pregnancy and the Postnatal Period*. Washington: ACOG.

American College of Sports Medicine (1986). *Guidelines for Exercise Testing and Prescription* (3rd ed.). Philadelphia: Lea and Feibiger.

American College of Sports Medicine (1991). *Guidelines for Exercise Testing and Prescription* (4th ed.). Philadelphia: Lea and Feibiger.

American College of Sports Medicine (1993). *Resource Manual for Guidelines for Exercise Testing and Prescription* (2nd ed.). Philadelphia: Lea and Feibiger.

American College of Sports Medicine (ACSM) (1995). ACSM Position stand on osteoporosis and exercise. *Medicine and Science in Sports and Exercise*, **27**, i-vii.

American Diabetes Association (1990). Diabetes mellitus and exercise: Position statement. *Diabetes Care*, **13**, 804–805.

American Heart Association (1984). *Exercise and Your Heart*. New York: American Heart Association.

American Heart Association (1991). *Exercise Standards: A Statement for Health Professionals from the American Heart Association*. Dallas: American Heart Association.

American Heart Association (1995). *Heart and Stroke Facts: 1996 Statistical Supplement*. Dallas: American Heart Association.

American Heart Association (1997). *Heart and Stroke Statistical Update*. Dallas: American Heart Association.

American Medical Association Council on Scientific Affairs (1981). Physician-supervised exercise programs in rehabilitation of patients with coronary heart disease. *Journal of the American Medical Association*, **245**, 1463–1465.

Anderson, M.K. and Hall, S.J. (1995). *Sports Injury Management*. London: Williams and Wilkins.

Anderson, S.D., Daviskas, E. and Smith, C.M. (1989). Exercise-induced asthma: A difference in opinion regarding the stimulus. *Allergy Proceedings*, **10**, 215–226.

Andrew, M., Carter, C., O'Brodovich, H. and Heigenhauser, G. (1986). Increases in factor VIII complex and fibrinolytic activity are dependent upon exercise intensity. *Journal of Applied Physiology*, **60**, 1917–1922.

Artal, R., Wiswell, R., Romen, Y. and Dorey, F. (1986). Pulmonary responses to exercise in pregnancy. *American Journal of Obstetrics and Gynecology*, **154**, 378–383.

Åstrand, P.O. (1992). Why exercise? *Medicine and Science in Sports and Exercise*, **24**, 153–162.

Åstrand, P.O. and Grimby, G. (eds) (1986). Physical activity in health and disease. *Acta Medica Scandinavica Supplementum*, **711**.

Astrup, T. (1973). The effects of physical activity on blood coagulation and fibrinolysis. In *Exercise Testing and Training in Coronary Heart Disease*, Naughton, J. and Hellerstein, H.J. (eds). New York: Academic Press; 169–192.

Atkinson, R.L. and Walberg-Rankin, J. (1994). Physical activity, fitness and severe obesity. In *Physical Activity, Fitness and Health. International Proceedings and Consensus Statement*, Bouchard, C., Shephard, R.J. and Stephens, T. (eds). Champaign, IL: Human Kinetics.

Badenhop, D.T. (1995). The therapeutic role of exercise in patients with orthotopic heart transplant. *Medicine and Science in Sports and Exercise*, 27(7), 975–985.

Barnard, R.J. (1975). Long-term effects of exercise on cardiac function. *Exercise and Sport Science Reviews*, 3, 113–133.

Benbassat, J. and Froom, P.F. (1986). Blood pressure response to exercise as a predictor of hypertension. *Archives of Internal Medicine*, **146**, 2053–2055.

Bjorntorp, P. (1974). Effects of age, sex and clinical conditions on adipose tissue cellularity in man. *Metabolism*, 23, 1091.

Bjorntorp, P. (1978). Physical training in the treatment of obesity. *International Journal of Obesity*, 2, 149–156.

Bjorntorp, P. (1983). Physiological and clinical aspects of exercise in obese patients. *Exercise and Sport Sciences Reviews*, 11, 159–180.

Blair, S.N. (1994). Physical activity, fitness and coronary heart disease. In *Physical Activity, Fitness and Health. International Proceedings and Consensus Statement*. Bouchard, C., Shephard, R.J. and Stephens, T. (eds). Champaign, IL: Human Kinetics.

Blair, S.N. (1997). British Association of Sport and Exercise Sciences Conference Keynote Presentation. York, 1997.

Blair, S.N., Goodyear, N.N., Gibbons, L.W. and Cooper, K.H. (1984). Physical fitness and incidence of hypertension in healthy normotensive men and women. *Journal of the American Medical Association*, 252, 487–490.

Blair, S.N., Kohl, H.W., Barlow, C.E., Paffenbarger, R.S., Gibbons, L.W. and Macera, C.A. (1995). Changes in physical fitness and all-cause mortality: a prospective study of healthy and unhealthy men. *Journal of the American Medical Association*, 273 (14), 1093–1098.

Blair, S.N., Kampert, J.B., Kohl, H.W., Barlow, C.E., Macera, C.A., Paffenbarger, R.S. and Gibbons, L.W. (1996). Influences of cardiorespiratory fitness and other precursors on cardiovascular disease and other all-cause mortality in men and women. *Journal of the American Medical Association*, 276(3), 205–210.

Bloor, C. M. and Leon, A. S. (1970). Interaction of age and exercise on the heart and its blood supply. *Laboratory Investigations.*, **22**, 16.

Bloor, C.M., White, F.C. and Saunders, T.M. (1984). Effects of exercise on collateral development in myocardial ischemia in pigs. *Journal of Applied Physiology*, 56, 656–665.

Blumenthal, S., Epps, R.P., Heavenrich, R., Lauer, R.M., Leiberman, E., Mirkin, B., Mitchell. S.C., Naito, V.B., O'Hare, D., Smith, W.M., Tarazi, R.C. and Upson, D. (1977). Report of the task force on blood pressure control in children. *Pediatrics*, 59 (5), Part 2.

Blumenthal, J., Williams, R., Williams, R. and Wallace, A. (1980). Effects of exercise on Type A (coronary prone) behaviour pattern. *Psychosomatic Medicine*, 42, 289–296.

Blumgart, H.L., Schlesinger, M.J. and Davis, D. (1940). Studies on relation of clinical manifestations of angina pectoris, coronary thrombosis and myocardial infarction to pathogenic findings with particular reference to significance of collateral circulation. *American Heart Journal*, 19, 1–91.

Boas, S.R. (1997). Exercise recommendations for individuals with cystic fibrosis. *Sports Medicine*, 14, 17–37.

Boileau, R.A., Buskirk, E.R. Horstman, P.H., Mendez, J. and Nicholas, W.C. (1971). Body composition changes in obese and lean men during physical conditioning. *Medicine and Science in Sport*, 3 (4), 183–189.

Boren, A.P., Campagna, L., Gilchrist, D., Young, C. and Beresford, P. (1992). Substrate and endocrine responses during exercise at selected stages of pregnancy. *Journal of Applied Physiology*, 73, 134–142.

Bouchard, C., Shephard, R.J. and Stephens, T. (eds) (1993). *Physical Activity, Fitness and Health Consensus Statement*. Champaign, IL: Human Kinetics.

Bouchard, C., Shephard, R.J. and Stephens, T. (eds) (1994). *Physical Activity, Fitness and Health. Consensus Statement*. Champaign, IL: Human Kinetics.

Boyer, J.L. and Kasch, F.W. (1970) Exercise therapy in hypertensive men. *Journal of the American Medical Association*, 211, 1668–71.

Braun, B., Zimmerman, M.B. and Kretchmer, N. (1995). Effects of exercise intensity on insulin sensitivity in women with non-insulin dependent diabetes mellitus. *Journal of Applied Physiology*, 78, 300–306.

Brewer, V., Meyer, B.M., Keele, M.S., Upton, J. and Hagan, R.D. (1983). Role of exercise in prevention of involutional bone loss. *Medicine and Science in Sports and Exercise, 15,* 445–449.

British Cardiac Society (1987). Report of the British Cardiac Society working group on coronary disease prevention.

British Heart Foundation (1986). Reducing the risk of a heart attack. *Heart Research Series, 14,* 5–78.

Brook, C.G.D. (1972). Evidence for a sensitive period in adipose cell replication in man. *Lancet, 2,* 624.

Brooks, G.A., Fahey, T.D. and White, T.P. (1996). *Exercise Physiology: Human energetics and its application* (2nd ed.). London: Mayfield Publishing Company.

Burgess-Wilson, E.L., Green, S., Heptinstall, S., and Mitchell, J.R.A. (1984). Spontaneous platelet aggregation in whole blood: Dependence upon age and haematocrit. *Lancet, 2,* 1213.

Butler, J.R. (1987) *An Apple a Day.* Canterbury: Health Services Research Unit, University of Kent at Canterbury.

Carpenter, M.W. (1994). Physical activity, fitness and health of the pregnant mother and fetus. In *Physical Activity, Fitness and Health. International Proceedings and Consensus Statement,* Bouchard, C., Shephard, R.J. and Stephens, T. (eds). Champaign, IL: Human Kinetics.

Carpenter, M.W., Sady, S.P., Sady, M.A., Haydon, B., Coustan, D.R., and Thompson, P.D. (1990). Effect of maternal weight gain during pregnancy on exercise performance. *Journal of Applied Physiology,* 68 (7), 1173–1176.

Castelli, W.P., Garrison, R.J., Wilson, P.W.F., Abbott, R.D., Kalousdian, S. and Kanel, W.B. (1986) Incidence of coronary heart disease and lipoprotein cholesterol levels. The Framingham Study. *Journal of the American Medical Association,* 256, 2835–2838.

Chandler, K.D., Leury, B.J., Bird, A.R. and Bell, A.W. (1985). Effects of under-nutrition and exercise during late pregnancy on uterine, foetal and uteroplacental metabolism in the ewe. *British Journal of Nutrition, 53,* 625–635.

Chandrashekar, Y. and Anand, L.C. (1991). Exercise as a coronary protection factor. *American Heart Journal,* 122, 1723–1739.

Charney, H.C. (1976). Childhood antecedents of adult obesity. *New England Journal of Medicine,* 195, 6.

Chirico, A.M. and Stunfard, A.J. (1976) Physical activity and human obesity. *New England Journal of Medicine,* 263, 935.

Choquette, G. and Ferguson, R.J. (1973). Blood pressure reduction in 'borderline' hypertensives following physical training. *Canadian Medical Association Journal.* 108, 699–703.

Clapp, J.F. (1991). The changing thermal responses to endurance exercise during pregnancy. *American Journal of Obstetrics and Gynecology,* 165, 1684–1689.

Clapp, J.F. and Dickstein, S. (1984). Endurance exercise and pregnancy outcome. *Medicine and Science in Sports and Exercise, 16,* 556–562.

Clapp, J.F, and Little, K.D. (1995). Effect of recreational exercise on pregnant weight gain and subcutaneous fat deposition. *Medicine and Science in Sports and Exercise,* 27, 87–94.

Clapp, J.F, Wesley, M. and Sleamaker, R.H. (1987). Thermoregulatory and metabolic responses to jogging prior to and during pregnancy. *Medicine and Science in Sports and Exercise.* 19, 124–130.

Clapp, J.F., Rokey, R., Treadway, J.L., Carpenter, M.W., Artal, R.M. and Warnes, C. (1992). Exercise in pregnancy, *Medicine and Science in Sports and Exercise,* 24 (6), S294–300.

Cohen, G.C., Prior, J.C., Vigna, Y. and Pride, S.M. (1989). Intense exercise during the first two trimesters of unapparent pregnancy. *Physician and Sportsmedicine,* 17, 87–94.

Connor, J.F., LaCamera, F., Swanick, E.J., Oldham, M.J., Holzaepfel, D.W. and Lyczkowskyi, O. (1976). Effects of exercise on coronary collaterialisation, angiographic studies of six patients in a supervised exercise programme. *Medicine and Science in Sports and Exercise,* 8 (3), 145–151.

Cooper, C.B. (1995). Determining the role of exercise in patients with chronic pulmonary disease. *Medicine and Science in Sports and Exercise,* 27(2), 147–157.

Coplan, N.L., Gleim, G.W. and Nicholas, J.A. (1988). Exercise and sudden cardiac death. *American Heart Journal,* 53, 207–212.

Corbin, C.B. and Pletcher, P. (1986). Diet and physical activity patterns of obese and non-obese elementary school children. *Research Quarterly,* 39, 922–928.

Coronary Prevention Group (UK) (1987) *Exercise-Heart-Health.* Conference Report. London: Health Education Council and Sports Council.

Cox, M.H. (1997). Exercise for coronary artery disease. *Physician and Sportsmedicine,* 25(12), 27–32.

Cowan, G.O. (1983). Influence of exercise on high density lipoprotein. *American Journal of Cardiology,* 52 (4), 138.

Currens, J.H. and White, P.D. (1961). Half a century of running: clinical, physiologic and autopsy findings in the case of Clarence DeMar (Mr Marathon). *New England Journal of Medicine* **265**, 988–993.

Dale, E., Mullinax, K.M. and Bryan, D.H. (1982). Exercise during pregnancy: effects on the foetus. *Canadian Journal of Applied Sports Science*, **7**, 98–103.

Dalsky, G.P., Stocke, K.S., Ehsani, A.A., Slatoplsky, E., Lee, W.C. and Birge, S.J. (1988). Weight bearing exercise training and lumbar bone mineral content in post-menopausal women. *Annals of Internal Medicine*, **108**, 824–828.

Davis, G.L., Abildgaard, C.F., Bernauer, E.M. and Britton, M. (1976). Fibrinolytic and hemostatic changes during and after maximal exercise in males. *Journal of Applied Physiology*, **40**, 287–292.

Davis, M.J. and Thomas, A. (1984). Thrombosis and acute coronary-artery lesions in sudden cardiac ischemic death. *New England Journal of Medicine*, **310**, 1137–1140.

Davis, M.G., Cooper, A.R. and Riddoch, C.J. (1998). Acute effects of three bouts of brisk walking per day on systolic and diastolic blood pressure. *Journal of Sports Sciences*, **16**, 44.

DeBusk, R.F., Haskell, W.L., Miller, N.H. *et al.* (1985). Medically directed at-home rehabilitation soon after clinically uncomplicated acute myocardial infarction: A new model for patient care. *American Journal of Cardiology*, **55**, 251.

DeBusk, R.F., Stenestrand, U., Sheehan, M. and Haskell, W.L. (1990). Training effects of long versus short bouts of exercise in healthy subjects. *American Journal of Cardiology*, **65**, 1010–1013.

Dela, F., Larsen, J.J., Mikines, K.J. *et al.* (1995). Insulin-stimulated muscle glucose clearance in patients with NIDDM. *Diabetes*, **44**, 1010–1020.

DiNubile, N.A. (1997a). Osteoarthritis. How to make exercise part of your treatment plan. *Physician and Sportsmedicine*, **25**, 47–56.

DiNubile, N.A (1997b). Exercise for osteoarthritis. *Physician and Sportsmedicine*, **25**, 57–58.

Donahoe, C.P., Lin, D.H., Kirschenbaum, D.S. and Keesey, R.L. (1984). Metabolic consequences of dieting and exercise in the treatment of obesity. *Journal of Consulting and Clinical Psychology*, **52**, 827–836.

Drinkwater, B.L. (1993). Exercise in the prevention of osteoporosis. In *Osteoporosis Proceedings*, Christiansen C. and Riis, B. (eds). Rodovre, Denmark: Osteopress Aps; 105–108.

Drinkwater, B.L. (1994). Physical activity, fitness and osteoporosis. In *Physical Activity, Fitness and Health. International Proceedings and Consensus Statement*, Bouchard C, Shephard, R.J. and Stephens, T. (eds). Champaign, IL: Human Kinetics.

Duncan, J.J., Gordon, N.F. and Scott, C.B. (1991). Women walking for health and fitness: How much is enough? *Journal of the American Medical Association*, **266**, 3295–3299.

Duncan, J.J., Farr, J.E., Upton, S.J., Hagon, R.D., Ogiesby, M.E. and Blair, S.N. (1985). The effects of aerobic exercise on plasma catecholamines and blood pressure in patients with mild essential hypertension. *Journal of the American Medical Association*, **254**, 2609–2613.

Eckstein, R.W. (1957). Effects of exercise on coronary heart narrowing and coronary collateral circulation. *Circulation Research*, **5**, 230–235.

Eichner, E.R. (1987). Antithrombotic effects of exercise. *American Family Physician*, **36**, 207–211.

Elwood, P.C., Renaud, S., Sharp, D.S., Beswick, A.D., O'Brien, J.R. and Yarnell, J.W.G. (1991). Ischemic heart disease and platelet aggregation. The Caerphilly collaborative heart disease study. *Circulation*, **83**, 38–44.

Enos, W.F., Holmes, R.H. and Beyer, J. (1953). Coronary disease amongst United States soldiers killed in action in Korea. *Journal of the American Medical Association*, **152**, 1090–1093.

Eriksson, B.O., Mellstrand, T., Peterson, L., Renstrom, P. and Svedmyr, N. (1990). *Sports Medicine: Health and Medication*, London: Guinness Publishing Ltd.

Erickson, S.M. and Sevier, T.L. (1997). Oseoporosis in active women. *Physician and Sportsmedicine*, **25**(11), 61–74.

Fagard, R.H. and Tipton, C.M. (1994). Physical activity, fitness and hypertension In *Physical Activity, Fitness and Health. International Proceedings and Consensus Statement*, Bouchard, C., Shephard, R.J. and Stephens, T. (eds). Champaign, IL: Human Kinetics.

Fentem, P.H. and Turnbull, N.B. (1987). Benefits of exercise for heart health: report on the scientific basis. In *Exercise – Heart – Health*. London: Coronary Prevention Group; 110–125.

Fentem, P.H., Bassey, E.J. and Turnbull, N.B. (1988) *The New Case for Exercise*. London: The Sports Council and the Health Education Authority.

Fentem, P.H., Turnbull, N.B. and Bassey, E.J. (1990). *Benefits of Exercise: the Evidence*. Manchester: Manchester University Press.

Ferguson, R.J., Petitelerc, R., Choquette, G., Chaniotis, L. Gauthier, P. Huot, R., Allard, C., Jankowski, L. and Campeau, L. (1974). Effects of physical training on treadmill capacity, collateral circulation and progression of coronary disease. *American Journal of Cardiology*, **34**, 764–769.

Fioretti, P., Genazzani, A., Aubert, M., Gragnoli, G. and Pupillo, A. (1970). Correlations between human chorionic somato-momotropin (lactogen), immunoreactive insulin, glucose and lipid fractions in plasma of pregnant women. *Obstetrics and Gynecology*, **77**, 745–751.

Folkins, C.M. and Amsterdam, E.A. (1977). Control and modification of stress emotions through chronic exercise. In *Exercise, Cardiovascular Health and Disease*, Amsterdam, E.A., Wilmore, J.H. and DeMaria, A.N. (eds). New York: Medical Books.

Folsom, A.R., Caspersen, C.J., Taylor, H.L. *et al.* (1985). Leisure time physical activity and its relationship to coronary risk factors in population-based sample. *American Journal of Epidemiology*, **121**, 570–579.

Freyder, S.C. (1989). Exercising whilst pregnant. *Journal of Orthopaedic and Sports Physical Therapy*, **10** (9), 358–365.

Friedman, M. and Rosenman, R.H. (1959). Association of specific overt behaviour patterns with blood and cardiovascular findings. *Journal of the American Medical Association*, **169**, 1286–1296.

Friedman, M. (1969). *Pathogens of Coronary Artery Disease*. New York: McGraw-Hill.

Friedman, M. and Rosenman, R.H (1974). *Type A Behaviour and Your Heart*. New York: Alfred A. Knopf.

Fries, J.F., Singh, G. and Morfield, D. (1994). Running and the development of disability with age. *Annals of Internal Medicine*, **121**(7), 502–509.

Fry, R.C. (1953). A comparative study of obese children selected on the basis of fat pads. *American Journal of Clinical Nutrition*, **1**, 453.

Furie, B. and Furie, B.C. (1992). Molecular and cellular biology of blood coagulation. *New England Journal of Medicine*, **326**, 800–806.

Giacca, A., Vranic, M., Davidson, J.K. and Lickley, H.L.A. (1991). Exercise and stress in diabetes mellitus. In *Clinical Diabetes Mellitus: A Problem Oriented Approach*, Davidson, J.K. (ed.). New York: Thieme-Stratton; 218–265.

Giacca, A., Qing Shi, Z., Marliss, E.B., Zinman, B. and Vranic, M. (1994). Physical activity, fitness and type 1 diabetes. In *Physical Activity, Fitness and Health. International Proceedings and Consensus Statement*, Bouchard, C., Shephard, R.J. and Stephens, T. (eds). Champaign, IL: Human Kinetics.

Gill, C. (1994). Aquanatal exercises: the midwives role. *British Journal of Midwifery*, **2**(6), 270–274.

Gilliam, T.B. and Burke, M.B. (1978) Effects of exercise on serum lipids and lipo-proteins in girls ages 8 to 10 years. *Artery*, **4**, 203.

Gleeson, P.B., Protas, E.J., LeBlanc, A.D., Scneider, V.S. and Evans, H.J. (1990). Effects of weight lifting on bone mineral density in pre-menopausal women. *Journal of Bone Mineral Research*, **5**, 153–158.

Goble, A., Hare, D., MacDonald, P., Oliver, R., Reid, M. and Worcester, M. (1991). Effect of early programmes of high and low intensity exercise on physical performance after transmural acute myocardial infarction. *British Heart Journal*, **65**, 126–131.

Goldberg, L. and Elliot, D.L. (1985). The effect of physical activity on lipid and lipoprotein levels. *Medical Clinics of North America*, **69** (1), 41–55.

Goldberg, A.P., Hagberg, J., Delemez, J.A., Camey, R.M., McKegitt, P.M., Ehsani, A.A. and Harter H.R. (1980) The metabolic and physiological effects of exercise training in hemodialysis patients. *American Journal of Clinical Nutrition*, **33**, 1620–1628.

Gong, H. Jr (1992). Breathing easy: Exercise despite asthma. *Physician and Sportsmedicine*, **20**(3), 159–167.

Goodman, D.S. (1988). Report of National Cholesterol Education Programme expert panel on detection, evaluation and treatment of high cholesterol in adults. *Archives of Internal Medicine*, **148**, 36.

Gordon, D.J., Wiztum, J.L, Hunninhake, D.B., Gates, S. and Gluck, C.J. (1983). Habitual physical activity and high density lipoprotein cholesterol in men with primary hypercholesterolemia. *Circulation*, **67**, 512–520.

Gorski, J., (1985). Exercise during pregnancy: maternal and foetal responses. A brief review. *Medicine and Science in Sports and Exercise*, **17** (4), 407–416.

Grundy, S.M. (1986) Cholesterol and coronary heart disease. *Journal of the American Medical Association*, **256**, 2849–2858.

Gudart, U., Berger, M. and Lefèbvre, P.J. (1994). Physical activity, fitness and non-insulin dependent diabetes mellitus. In *Physical Activity, Fitness and Health. International Proceedings and Consensus Statement*, Bouchard, C., Shephard, R.J. and Stephens, T. (eds). Champaign, IL: Human Kinetics.

Gwinap, G. (1971). Thickness of subcutaneous fat and activity of underlying muscles. *Annals of Internal Medicine,* **74,** 408.

Hagberg, J.M., Montain, S.J., Martin, W.H. *et al.* (1989). Effect of exercise training in 60–69 year old persons with essential hypertension. *American Journal of Cardiology,* **64,** 348–353.

Hadler, N.M. (1985). Osteoarthritis as a public health problem. *Clinics on Rheumatic Diseases,* **11**(2), 175–185.

Hall, D.C. and Kaufmann, D.A. (1987). Effects of aerobic and strength conditioning on pregnancy outcomes. *American Journal of Obstetrics and Gynecology,* **157,** 119–1203.

Hardman, A.E. (1996). Exercise in the prevention of atherosclerotic, metabolic and hypertensive diseases: A review. *Journal of Sports Sciences,* **14**(3), 201–218.

Hardman, A.E. *et al.* (1998). Loss of lipoprotein lipase activity with detraining BASES Annual Conference, Physiology Keynote presentation. Leeds: BASES.

Hartung, G.H. (1984). Diet and exercise and the regulation of plasma lipids and lipoproteins in patients at risk of coronary disease. *Sports Medicine* **1,** 413–418.

Haskell, W.L. (1978). Cardiovascular complications during exercise training of cardiac patients. *Circulation,* **57,** 920–924.

Haskell, W. L. (1984a) The influence of exercise on the concentrations of triglyceride and cholesterol in human plasma. *Exercise and Sport Sciences Reviews,* **12,** 205–244.

Haskell, W.L. (1984b). Exercise induced changes in plasma lipid and lipoprotein levels. *Preventive Medicine* **13,** 23–36.

Haskell WL (1994). The efficacy and safety of exercise programs in cardiac rehabilitation. *Medicine and Science in Sports and Exercise,* **26**(7), 815–823.

Hatch, M.C., Hu, X., McLean, D.E., Levin, B., Begg, M., Reuss, L. and Susser, M. (1993). Maternal exercise during pregnancy, physical fitness and fetal growth. *American Journal of Epidemiology,* **137,** 1105–1114.

Health of the Nation (1993). *A strategy for Health in England.* London: HMSO.

Heath. G.W., Leonard, B.E., Wilson, R.H., Kendrick, J.S. and Powell, K.E. (1987). Community-based exercise intervention: Zuni diabetes project. *Diabetes Care,* **10,** 579–583.

Heffron, M., Davey, R. and Cochrane, T. (1997). Weight-training and bone mass in post-menopausal women. *Sports, Exercise and Injury,* **3,** 143–149.

Helmrich, S.P., Ragland, D.R., Leung, R.W. and Paffenbarger, R.S. (1991). Physical activity and reduced occurrence of non-insulin dependent diabetes mellitus. *New England Journal of Medicine,* **325,** 147–152.

Hill, J.O., Drougas, H.J. and Peters, J.C. (1994). Physical activity, fitness and moderate obesity. In *Physical Activity, Fitness and Health. International Proceedings and Consensus Statement,* Bouchard, C., Shephard, R.J. and Stephens, T. (eds). Champaign, IL: Human Kinetics.

Hirsch, J. (1972). Can we modify the number of adipose cells? *Postgraduate Medicine,* **51,** 83–86.

Hirsch, J. and Batchelor, B.R. (1976). Adipose cellularity in human obesity. *Clinics in Endocrinology and Metabolism,* **5,** 299.

Hollmann, W. (1991). Physical fitness; an introduction. In *Sport for All,* Oja, P. and Telama, R. (eds). New York: Elsevier.

Holloszy, J.O. (1983). Exercise, health and aging: a need for more information. *Medicine and Science in Sports and Exercise,* **15,** 1.

Holness, M.J., Changani, K.K. and Sugden, M.C. (1991). Progressive suppression of muscle glucose utilization during pregnancy. *Biochemical Journal,* **280,** 549–552.

Horan, M.J. and Lenfant, C. (1990). Epidemiology of blood pressure and predictors of hypertension. *Hypertension,* **15**(Suppl. I), I25–I28.

Horan, M.J. and Mockrin, S.C. (1990). Hypertension research: the next five years. *Hypertension,* **15**(Suppl. I), I29–I32.

Howell, D.S. and Manicourt, D.H. (1988). The connective tissues: structure, function and metabolism. In *Primer on the Rheumatic Diseases* (9th ed.), Schuacher, H.R. Jr, Kippel, J.H. and Robinson, D.R. (eds). Atlanta, GA: Arthritis Foundation.

Howley, E.T. and Franks, B.D. (1997). *Health Fitness Instructor's Handbook* (3rd ed.). Champaign, IL: Human Kinetics.

Huftel, M.A., Gaddy, J.N. and Busse, W.W. (1991). Finding and managing asthma in competitive athletes. *Journal of Respiratory Diseases,* **12,** 1110–1112.

Hutchinson, R.G. (1985) *Coronary Prevention: A Clinical Guide Year Book.* Chicago: Medical Publications Inc.

Huttunen, J.K., Lansimies, E., Voulilainen, E., Ehnholm, C., Hietanen, E., Penttila, I., Sitonen, O. and Rauramaa, R. (1979). Effect of moderate physical exercise on serum lipoproteins. A controlled clinical trial with special reference to serum high density lipoproteins. *Circulation*, **60**, 1220–1229.

Hyers, T.M., Martin, B.J., Pratt, D.S., Dreisin, R.B. and Franks, J.J. (1980). Enhanced thrombin and plasmin activity with exercise in man. *Journal of Applied Physiology*, **48** (5), 821–825.

Hytten, F.E. and Paintin, D.B. (1963) Increase in plasma volume during normal pregnancy. *Journal of Obstetrics and Gynaecology of the British Commonwealth*, **70**, 402.

Ike, R.W., Lampman, R.M. and Castor, C.W. (1989). Arthritis and aerobic exercise: a review. *Physician and Sportsmedicine*, **17**(2), 128–138.

Ivy, J.L. (1997). Role of exercise training in the prevention and treatment of insulin resistance and non-insulin-dependent diabetes mellitus. *Sports Medicine*, **24**(5), 321–336

Johnson, M.L., Burke, B.S. and Mayer, J. (1956). Relative importance of inactivity and overeating in the energy balance of obese high school girls. *American Journal of Clinical Nutrition*, **4**, 37.

Jovanovic-Peterson, L., Durak, E.P. and Peterson, M. (1989). Randomized trial of diet versus diet plus cardiovascular conditioning on glucose levels in gestational diabetes. *American Journal of Obstetrics and Gynecology*, **161**, 415.

Joye, K., DeMaria, A.N., Giddens, J., Kaku, R., Amsterdam, E., Mason, D.T. and Lee, G. (1978) Exercise induced decrease in platelet aggregation: comparison between normals and coronary patients showing similar physical activity related effects. *American Journal of Cardiology*, **41**, 432.

Kannel, W.B. and Dawber, T.R. (1972). Atherosclerosis as a pediatric problem. *Journal of Pediatrics*, **80**, 544–554.

Kannel, W.B., Wilson, P. and Blair, S.N. (1985). Epidemiological assessment of the role of physical activity and fitness in the development of cardiovascular disease. *American Heart Journal*, **109** (4), 876–885.

Kasch, F.W. (1976) Effects of exercise on the aging process. *Physician and Sportsmedicine*, **4**, 64.

Kasch, F.W. and Wallace, J.P. (1976). Physiological variables during 10 years of endurance exercise. *Medicine and Science in Sports*, **5**, 5–8.

Katch, F.I. (1969). Effects of physical training on body composition and diet of females. *Research Quarterly*, **40**, 99.

Katch, F.I. (1984). Effects of sit-up exercise training on adipose cell size and adiposity. *Research Quarterly for Exercise and Sport*, **55** (3), 242–247.

Kelemen, M.H., Stewart, K.J., Gillan, R.E. *et al.* (1981). Circuit weight training in cardiac patients. *Journal of the American College of Cardiology*, **7**, 38–42.

Kiyonaga, A., Arakawa, K., Tanaka, H. and Shindo, M. (1984). Blood pressure and hormonal responses to aerobic exercise. *Hypertension*, **7**, 125–131.

Klinger, K.W. (1985). Genetics of cystic fibrosis. *Seminars in Respiratory Medicine*, **6**, 243–251.

Kovar, P.A., Allegrante, J.P. and MacKenzie, C.R. (1992). Supervised fitness walking in patients with osteoarthritis of the knee: a randomized, controlled trial. *Annals of Internal Medicine*, **116**(7), 529–534.

Kramsch, D.M. (1981). Reduction of coronary atherosclerosis by moderate conditioning exercise in monkeys on an atherogenic diet. *New England Journal of Medicine*, **305**, 1483–1489.

Kujala, U.M., Kettunen, J. and Paananen, H. (1995). Knee osteoarthritis in former runners, soccer players, weight lifters and shooters. *Arthritis and Rheumatism*, **38**(4), 539–546.

Kukkonen, K., Pauramaa, R., Voutilainen, E. and Lansimies, E. (1982) Physical training of middle-aged men with borderline hypertension. *Annals of Clinical Research*, **14** (Suppl. 34), 139–145.

Laakso, M., Edelman S.V., Olefsky, J.M. *et al.* (1990). Kinetics of in vivo muscle insulin-mediated glucose uptake in human obesity. *Diabetes*, **39**, 965–974.

Laakso, M., Edelman S.V., Brechtel, G. *et al.* (1992). Impaired insulin mediated skeletal muscle blood flow in patients with NIDDM. *Diabetes*, **41**, 1076–1083.

Laiard-Meeter, K, van de Ley, G, Bom, T and Wladimiroff, J.W. (1979). Cardiocirculatory adjustments during pregnancy – an echocardiographic study. *Clinics in Cardiology*, **2**, 328–332.

Lane, N.E., Bloch, D.A., Jones, H.H. *et al.* (1986). Long distance running, bone density and osteoarthritis. *Journal of the American Medical Association*, **255**, 1147.

Laughlin, M.H., McAllister, R.M. and Delp, M.D. (1994). Physical activity and the microcirculation in cardiac and skeletal muscle. In *Physical Activity, Fitness and Health. International Proceedings and Consensus Statement*, Bouchard, C., Shephard, R.J. and Stephens, T. (eds). Champaign, IL: Human Kinetics.

Ledwidge, B. (1980) Run for your mind: aerobic exercise as a means of alleviating anxiety and depression. *Canadian Journal of Behavioural Science*, **12**, 126–139.

Lees, M.M., Taylor, S.H., Scott, D.B. and Keer, M.G. (1967). A study of cardiac output at rest throughout pregnancy. *Journal of Obstetrics and Gynaecology of the British Commonwealth,* **74**, 3.

Lefèbvre, P.J., Pirnay, F., Pallikarakis, N., Krzentowski, G., Jandrain, B., Mosora, F., Lacroix, M. and Luyckx, A.S. (1986). Metabolic availability of carbohydrates ingested during, before or after muscular exercise. *Diabetes Metabolism Review,* **1**, 483–500.

Leon, A.S., Conrad, J. Hunninghake, D.B. and Serfass, R. (1979). Effects of a vigorous walking program on body composition and carbohydrate and lipid metabolism of obese young men. *American Journal of Clinical Nutrition,* **32**, 1776–1787.

Linder, C.W. and DuRant, R.H. (1982). Exercise, serum lipids and cardiovascular disease risk factors in children. *Pediatric Clinics of North America,* **29**, 1341–1354.

Ljunger, H. and Bergqvist, D. (1984). Decreased fibrinolytic activity in human atherosclerotic vessels. *Atherosclerosis,* **50**, 113–116.

Lokey, E.A., Tran, V., Wells, C.L., Myers, B.C. and Tran, A.C. (1991). Effects of physical exercise on pregnancy outcomes: a meta-analytic review. *Medicine and Science in Sports and Exercise,* **23**, 1234–1239.

Long, B.C. (1983). Aerobic conditioning and stress reduction: participation or conditioning? *Human Movement Science,* **2**, 171–186.

Longo, L.D. (1983). Maternal blood volume and cardiac output during pregnancy: A hypothesis of endocrinologic control. *American Journal of Physiology,* **245** R720–R729.

Looker, A.C., Johnston C.C., Wahner H.W. *et al.* (1995). Prevalence of low femoral bone density in older U.S. women from NHANES III. *Journal of Bone Mineral Research,* **10**(5), 796–802.

Lotgering, F.K., Gilbert, R.D. and Longo, L.D. (1983). Exercise responses in pregnant sheep. Oxygen consumption, uterine blood flow and blood volume. *Journal of Applied Physiology,* **55**, 834–841.

Lund, C.J. and Donovan, J.C. (1967). Blood volume during pregnancy. *American Journal of Obstetrics and Gynecology,* **98** (23), 393–403.

MacHeath, J. (1984). *Activity, Health and Fitness in Old Age.* London: St Martin's Press.

MacKeen, P.C., Franklin, B.A., Nicholas, W.C. and Buskirk, E.R. (1983). Body composition, physical work capacity and physical activity habits at 18–month follow-up of middle-aged women

participating in an exercise intervention program. *International Journal of Obesity,* **7**, 61–71.

Maheux, P., Jeppensen, J., Sheu, W.H., Hollenbeck, C.B., Clinkingbeard, C., Greenfield, M.S., Chen, Y.D. and Reaven, G.M. (1994). Additive effects of obesity, hypertension, and type 2 diabetes on insulin resistance. *Hypertension,* **24**(6), 695–698.

Manninen, V. *et al.* (1988). Lipid alterations and decline in the incidence of coronary heart disease in the Helsinki study. *Journal of the American Medical Association,* **260**, 641.

Manson, J.E., Rimm, E.B., Stampfer, M.J., Colditz, G.A., Willett, W.C., Krolewski, A.S., Rosner, B., Hennekens, C.H. and Speizer, F.E. (1991). Physical activity and incidence of non-insulin dependent diabetes mellitus in women. *Lancet,* **338** (8770), 774–778.

Mayer, J. (1980). *Overweight: Causes, Cost and Control.* Englewood Cliffs, NJ: Prentice Hall.

Mayer, J. and Thomas, D.W. (1967). Regulation of food intake and obesity. *Science,* **156**, 328.

McFadden, E.R. Jr (1995). Exercise induced airway obstruction. *Clinical Chest Medicine,* **16**, 671–682.

McMurray, R.G., Berry, M.J. and Katz, V. (1990). The beta-endorphin responses of pregnant women during aerobic exercise in water. *Medicine and Science in Sports and Exercise,* **22**, 298–303.

McNamara, J.J., Molot, M.A., Stremple, J.F. and Cutting, R.T. (1971) Coronary artery disease in combat casualties in Vietnam. *Journal of the American Medical Association,* **216**, 1185–1187.

Meade, T.W., Chakrabarti, R., Haines, A.P., North, W.R.S. and Stirling, Y. (1979). Characteristics affecting fibrinolytic activity and plasma fibrinogen concentration. *British Medical Journal,* **278** (i), 153–156.

Meade, T.W., Brozovic, M., Chakrabarti, R.R., Haines, A.P., Imeson, J.D., Mellows, S., Miller, G.J., North, W.R.S., Stirling, Y. and Thompson, S.G. (1986). Haemostatic function and ischemic heart disease: Principal results of the Northwick Park heart study. *Lancet,* **331**, 533–537.

Melton, L.J. III. (1995). How many women have osteoporosis now? *Journal of Bone Mineral Research,* **10**(2), 175–177.

Mezzapelli, J., Motola, M.F., Scanchter, C.L., and McKenzie, K. (1991). Effects of metabolic alterations due to exercise on maternal blood glucose, lactate and foetal outcome in rat. *Medicine and Science in Sports and Exercise,* **23**, S169.

Milkines, K.J., Farrell, P.A., Sonne, B., Tronier, B. and Balbo, H. (1988). Post exercise dose response relationship between plasma glucose and insulin secretion. *American Journal of Physiology*, **63**(3), 988–999.

Miller, W.J., Sherman, W.M. and Ivy, J.L. (1984). Effect of strength training on glucose tolerance and post-glucose insulin response. *Medicine and Science in Sports and Exercise*, **16**, 539–543.

Mink, B.D. (1997). Exercise and chronic obstructive pulmonary disease. Modest fitness gains pay big dividends. *Physician and Sportsmedicine*, **25**(11), 43–57.

Mole, P.A., Stern, J.S., Schultz, C.L., Bernauer, E.M. and Holcomb, B.J. (1989). Exercise reverses depressed metabolic rate produced by severe caloric restriction. *Medicine and Science in Sports and Exercise*, **21** (1), 29–33.

Moore, S. (1994). Physical activity, fitness and atherosclerosis. In *Physical Activity, Fitness and Health. International Proceedings and Consensus Statement*, Bouchard, C., Shephard, R.J. and Stephens, T. (eds). Champaign, IL: Human Kinetics.

Morris, N., Osborn, S. and Wright, H. (1956). Effective uterine blood flow during exercise in normal and pre-eclamptic pregnancies. *Lancet*, **271**, 481–484.

Morris, J.N., Everitt, M.G. and Senunence, A.M. (1987) Exercise and heart disease. In *Exercise Benefits, Limits and Adaptations*, Macleod, D., Maughan, R., Nimmo, M., Reilly, T. and Williams, C. (eds). London: E & FN Spon; 4–17.

Morris, J.N. (1994). Exercise in the prevention of coronary heart disease: today's best buy in public health. *Medicine and Science in Sports and Exercise*, **26** (7), 807–814.

National Diabetes Data Group (1979). Classification and diagnosis of Diabetes and other categories of glucose intolerance. *Diabetes*, **28**, 1039–1057.

National Institutes of Health Consensus Development Conference Statement (1985). Lowering blood cholesterol to prevent heart disease. *Journal of the American Medical Association*, **253**, 2080.

Newton, P.M., Mow, V.C. and Gardener, T.R. (1997). The effect of lifelong exercise on canine articular cartilage. *American Journal of Sports Medicine*, **25**(3), 282–287.

Nizankowska-Blaz, T. and Abramowicz, T. (1983). Effects of intensive physical training on serum lipids and lipoproteins. *Acta Pediatrica Scandinavica*, **72**, 357–359.

Noakes, T.D., Opie, L.H. and Rose, A.G. (1984) Marathon running and immunity to coronary heart disease: Fact versus Fiction. *Clinics in Sports Medicine*, **3** (2), 527–543.

Noland, M. and Kearney, J.T. (1978). Anthropometric and densitrometric responses of women to specific and general exercises. *Research Quarterly*, **49**, 322.

Nordemar, R., Ekblom, B., Zachrisson, L. and Lundqvist (1981). Physical training in rheumatoid arthritis: a controlled long term study (I and II). *Scandinavian Journal of Rheumatology*, **10**, 17–30.

Oldridge, N.B., Guyatt, M.E., Fisher, M.E. and Rimm, A.A. (1988). Cardiac rehabilitation after myocardial infarction: combined exercise and randomized clinical trials. *Journal of the American Medical Association*, **260**, 945–950.

Olefsky, J.M. (1976). The insulin receptor: Its role in insulin resistance in obesity and diabetes. *Diabetes*, **25**, 1154–1164.

Olefsky, J.M. and Reaven, G.M. (1974). Decreased insulin binding to lymphocytes from diabetic patients. *Journal of Clinical Investigation*, **54**, 1323–1328.

Pace, P.J., Webster, J. and Garrow, J.S. (1986). Exercise and obesity. *Sports Medicine*, **3**, 89–113.

Paffenbarger, R.S., Hyde, R.T., Wing, A.L. and Steinmetz, C.M. (1984). A natural history of athleticism and cardiovascular health. *Journal of the American Medical Association*, **252,** 491–495.

Panush, R.S. and Brown, D.G. (1987). Exercise and arthritis. *Sports Medicine*, **4**, 54.

Peckos, P.S. (1953). Caloric intake in relation to physique in children. *Science*, **117,** 631.

Pescatello, L.S., Fargo, A.E., Leach, C.N. and Scherzer, H.H. (1991). Short-term effect of dynamic exercise on arterial blood pressure. *Circulation*, **83**, 1557–1561.

Pomerance, J.J., Gluck, L. and Lynch, V.A. (1974). Physical fitness in pregnancy: Its effect on pregnancy outcome. *American Journal of Obstetrics and Gynecology*, **119**, 867–876.

Powell, K.E., Thompson, P.D., Caspersen, C.J. and Kendrick, J.S. (1987). Physical activity and the incidence of coronary heart disease. *Annual Review of Public Health*, **8**, 253–287.

Qu Xia (1990). Morphological study of myocardial capillaries in endurance trained rats. *British Journal of Sports Medicine*, **24** (2), 113–116.

Rauramaa, R. and Salonen, J.T. (1994). Physical activity, fibrinolysis and platelet aggregability. In *Physical Activity, Fitness and Health. Inter-*

national *Proceedings and Consensus Statement,* Bouchard, C., Shephard, R.J. and Stephens, T. (eds). Champaign, IL: Human Kinetics.

Rauramaa, R., Salonen, J.T., Seppanen, K., Salonen, R., Venalainen, J.M., Ihanainen, M. and Rissanen, V. (1986). Inhibition of platelet aggregability by moderate intensity physical exercise: A randomised clinical trial in overweight men. *Circulation,* **74**, 939–944.

Ray, W.A., Griffin, M.R. and Baugh, D.K. (1990). Mortality following hip fracture before and after implementation of the prospective payment system. *Archives of Internal Medicine,* **150**(10), 2109–2114.

Reaven, G.M. (1994). Syndrome X; 6 years later. *Journal of International Medicine Supplementum,* **736**, 13–22.

Reaven, G.M. and Laws, A. (1994). Insulin resistance, compensatory hyperinsulinaemia, and coronary heart disease. *Diabetologia,* **37**(9), 948–952.

Reaven, P.D., Barrett-Connor, E. and Edelstein, S. (1991). Relation between leisure-time physical activity and blood pressure in older women. *Circulation,* **83**, 559–565.

Rikkers, R. (1986) *Seniors on the Move.* Champaign, IL: Human Kinetics.

Roberts, W.C. (1984). An agent with lipid lowering, antihypertensive, positive, inotropic, negative chronotropic, vasodilating, diuretic, anorexigenic, weight reducing, cathartic, hypoglycemic, tranquilising, hypnotic and antidepressive qualities. *American Journal of Cardiology,* **53** (1), 261.

Rodnick, K.J., Haskell, W.L., Swislocki, A.L.M., Foley, J.E. and Reaven, G.M. (1987). Improved insulin action in muscle, liver and adipose tissue in physically trained human subjects. *American Journal of Physiology,* **235**, E489–495.

Rognum, T.O., Rodahl, K. and Opstad, P.K. (1982). Regional differences in the lipolytic response of the subcutaneous fat depots to prolonged exercise and severe energy deficiency. *European Journal of Applied Physiology,* **49,** 401.

Roman, O. Camuizzi, A.L., Villalon, E. and Kienner, C. (1984). Physical training program in arterial hypertension: a long term prospective follow-up. *Cardiology,* **67,** 230–243.

Rose, D.J., Bader, M.E., Bader, R.A. and Braunwald, E. (1956). Catheterization studies of cardiac hemodynamics in normal pregnant women with reference to left ventricular work. *American Journal of Obstetrics and Gynecology,* **72**, 2.

Rotkis, T.C., Boyden, T.W., Parmenter, R.W., Stanforth, P. and Wilmore, J.H. (1980). High density lipoprotein cholesterol and body composition of female runners. *Metabolism, Clinical and Experimental,* **30**(10), 994–995.

Rubler, S., Damani, P.M. and Pinto, E.R. (1977). Cardiac size and performance during pregnancy estimated with echocardiography. *American Journal of Cardiology,* **40**, 534–540.

Ruderman, N.B., Ganda, O.P. and Johansen, K. (1979). The effect of physical training on glucose tolerance and plasma lipids in maturity-onset diabetes. *Diabetes,* **28** (Supplement), 89–92.

Salans, L.B., Cushman, S.W. and Weismann, R. E. (1973). Studies of human adipose tissue, adipose cell size and number in non-obese and obese. patients. *Journal of Clinical Investigation,* **52,** 929.

Salonen, J.T., Puska, P. and Tuomilcht, J. (1982). Physical activity and risk of myocardial infarction, cerebral stroke and death. *American Journal of Epidemiology,* **115** (4), 526.

Schade, M., Hellebrandt, F.A., Waterland, J.C. and Carns, M.C. (1962). Spot reducing in overweight college women. *Research Quarterly,* **33,** 461–71.

Schaible, T., Pehpargkul, S. and Scheuer, J. (1981). Cardiac responses to exercise in male and female rats. *Journal of Applied Physiology,* **50**, 112.

Scheuer, J. (1982). Effects of physical training on myocardial vascularity and perfusion. *Circulation,* **66**, 491–495.

Schiesinger, M.J. (1938). An injection plus dissection study of coronary artery occlusions and anastomoses. *American Heart Journal,* **15**, 528–568.

Schneider, S.H., Kim, H.C., Khachadurian, A.K. and Ruderman, N.B. (1988). Impaired fibrinolytic response to exercise in type II diabetes: Effects of exercise and physical training. *Metabolism,* **37**, 924–929.

Seals, D.R. and Hagberg, J.M. (1984). The effect of exercise training on human hypertension: a review. *Medicine and Science in Sports and Exercise,* **16,** 107–115.

Segal, K.R. and Pi-Sunyer, F.X. (1989). Exercise and obesity. *Medical Clinics of North America,* **73** (1), 217–236.

Shangold, M.M. (1994). Exercise during pregnancy in the 90's. *Sports Medicine Digest,* **16**(12).

Shephard, R.J. (1976). Exercise and chronic obstructive lung disease. *Exercise and Sport Science Reviews,* **4**, 263–296.

Shephard, R.J. (1994). *Aerobic Fitness and Health.* Champaign, IL, Human Kinetics.

Shephard, R.J. (1997). What is the optimal type of physical activity to enhance health? *British Journal of Sports Medicine*, **31**, 277–284.

Sims, E.A.H. (1974). Studies in human hyperphagia. In *Treatment and Management of Obesity*, Bray, G.A. and J.E. Bethune, J.E. (eds). New York: Harper & Row.

Smith, E.L., Smith, K.A. and Gilligan, C. (1990). Exercise fitness and osteoporosis. In *Exercise, Fitness and Health*, Bouchard, C., Shephard, R.J., Stephens, T., Sutton, J. and McPherson, B. (eds). Champaign, IL: Human Kinetics.

Sonnenberg, G.E., Kemmer, F.W. and Berger, M. (1990). Exercise in type 1 (insulin-dependent) diabetic patients treated with continuous subcutaneous insulin infusion. *Diabetologia*, **33**, 696–703.

Sparling M, Cantwell J, Dolan R and Niederman R (1990). Strength training in a cardiac rehabilitation programme. A six-month follow-up. *Archives of Physical Medicine and Rehabilitation*, **71**, 148.

Spector, T.D. (1990). Rheumatoid arthritis. *Rheumatic Disease Clinics of North America*, **16**(3), 513.

Sports Council/Health Education Authority (1992). *Allied Dunbar National Fitness Survey*. London: Sports Council/HEA.

Squires, R.W. (1983). Cardiac rehabilitation issues for heart transplantation patients. *Journal of Cardiopulmonary Rehabilitation*, **10**, 159–168.

Sternfeld, B., Quesenberry, C.P., Eskenazi, B. and Newman, L.A. (1995). Exercise during pregnancy and pregnancy outcome. *Medicine and Science in Sports and Exercise*, **27** (5), 634–640.

Stevenson, J.A.F., Feleki, V., Rechnitzer, P. and Beaton, J.R. (1964). Effect of exercise on coronary tree size in the rat. *Circulation Research*, **15**, 265–269.

Stone, M.C. and Thorpe, J.M. (1985). Plasma fibrinogen – a major coronary risk factor. *Journal of the Royal College of General Practitioners*, **35**, 565–569.

Stratton, J.R., Chandler, W.L., Schwartz, R.S., Cerqveira, M.D., Levy, W.L., Kahn, S.E., Larson, V.G., Cain, K.C., Beard, J.C. and Abrass, I.B. (1991). Effects of physical conditioning on fibrinolytic variables. *Circulation*, **83**, 1692–1697.

Strauzenberg, S.E. (1981) Sport in old age; advantages and risks. *Journal of Sports Medicine and Physical Fitness*, **21** (4), 309–319.

Synder, D.K. and Caruth, B.R. (1984). Current controversies: exercising during pregnancy. *Journal of Adolescent Health Care*, **5**, 34–36.

Takada, A. and Takada, Y. (1988). Physiology of plasminogen: with special reference to activation and degradation. *Haemostasis*, **18** (Supplement 1), 25–35.

Tan, R.A. and Spector, S.L. (1998). Exercise induced asthma *Sports Medicine*, **25**(1), 1–6.

Taunton, J.E., Martin, A.D., Rhodes, E.C., Wolski, L.A., Donelly, M. and Elliot, J. (1997). Exercise for the older woman: choosing the right prescription. *British Journal of Sports Medicine*, **31**, 5–10.

Tepperman, J. and Pearlman, D. (1961). Effects of exercise and anemia on coronary arteries of small animals as revealed by the corrosion-cast technique. *Circulation Research*, **9**, 576–584.

Tharp, G.D. and Wagner, C.T. (1982). Chronic exercise and cardiac vascularisation. *European Journal of Applied Physiology*, **48**, 97.

Thorland, W.G. and Gilliam, T.B. (1981) Comparison of serum lipids between habitually high and low active preadolescent males. *Medicine and Science in Sports and Exercise*, **13**, 316–321.

Thornton, E. W. (ed.) (1984). *Exercise and Aging: An unproven relationship*. Liverpool: Liverpool University Press.

Thompson, P.D. and Fahrenbach, M.C. (1994) Risks of exercising: cardiovascular including sudden cardiac death. In *Physical Activity, Fitness and Health. International Proceedings and Consensus Statement*, Bouchard, C., Shephard, R.J. and Stephens, T. (eds). Champaign, IL: Human Kinetics.

Thompson, P.D., Cullinane, E.M., Sady, S.P., Flynn, M.S., Chenevert, C.B. and Herbert, P.N. (1991). High density lipoprotein metabolism in endurance athletes and sedentary men. *Circulation*, **84**, 140–152.

Tipton, C.M. (1984). Exercise training and hypertension. *Exercise and Sport Science Reviews*, vol. 12. Baltimore: Waverly Press; 245–306.

Tipton, C.M. (1991). Exercise training and hypertension: An update. *Exercise, Sport Science Reviews*, vol. 19. Baltimore: Waverly Press; 447–505.

Trip, M.D., Cats, V.M., van Capelle, F.J.L. and Vreeken, J. (1990). Platelet hyperreactivity and prognosis in survivors of myocardial infarction. *New England Journal of Medicine*, **302**, 1424–1425.

Udall, J.G. (1978). Interaction of maternal and neonatal obesity. *Pediatrics*, **62**, 17.

Ueland, K., Novy, M.J., Peterson, E.N. and Metcalfe, J. (1969). Maternal cardiovascular dynamics. *American Journal of Obstetrics and Gynecology*, **104**, 6.

Valimaki, I., Hursti, M.L., Pihiaskoski, L. and Viikari, J. (1980). Exercise performance and serum lipids in relation to physical activity in school children. *International Journal of Sports Medicine*, **1**, 132–138.

Van Camp, S.P. and Peterson, R.A. (1986). Cardiovascular complications of outpatient cardiac rehabilitation programmes. *Journal of the American Medical Association*, **256**, 1160–1163.

Vanderport, M. and McComas, A.J. (1986). Contractile changes in opposing muscles of the human ankle joint with ageing. *Journal of Applied Physiology*, **61**, 361–367.

Varassi, G., Bazzano, C. and Edwards, W.T. (1989). Effects of physical activity on maternal plasma beta-endorphin levels and perception of labour pain. *American Journal of Obstetrics and Gynecology*, **180**, 707–712.

Vinten, J. and Galbo, H. (1983). Effect of physical training on transport and metabolism of glucose in adipocytes. *American Journal of Physiology*, **244** (2), E129.

Vogt, A. and Straub, P.W. (1979). Lack of fibrin formation in exercise induced activation of coagulation. *American Journal of Physiology*, **236** (4), H577–9.

Voy, R.O. (1986). The U.S. Olympic Committee experience with exercise induced bronchospasm – 1984. *Medicine and Science in Sports and Exercise*, **18**, 328–330.

Vranic, M., Wasserman, D. and Bukowiecki, L. (1990). Metabolic implications of exercise and physical fitness in physiology and diabetes. In *Diabetes mellitus: Theory and practice*, Rifkin, H. and Porte, D. Jr (eds). New York: Elsevier Science; 198–219.

Wake, J. (1998). Exercise for stroke survivors. *Exercise*. Jan and Feb edition.

Wallberg-Henriksson, H., Rincon, J. and Zierath, J.R. (1998). Exercise in the management of non-insulin-dependent diabetes mellitus. *Sports Medicine*, **25**(1), 25–35.

Walters, W.A.W., MacGregor, W.G. and Hills, M. (1966). Cardiac output at rest during pregnancy and the puerperium. *Clinical Science*, **30**, 1.

Wells, C.L. (1991). *Women, Sport and Performance*. Champaign, IL: Human Kinetics.

Whipp, B.J. and Casaburi, R. (1994). Physical activity, fitness and chronic lung disease. In *Physical Activity, Fitness and Health. International Proceedings and Consensus Statement*, Bouchard, C., Shephard, R.J. and Stephens, T. (eds). Champaign, IL: Human Kinetics.

Widhalm, K., Maxa, L. and Zyman, H. (1978). Effect of diet and exercise upon cholesterol and triglyceride control of plasma lipoproteins in overweight children. *European Journal of Pediatrics*, **127**, 121–126.

Wilhelmsen, L., Svarsdudd, K., Korsan-Bengsten, K., Larsson, B., Welin, L. and Tibblin, G. (1984). Fibrinogen as a risk factor for stroke and myocardial infarction. *New England Journal of Medicine*, **311**, 501–505.

Wilmore, J.H. (1983). Body composition in sport and exercise: directions for future research. *Medicine and Science in Sports and Exercise*, **15** (1), 21–31.

Wilson, M., Morganti, A., Zervoudakis, J., Letcher, K.L., Romney, B.M. *et al.* (1980). Blood pressure and the renin-aldosterone system and sex steroids throughout normal pregnancy. *American Journal of Medicine*, **68**, 97–104.

Wolf, P.A. and Kanel, W.B. (1986). Reduction of stroke through risk factor modification. *Seminars in Neurology*, **6**, 243–253.

Wolfe, L.A., Hall, P., Webb, K.A., Goodman, L., Monga, M. and McGrath, M.J. (1989). Prescription of aerobic exercise during pregnancy. *Sports Medicine*, **8** (5), 273–301.

Woo, R. and Pi-Sunyer, F.X. (1985). Effects of increased physical activity on voluntary food intake in lean women. *Metab. Clin. Exp.*, **34**, 836–41.

Woo, R., Garrow, J.S. and Pi-Sunyer, F.X. (1982a). Effects of exercise on spontaneous caloric intake in obesity. *American Journal of Clinical Nutrition*, **36**, 470–477.

Woo, R., Garrow, J.S. and Pi-Sunyer, F.X. (1982b). Voluntary food intake during prolonged exercise in obese women. *American Journal of Clinical Nutrition*, **36**, 478–484.

Wood, P.D. and Haskell, W.L. (1979). The effect of exercise on plasma high density lipoproteins. *Lipids*, **14** (4), 417–427.

Woolf-May, K., Bird, S. and Owen, A. (1997). The effects of an 18 week walking programme on cardiac function in previously sedentary or relatively inactive adults. *British Journal of Sports Medicine*, **31**(1), 48–53.

Wong, S.C. and McKenzie, D.C. (1989). Cardiorespiratory fitness during pregnancy and its effects on outcome. *International Journal of Sports Medicine*, **8**, 79–83.

Wood, P.D., Stefanick, M.L., Williams, P.T. and Haskell, W.L. (1991). The effects on plasma lipoproteins of a product weight-reducing diet, with or without exercise, in overweight men and women. *New England Journal of Medicine*, **325**, 461–466.

Work, J.A. (1989). Is weight training safe during pregnancy? *Physician and Sportsmedicine*, **17**, 257–259.

Wyatt, H.L. and Mitchell, J. (1978). Influences of physical conditioning and deconditioning on coronary vasculature of dogs. *Journal of Applied Physiology*, **45**, 619–635.

Young, J.C. and Treadway, J.L. (1992). The effect of prior exercise on oral glucose tolerance in late gestational women. *European Journal of Applied Physiology and Occupational Physiology*, **64** (5), 430–433.

Zavaroni, I., Dall'Aglio, E., Braschi, F. *et al.* (1986). Effect of age and environmental factors on glucose tolerance and insulin secretion in a worker population. *Journal of the American Geriatric Society*, **34**, 271–275.

Zierath, J.R. and Wallberg-Henriksson, H. (1992). Exercise training in obese diabetic patients: special considerations. *Sports Medicine*, **14**, 171–189.

Zoll, P.M. Wessler, S. and Schlesinger, M.J. (1951). Interarterial coronary anastomoses in the human heart with particular reference to anemia and relative anoxia. *Circulation*, **4**, 797–815.

Zuti, W.B. and Golding, L.A. (1976). Comparing diet and exercise as weight reducing tools. *Physician and Sportsmedicine*, **4**, 49–53.

ADDRESS

National Osteoporosis Society, PO Box 10, Radstock, Bath BA3 3YB, UK.

A review of movement terminology (planes, axes, rotations), terminology to describe body parts and positions, the types of muscular contractions (concentric, eccentric and isometric) and muscle roles related to function.

THE NEED FOR PRECISE TERMINOLOGY

When describing the movements of the body specific terminology is required to prevent confusion. For instance, if the exercise adviser/therapist was to record that Mr X experienced pain when he 'bent his elbow' the precise movement that caused the pain could be interpreted and visualised by another practitioner in a number of different ways: it could refer to the client bending his elbow so that his forearm came across his body, bending it to the side away from his body, out in front of his body or even behind his back. Clearly such confusions must be avoided when describing an individual's condition to another practitioner or when making notes that may be read at a later date. In order to prevent such confusion a specific vocabulary is used.

Likewise, to say simply that a muscle 'contracts' does not convey whether it produces movement or simply generates tension without associated movement. Because muscles fulfil many functions, an appropriate use of standard terminology is required to accurately describe the type of contraction occurring.

PLANES AND AXES

One method of accurately describing a movement is to use terminology which describes movements with reference to specific planes and axes. For this purpose there are three major planes (also referred to as the primary or cardinal planes): the *transverse* plane, the *sagittal* plane and the *frontal* or *lateral* plane (Figure 12.1). Each plane has a corresponding axis which passes perpendicularly through it. Movements may therefore be described as occurring in a plane and about an axis.

THE TRANSVERSE PLANE

The transverse plane can be visualised as passing horizontally through the body, dividing it into a top and bottom half. Passing through the plane, from the top of a person's head down to between the feet runs the *longitudinal,* or *vertical axis* (Figure 12.2).

To assist with the visualisation of the planes and axes and the movements that occur in them it helps to use models made of stiff cardboard or plasticine. A wire or pencil passing through the model can be used to represent the axis. If the pencil is spun in the transverse plane and longitudinal axis, the model would rotate about the axis rather like an ice skater performing a spin. Movements in the transverse plane about the longitudinal axis include rotating the head, twisting the body or moving the forearm across the body (Figure 12.3).

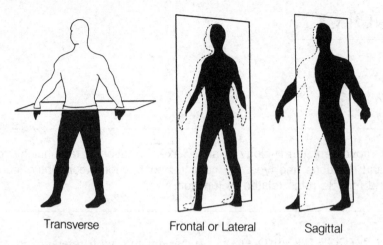

Figure 12.1   The three major planes. Each plane may be visualised as a pane of glass. A particular movement is said to be in that plane if it runs parallel to the pane of glass

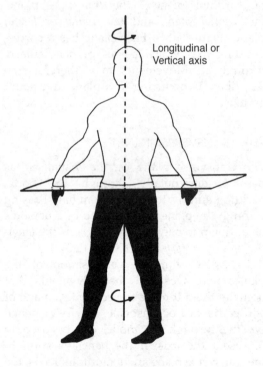

Transverse plane

Figure 12.2   Transverse plane and longitudinal axis

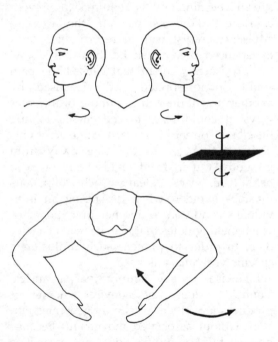

Figure 12.3   Movements in the transverse plane

THE SAGITTAL PLANE

A second plane, extending down the centre of the body and dividing it into left and right halves, is the sagittal plane. The sagittal plane's corresponding axis, the *bilateral axis*, passes through the body from one hip to another

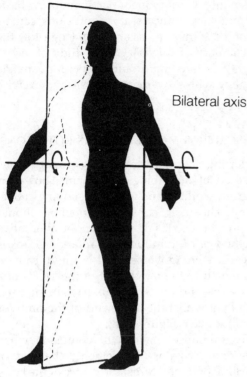

Bilateral axis

Sagittal plane

Figure 12.4 The sagittal plane

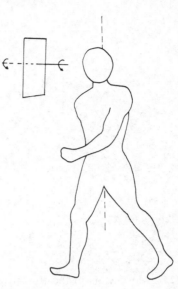

Figure 12.5 Movements in the sagittal plane

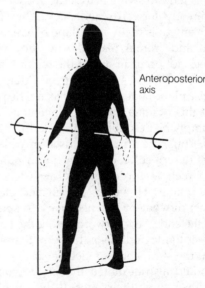

Anteroposterior axis

Figure 12.6 The frontal or lateral plane

(Figure 12.4). If the body were to rotate about this axis it would rotate forwards or backwards, as occurs in a somersault. The use of models may again help to aid visualisation of this movement. Basic movements in the sagittal plane include those of the legs when walking (Figure 12.5).

THE LATERAL PLANE

The third major plane passes through the body, dividing it into front and back halves, and is referred to as the frontal or lateral plane. Its corresponding *anteroposterior axis* runs through the body from front to back (Figure 12.6). Movements in this plane and about the anteroposterior axis are illustrated in Figure 12.7.

OTHER PLANES AND AXES

Although these planes and axes are useful as terms of reference, most of the movements made by the body fall between and across them. For instance, the arm action when walking is not quite in the sagittal plane because

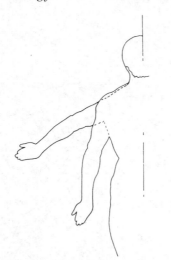

Figure 12.7 Movements in the frontal or lateral plane

the arms tend to swing across the body rather than directly forwards and back. Therefore, the movement is really in a plane between the sagittal and frontal planes. Any movement that does not occur in one of the major planes may be described as occurring in a diagonal or *oblique* plane about an *oblique* axis. The position of this oblique plane of movement may then simply be described relative to the major planes. Thus, the arm action used in walking may be described as occurring in an oblique plane which is approximately at 10° to the sagittal plane. However, to further clarify the exact movement it is necessary to specify that at the end of the forward swing the hands are closer to the midline of the body than they were at the start, and not vice versa.

It should also be noted that if the subject moves then so do the planes. If the subject is lying horizontal then the sagittal plane still extends forwards, dividing the body into left and right halves, the transverse plane still divides the body into top and bottom halves, and the frontal plane divides it into front and back halves. Most bodily movements are complex, involving many body parts which may be moving in slightly different planes. By systematically breaking down the move-

ment into its component parts and using basic terminology unnecessary confusions can be avoided. Thus a basic knowledge of the vocabulary of *kinesiology* (the study of movement) is an important asset for anyone dealing with movement analysis and exercise prescription.

DESCRIBING MOVEMENTS AS ROTATIONS

Referring to planes and axes provides one method of describing movements; however, there are others and when describing movements the most convenient method should always be used. For instance, an alternative method of description uses rotations. This is because the movement of a limb can be compared to the movement of the hands of a clock; one end can be visualised as being fixed at a joint whilst the other end of the limb (or bone) moves (Figure 12.8).

To minimise the risk of confusion when describing rotatory movements the end of the limb or bone nearest the centre of the body is referred to as the *proximal* end, whilst the end furthest from the centre of the body is described as being *distal*. So, when describing movements of the forearm, the ends of the radius and ulna that are nearest the elbow are proximal, and the ends furthest from the

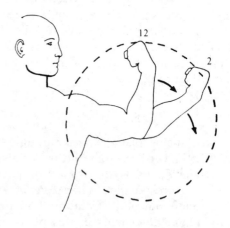

Figure 12.8 How rotatory movements may be described with reference to a clock face

elbow and nearest the hand are distal. Similarly, the top of the femur would be referred to as proximal whilst the foot would be considered distal. So, when relating the movement to a clock face it is usually the proximal end of the limb that is imagined to be at the centre of the clock face and the distal end of the limb to be at the periphery. In most movements the proximal end remains fixed and the distal end is seen to move. However, there are a few examples in which the positions are reversed and the distal end remains fixed (at the centre of the clock) whilst the proximal end moves.

To give a description of the movements in terms of rotation, it is first necessary to standardise the position of the imaginary clock because the action of raising a glass to one's lips may be seen as a clockwise rotation of the forearm in the sagittal plane when viewed from one side of the subject but as an anticlockwise action in the sagittal plane when viewed from the opposite side. Therefore, for all rotations in the sagittal plane the subject is viewed as looking to the right with the clock facing the observer (Figure 12.9). Even if the subject is not really being viewed from this angle when the movement is being described, the assessor must imagine viewing

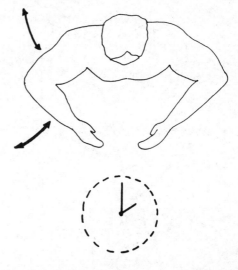

Figure 12.10 Describing clockwise and anticlockwise movements in the transverse plane

the movement from the subject's right side in order to describe the movement in the standard manner – the assessor must always 'see' the right-hand side of the subject.

Similarly, when describing movements in the transverse plane about the longitudinal axis, the assessor must visualise the movement from above with a clock at the foot of the subject, facing upwards (Figure 12.10). For rotations in the frontal plane about the anteroposterior axis the assessor must visualise the subject facing them with a clock above and behind them, also facing the assessor (Figure 12.11).

DESCRIBING BODY PARTS AND MOVEMENTS

Correct use of planes and axes will enable accurate description of the direction of a movement. This description can be enhanced by the use of a more extensive and specific vocabulary that refers to the types of movement possible within those planes. Common everyday expressions such as 'to bend' or 'to move' may be interpreted in a number of ways. To prevent this, those working in the

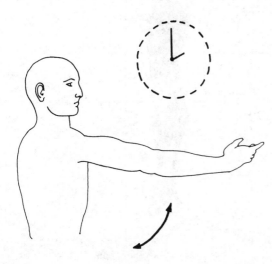

Figure 12.9 How clockwise and anticlockwise movements may be described in the sagittal plane

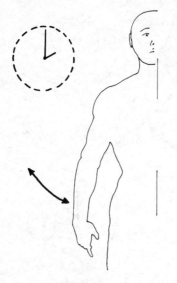

Figure 12.11 How clockwise and anticlockwise movements may be described in the frontal or lateral plane

fields of exercise prescription and exercise therapy should have a basic kinesiological vocabulary which will enable them to describe movements accurately. Common terms used to describe forms of movement include flexion, extension, abduction, adduction, elevation, depression, eversion, inversion, supination and pronation. Other standardised terms may also required to describe precisely the body part that is being moved – in this context anterior, posterior, lateral, medial, distal, proximal, superior, inferior, deep and superficial may be utilised. When these terms are used in conjunction with the planes and axes described earlier, any movement can be precisely described.

A starting point is needed as a frame of reference. In kinesiology the starting point is the *anatomical position* (Figure 12.12). Many movements need to be visualised as beginning from the anatomical position even if in reality they have not. This helps to clarify the description of certain movements.

LATERAL AND MEDIAL

The term *lateral* refers to the body part furthest from the midline of the body, whereas *medial* refers to the body part nearest the midline of the body (Figure 12.13). Hence particular

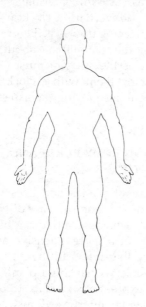

Figure 12.12 The anatomical position

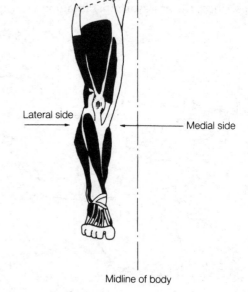

Lateral side ⟷ Medial side

Midline of body

Figure 12.13 Use of the terms lateral and medial

ligaments in the knee are referred to as being lateral ligaments (positioned down the outer side of the knee) and medial ligaments (positioned down the inner side of the knee). Similarly, the foot may be described as having a lateral border and a medial border.

DISTAL AND PROXIMAL

When referring to part of the limbs of the body the term *distal* refers to the part furthest way from the centre of the body and *proximal* refers to the part nearest the centre. This can be illustrated using the example of the radius and ulna of the forearm. The distal ends of these bones form part of the wrist joint, their proximal ends form part of the elbow joint.

ANTERIOR AND POSTERIOR

Anterior refers to the body part nearest the front of the body, *posterior* refers to the body part nearest the back or dorsal side of the body.

SUPERIOR AND INFERIOR

Superior parts are nearest the head, *inferior* parts lie furthest away from the head. Internal structures such as arteries are often named using this criterion.

DEEP AND SUPERFICIAL

Deep refers to the part furthest from the surface of the body whilst *superficial* refers a part near the surface. Thus a muscle may be described as having superficial fibres and deep fibres. Alternatively, muscle damage may be described as deep or superficial.

FLEXION AND EXTENSION

A movement which reduces the angle of a join is termed *flexion*. A simple flexion movement in the sagittal plane is shown in Figure 12.14. Other examples include hip flexion

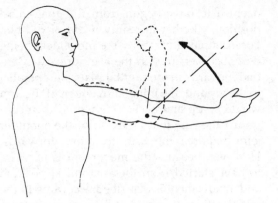

Figure 12.14   Flexion of the elbow joint

(lifting the thigh whilst walking), flexing the knee, flexion of the back (leaning forward) and dorsal flexion of the ankle.

Movement of the arm about the shoulder joint is a little more difficult to define since it is not very clear when the angle of the joint is decreasing. However, as with all other movements in the sagittal plane (except the knee) a forward movement from the anatomical position is referred to as flexion. Raising the arm from the anatomical position is considered to be shoulder flexion (Figure 12.15).

With such a movement it is important to remember the rule that the movement is

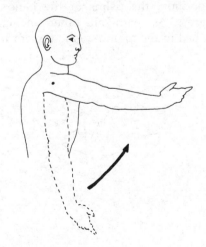

Figure 12.15   Shoulder flexion

deemed to have begun from the anatomical position, whether in reality it did or did not. For example, if in reality the movement being described began with the arm already extended forwards in the sagittal plane and parallel to the ground, the initial movement of the arm would be up and back. This would then contradict the rule that a flexion of the shoulder joint requires the arm to move forwards. However, because the movement is *imagined* to have started from the anatomical position and a movement is described according to the initial action, it would still be referred to as shoulder flexion and thus would not contravene the rule.

The opposite of flexion is *extension*; any movement that increases the angle at a joint is therefore referred to as an extension movement. Extending the ankle, knee and hip all occur in the sagittal plane whilst walking as the foot pushes against the ground and the leg straightens (note the imprecise nature of non-scientific vocabulary: 'leg straightens'). Lowering the arm and straightening the elbow are also extension movements (Figure 12.16).

In the sagittal plane the movement of the fingers may be considered in a similar manner to the movement of the limbs and trunk. This consistency is ensured since, in the anatomical position, the palms of the hands face forwards. As with all other movements described in the sagittal plane (except that at the knee joint) the 'bending' of the fingers is referred to as flexion and their straightening as extension. Movements of the foot at the ankle joint in the sagittal plane may also be described using the terms flexion or extension – or the more specific terms of dorsiflexion and plantar flexion are applied to describe ankle flexion and ankle extension respectively. *Dorsiflexion* is the ankle movement that brings the toes nearer to the knees, *plantar flexion* refers to the ankle movement that occurs when someone 'points' their toes or stands on the balls of their feet.

The term *hyperextension* is often used to refer to an extension movement that is beyond the normal anatomical position. Hyperextending the back would result in a participant 'leaning' backwards (Figure 12.17). Some individuals will also exhibit an ability to hyperextend other joints beyond the 'normal' expected range of movement, in which case the term hyperextension may again be applied.

It can be seen from the diagrams that flexion and extension movements may also be described as rotations in the various planes. This alternative mode of description is covered in a later section.

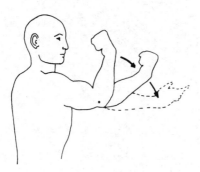

Figure 12.16 Extension of the elbow

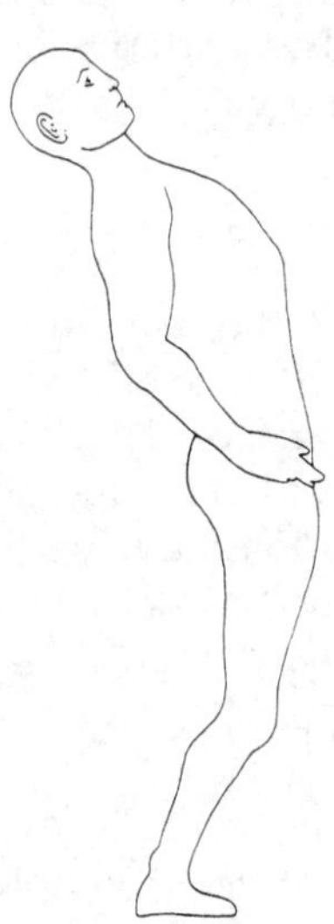

Figure 12.17 Hyperextension of the back

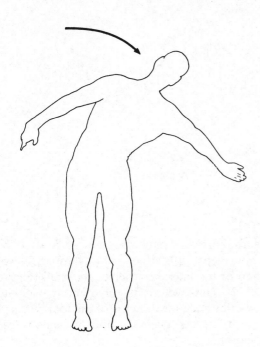

Figure 12.18 Lateral flexion of the spine

LATERAL FLEXION

Flexion movements also occur in the frontal plane. For example, bending to the side may be described as a *lateral flexion* of the trunk (Figure 12.18). Bending to the right, decreasing the angle of the trunk on that side, is called 'right lateral flexion of the trunk'; bending to the left would be 'left lateral flexion of the trunk'. The terms left and right lateral flexion may also be used to describe movements of the neck in the frontal plane.

ABDUCTION AND ADDUCTION

These are terms used to describe movements in the frontal plane about the anteroposterior axis. In order to describe these movements it is first necessary to visualise the body in the anatomical position with a 'midline' running down the centre from the top of the head to the floor. Beginning in the anatomical position, any movement of a body part away from the midline of the body is referred to as *abduction* whereas any movement towards the midline

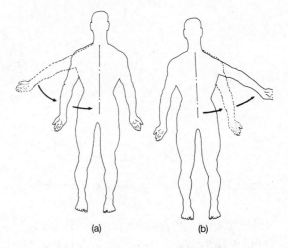

Figure 12.19 (a) Adduction and (b) abduction of the arm at the shoulder joint

of the body is referred to as *adduction* (Figure 12.19).

As with the flexion movements in the sagittal plane, movements in the frontal plane must be envisaged as starting from the anatomical position. Thus when crossing the feet (left leg over right leg) the left foot will initially move to the subject's right, towards the midline of the body, cross the midline of the body and then continue moving to their right away from the midline of the body. However, because the movement is envisaged to have started from the anatomical position and the initial movement is clearly towards the midline of the body and hence an adduction, the entire movement, regardless of where it was initiated, is referred to as an adduction. The movement of the arms in the frontal plane may be described in a similar manner.

The movements of the fingers in the frontal plane are considered separately to those of the limbs or trunk. When describing movement of the fingers in the frontal plane a midline is imagined running through the middle finger of the hand. Any movement of the digits away from the middle finger is referred to as abduction, movement towards the middle finger as adduction (Figure 12.20).

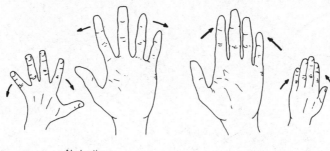

Figure 12.20 Abduction and adduction of the fingers

HORIZONTAL EXTENSION (HORIZONTAL ABDUCTION) AND HORIZONTAL FLEXION (HORIZONTAL ADDUCTION)

These movements are performed in the transverse plane and, unlike most other actions, cannot be performed directly from the anatomical position. To perform these movements the limb must first be abducted or flexed until it is in a horizontal position. Horizontal extension and horizontal flexion may be performed by both the upper and the lower limbs. However, strength and flexibility are required to perform such movements with the lower limbs: without assistance, many individuals will only be able to perform them with the upper limbs. *Horizontal extension* (horizontal abduction) is a movement of the limb in the transverse plane away from the midline of the body. *Horizontal flexion* (horizontal adduction) refers to a movement of the limb in the transverse plane towards the midline of the body (Figure 12.21).

ELEVATION AND DEPRESSION

The terms elevation and depression are commonly used to describe movements of the shoulder, the simplest example being 'shrugging' the shoulders. In such an action, the upward movement of the shoulders is referred to as *elevation* and the downward movement is known as *depression*. Elevation

and depression may also be used to describe movements of the foot – for example, 'elevation of the lateral border of the foot' (Figure 12.22). However, it is often more usual to describe such movements of the foot with the specific terms 'eversion' and 'inversion' (see below).

EVERSION AND INVERSION

These are terms commonly used to describe movements of the foot. *Eversion* refers to

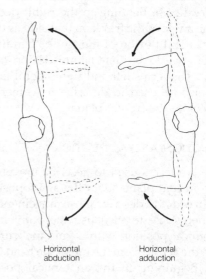

Horizontal abduction

Horizontal adduction

Figure 12.21 Horizontal extension (horizontal abduction) and horizontal flexion (horizontal adduction) of the elbows in the transverse plane

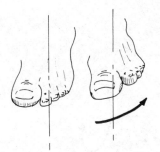

Figure 12.22   Elevation of the lateral border of the foot

raising of the lateral border such that, if standing, the weight is placed on the medial border of the foot. The opposite to eversion is *inversion*, in which the medial border is raised and weight is placed on the lateral border of the foot.

SUPINATION AND PRONATION

These are somewhat more complex movements and their exact meaning will depend upon the body part being moved and the plane in which it is being moved. *Pronation* of the arm is best illustrated by considering the subject to be in the anatomical position and then his or her hands turning so that the palms face backwards rather than forwards. This is achieved by rotating or twisting the right hand anticlockwise and the left hand clockwise (for movements in the transverse plane imagine the clock at the feet of the subject and viewing the movement from above their head). The opposite to pronation is *supination*.

Supination describes the action used to tighten a screw (if using the right hand), whereas a pronating action with the right hand would loosen the screw.

The terms pronation and supination are also often used to describe movements of the foot. In this case the movement occurs in an oblique plane. Pronation of the foot is used to describe the combination of moving the toes away from the middle of the body and

raising the lateral border so that the weight tends to be placed on the medial side of the foot. Supination refers to the opposite action – that of moving the toes closer to the midline of the body and raising the medial border such that the weight is placed on the lateral border of the foot.

CLOCKWISE AND ANTICLOCKWISE ROTATIONS

Such terms may be effectively used to describe twisting movements such as rotating the spine in the transverse plane (Figure 12.23). However, when describing such movements it must be remembered that the movement has to be 'viewed' from above the subject. The use of the terms clockwise and anticlockwise rotations may also be used to describe flexion and extension movements in the sagittal, frontal and oblique planes, thereby providing an alternative mode of description. Similarly, certain movements of the arms and legs may also be described as inward and outward rotations. Thus, if starting from the anatomical position, a clockwise rotation of the right limbs would be described as an outward

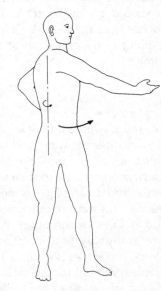

Figure 12.23   Anticlockwise rotation of the spine

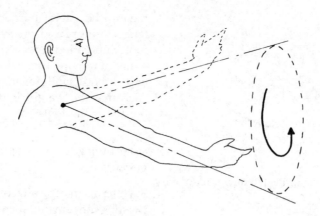

Figure 12.24 Circumduction of the shoulder joint

rotation. Conversely, an outward rotation of the left limbs would require an anticlockwise rotation. Inward rotations would therefore be achieved by a clockwise rotation of the left limbs and an anticlockwise rotation of the right.

CIRCUMDUCTION

Circumduction refers to a rotary movement of a body part so that its movement traces a cone. An example would be the circumduction of the shoulder joint (Figure 12.24) where the arm rotates from the shoulder joint (which forms the point of the cone) whilst the hand traces a circle.

SUMMARY

In practice, any movement may be described in a number of different ways and it is up to the individual to use the most appropriate in terms of clarity. Correct use of such terms will allow precise and unambiguous description of movements. This form of movement terminology also enables classification of muscles and muscle groups by function (hip flexors, elbow flexors, ankle flexors, etc.). This provides a simple, practical means of description to use instead of, or as well as, their Latin names, depending upon circumstances.

TYPES OF MUSCLE ACTION AND TERMINOLOGY

Muscles fulfil many roles – some obvious, others not so obvious. They contract to initiate movement of the whole body or a body part, regulate movement that is being caused by another force, or even to prevent movement that is being caused by another muscle or an external force such as gravity. Basic co-ordinated movements require many muscles to contribute in a variety of ways to produce the desired action. To gain an understanding of the complex and varied roles that muscles fulfil in movement sequences it is first necessary to review their functions in isolation – always remembering that muscles work in co-ordinated groups rather than separately.

When an appropriate nerve impulse is sent to a muscle, tension builds up in that muscle. This process is more commonly described as a *muscular contraction* (for details of the process of muscle contraction see one of the exercise physiology texts listed at the end of this chapter). Muscles may contract in a number of different ways depending upon the function they are fulfilling. If there is a change in the length of the muscle, and hence the build up of tension is associated with movement, the contraction is described as being *dynamic*. Alternatively, if tension builds up in the muscle but its length remains unaltered (and there is therefore no movement), the contraction is described as *static* or *isometric*. The different types of muscle contraction may be classified as:

- concentric;
- eccentric; or
- static (isometric).

CONCENTRIC CONTRACTIONS

A concentric contraction is a dynamic contraction during which the muscle shortens. It may be *isotonic* ('isoinertial' is the term preferred by some authorities; Abernethy *et al.*, 1995) or *isokinetic*. A muscle contraction is said to be concentric when the resulting tension in the muscle causes it to shorten and cause movement.

Isotonic contraction

The term isotonic means 'same tension'. With this form of contraction, the speed of the resulting movement will vary owing to various physiological and biomechanical factors. For example, the movement may be relatively slow in the early stages of its initiation, quite rapid during the middle phase, and then slow towards the end. Many body and limb movements will fall into this category. Such movements occur when the tension in the muscle, and thus the force of contraction, exceeds that of an opposing force or resistance applied to it. The resistance (or opposing force) may be the weight of a limb or of an object that the individual is attempting to lift. If the force of the contraction exceeds that of the resistance, the muscle will shorten and cause movement. For example, the hip flexors contract to raise the leg in the process of walking; the biceps contracts when raising a glass to one's mouth. The change in speed during the movement is attributable to a number of factors, including differences in the strength of the muscle at different lengths, changes in the effective angle of pull of the muscle on the bones during the movement, and the general inertia of the part providing the resistance.

Isokinetic contractions

Concentric isokinetic contractions are in many respects similar to isotonic contractions. However, during an isokinetic contraction the speed of the movement remains constant; 'isokinetic' means 'same speed'. This is achieved by altering the tension in the muscle during the movement or by providing an accommodating resistance which enables a constant speed to be produced throughout the range of movement. Isokinetic machines can dictate the speed of contraction and measure the force of contraction very precisely. A less precise form of accommodating resistance can be applied by an assistant.

ECCENTRIC CONTRACTIONS

Eccentric contractions occur when tension is present in the muscle but it is forced to lengthen, rather than shorten, by an opposing force. This occurs when the muscle is already in a shortened or semi-shortened state and the force generated is less than that of an opposing external force. In such movements the opposing force causes the muscle to lengthen, despite the muscle generating a force which would otherwise have caused it to shorten. Eccentric contractions are commonly used to regulate movements caused by external forces such as gravity – as in lowering an object onto a table. Here the movement is caused by the force of gravity but the eccentric contractions of the biceps control the lowering action. By generating a tension in the biceps that is slightly less than that of the external force (gravity acting upon the arm and object being held) the muscle slowly lengthens, gradually lowering the object. If the biceps did not contract eccentrically the arm holding the object would fall in an uncontrolled manner. Another example of eccentric contraction occurs when lowering oneself into a chair: the eccentric contractions of the hip and leg extensors permit a controlled lowering action. If the eccentric contractions did not take place we would simply fall into the chair rather than lowering ourselves in a controlled manner.

Eccentric contractions during walking

A similar form of eccentric contraction occurs when someone walks or runs. When the foot strikes the ground and begins to take the weight of the body, the hip and knee joints tend to flex. If this flexion were not checked we would simply collapse onto the floor. To prevent this, the hip and knee extensors contract to oppose the flexion movement. In the early stages of this 'checking' process the amount of force generated by the contraction of hip and knee extensors is insufficient to instantly halt the movement. Hence the hip and knee extensors lengthen despite the tension being generated in them, and thus the hip and knee joints continue to flex (albeit at a decelerating rate). The hip and knee extensor muscles can therefore be said to be working eccentrically. A fraction of a second later in the movement, as the muscular contractions of the knee extensors continue, they exceed the force of gravity, causing the downward (flexion) movement to be slowed and eventually stopped. The flexion movement is then stopped for an instant and as the force of the muscular contractions continue to exceed that of gravity the extensor muscles start to shorten and cause the leg to straighten. Hence, when walking, the hip and knee extensors will work eccentrically to check the downward movement caused by gravity as the weight is placed on the leg, the movement (flexion) will be stopped for an instant and the extensors will then start to work concentrically as their force of contraction exceeds that of gravity, and they shorten, causing the hip and knee to be extended. Eccentric contractions can be very stressful on the muscles and are associated with muscular soreness 24–48 hours after exercise (delayed

onset of muscular soreness; DOMS). It is commonly experienced after unfamiliar exercises such as a new weight training exercise, circuit training or downhill running.

Eccentric contractions can also be produced using isokinetic devices.

STATIC (ISOMETRIC) CONTRACTIONS

If the resistance or opposing force applied to a muscle is equal to the force of contraction that the muscle is generating, then, although tension is present in the muscle, no movement will take place. This form of muscle contraction is referred to as a static or isometric contraction. Many muscles and muscle groups function in this manner. For example, although the muscles of the torso may be used to move the body they also spend much of their time maintaining the torso in a relatively fixed position, combating the force of gravity and retaining the posture. Other muscles may work in a similar manner to prevent unwanted movement caused either by external forces such as gravity or by the action of other muscles that may be contracting dynamically. Consequently, although an activity such as walking occurs through the dynamic contraction of various muscles, the activity also requires numerous other muscles to contract isometrically in order to maintain body posture during the activity.

RANGE OF MOVEMENT

The movement of a limb or body part may be described according to its motion within the *full range of movement* that the joint can produce – from the position where it is fully flexed to the position where it is fully extended, or from the position of maximal abduction to maximal adduction and so on, depending on the specific movement being considered. The *outer range of movement* of a joint is the movement in the region where the muscle causing the movement is close to its longest possible length. Conversely, the *inner range of movement*

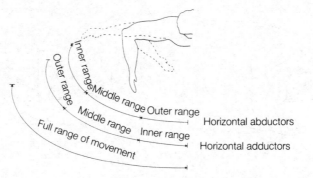

Figure 12.25 The movement at the elbow joint may be described in terms of its inner, middle, outer and full range

of a joint corresponds to movement in the range where the muscle causing the movement is almost fully shortened. The *middle range of movement* lies between the two (Figure 12.25).

In a further example – that of elbow flexion and extension – movement from a fully extended to a partially flexed position is described as its outer range of movement because during the motion the biceps is close to being at its maximum length. As the flexion continues the biceps moves the elbow through its middle range into its inner range of movement, at which point it is close to being fully shortened. Conversely, the extension movement caused by the triceps muscle would be described in the following manner: the initial movement from the fully flexed position (when the triceps is close to its maximum length) is its outer range and the region during which the elbow is almost fully extended and the triceps is fully contracted is its inner range. In this way the description of a range of movement at a joint depends upon the muscles that are acting to cause the movement.

THE VARIED ROLES THAT MUSCLES FULFIL

Having briefly covered the different forms of muscle contraction it is now possible to discuss the various roles of muscles and the functions they fulfil in initiating, controlling and preventing movement. Muscles may be considered as:

- agonists or movers;
- antagonists;
- fixators, including stabilisers and supporters;
- regulators;
- neutralisers;
- synergists.

However, it must be remembered that in different circumstances a muscle or muscle group may fulfil many roles, even during what may at first appear to be the same movement. For instance, the biceps of the arm may be considered as an agonist when lifting an object, a regulator when lowering it, a supporter when holding it steady and an antagonist when the elbow is being extended by the triceps. If the movement shown in Figure 12.26 is considered, the initial flexion is caused by the biceps acting as an agonist whilst the triceps remains relaxed and lengthens, thereby being by definition an antagonist. However, once the forearm has passed the vertical the movement would automatically continue under the force of gravity but may need to be controlled by the eccentric contraction of the triceps, which would then be acting as a regulator. The reverse movement, during which the elbow was extended, would initially

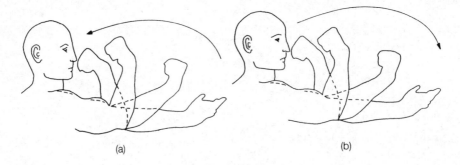

(a)   (b)

Figure 12.26 The roles which muscles fulfil may alter during a single movement. (a) The biceps acts as agonist and the triceps as antagonist until the movement reaches the vertical, whereupon gravity continues the movement and the triceps works eccentrically as a regulator. (b) The triceps acts an agonist and the biceps as an antagonist during the early phase of the movement; once beyond the vertical gravity will continue the movement and the biceps works eccentrically as a regulator

involve the triceps working as the agonist and the biceps remaining relaxed and lengthened, thereby being the antagonist. In the second phase of the movement the biceps may be required to act as regulator in order to control the lowering movement. This example also serves to illustrate the fact that muscles usually work in pairs or groups, not singularly. This requires complex co-ordination and co-operation between muscle groups. Failure to achieve this co-ordination will result in unco-ordinated and/or impeded movement.

When describing a movement and relating it to the muscle groups involved it is important to ask a number of questions:

- Is the movement being caused by muscular contraction or gravity?
- If the movement is being caused by gravity, is it being regulated by eccentric muscular contractions?
- Which joints are involved, and which muscle groups are active during the movement?

Another factor to be considered is whether any other muscle groups are involved in stabilising either the joint or other parts of the body during the movement.

AGONISTS

Agonists are muscles that cause a movement; they are therefore sometimes also described as *movers*. When flexing the elbow from the anatomical position in the sagittal plane the elbow flexors would be referred to as the agonists, with the major muscle involved being the biceps brachii: in such an action the biceps brachii may thus be referred to as the prime mover. Other examples of agonists include the hip flexors, when raising the leg upwards and forwards during walking, or the knee and ankle extensors during walking when pushing against the ground.

ANTAGONISTS

An *antagonist* is a muscle that opposes a movement if it contracts. In order to permit a free movement the antagonist must relax and lengthen. If it does not, as can happen in certain neuromuscular disorders such as spasticity, the movement will be impeded. Examples of antagonists include the elbow extensors (triceps brachii) when the elbow is flexing, and the ankle extensors (such as the gastrocnemius) when the ankle is being flexed.

FIXATORS

A *fixator* is a muscle which contracts to prevent unwanted movement. There are two classes of fixator: *stabilisers* and *supporters*. Stabilisers contract to prevent movement that would occur due to the contraction of another muscle, whereas supporters contract to prevent movement that would occur due to an external force such as gravity.

Stabilisers

A stabiliser prevents an unwanted movement that may be caused by the active contraction of another muscle. Movement may be brought about by shortening muscle groups attached to bones. Often the desired action will be movement in a joint at the distal end of the bone but movement of the joint at the proximal end of the bone may reduce the effectiveness of the action. Therefore a stabilising muscle may contract to hold the proximal end of the bone in position. During many actions a limited amount of movement is necessary at the proximal end of the bone and hence stabilisers will often work both isometrically and isotonically to achieve the desired effect. The stabilising action of muscles operate at an unconscious level and illustrate the complexity of co-ordinated movement.

Supporters

In contrast to a stabiliser, which fixes a bone in position and opposes a movement that would occur due to the action of another muscle, a supporter fixes a body part in position against an external force such as gravity. This requires the muscle to contract statically, opposing the force of gravity with an equal force. Many muscles work in this manner to maintain posture and body position, especially those of the back.

REGULATORS

A regulator muscle controls a movement caused by the force of gravity. In doing so it must contract eccentrically. Examples of regulating actions include lowering a heavy pan or weight onto a table or lowering oneself into a chair. If the muscles did not contract eccentrically to control/regulate the movement, one would fall into the chair in an uncontrolled manner or lower the pan too rapidly.

NEUTRALISERS

A neutraliser contracts to prevent the unwanted action of another muscle whilst permitting the desired action of that muscle. An example of this can be seen with the biceps brachii. This muscle not only flexes the elbow but can also supinate the forearm (when turning a door handle or tightening a screw (with the right hand) the desired action would be that of supination). If the action of forearm flexion were to occur at the same time as supination it would prove to be most inconvenient, pulling the hand away as it turned. To prevent forearm flexion the elbow extensors (triceps brachii) also contract, neutralising the unwanted flexion movement whilst permitting the desired supination. Another example would be that of moving from a lying to a sitting position in bed. To sit up a number of abdominal muscles are involved, including the right and left external obliques. Depending upon which other muscles contract at the same time, the contraction of the external obliques can result in flexion, lateral flexion or rotation. If the external obliques were to contract separately then the right external obliques would cause the body to rotate to the left whilst the left external obliques would cause the body to rotate to the right. This rotary action is really a combination of forward flexion and rotation. However, if both the left and right external obliques contract together they neutralise their opposing rotary actions and permit the desired forward flexion of the trunk.

SYNERGISTS

Synergists are muscles which operate in a complex manner to assist in movement. They work at an unconscious level and make the actions of the agonists stronger. Synergists often act to prevent unwanted movement, steady the actions caused by the agonists and help to maintain a muscle at its optimum length.

THE MAJOR MUSCLE GROUPS AND THEIR ACTIONS

The human body contains over 600 muscles which act on the 206 bones of the skeleton to stabilise it and produce effective movement. The muscles affect the actions at more than 200 joints or articulations. To describe such actions in detail would require a separate text, and the aim here is to present a brief overview of these aspects rather than an in-depth study. This overview should provide exercise advisers, therapists and other health professionals with a suitable basic background and insight into the topic from which they may pursue the subject in greater detail. In summary, this section presents a basic coverage of the muscles that are used in the major movements of the limbs. These movements are those which are most likely to be incorporated into an exercise programme.

It should be remembered that body movements are complex, involving many muscles which fulfil many roles. Indeed, the exact role which a muscle fulfils at any one time may depend upon many factors.

- The fibres that are contracting within the muscle. In certain muscles the contraction of different parts of the same muscle can produce different results and, in addition, the number of fibres contracting within the muscle will influence the amount of force it generates.
- Other muscles are that contracting at the same time. These may be assisting with the movement, opposing it, or stabilising a joint or body part during the movement.

- The external forces that are acting upon the body.
- The position of the body part when the muscle contracts.

Such differences can have a profound effect upon the resulting action, making the study of the topic far from simple. It should also be realised that some muscles extend over two joints and thus their actions will affect the movements at more than one joint, complicating the subject still further.

In order to assist with the coverage of the major muscle groups and their actions a labelled skeleton is presented in Figure 12.27 and the positions of a selection of the major muscles of the body are illustrated in Figure 12.28. For the sake of clarity, Figure 12.28 illustrates only the major superficial muscle groups and not the deeper muscles, which are positioned behind those illustrated. For more detailed information on the specific actions of particular muscles the reader should refer to the recommended further reading.

MOVEMENTS OF THE HIP

Two of the major muscle groups involved with movements of the hip are the quadriceps femoris and hamstrings. The quadriceps femoris consists of four distinct parts: rectus femoris, vastus lateralis, vastus medialis and vastus intermedius. The functions of these constituent parts differ, and they are therefore described separately in this section. Likewise the actions of the three constituent muscles of the hamstring muscle group (the biceps femoris, semitendinosus and semimembranosus) are also described separately.

Hip flexion

Psoas, iliacus (also stabilises hip), sartorius, rectus femoris, pectineus, tensor fasciae latae, gluteus medius (anterior fibres), gluteus minimus (anterior fibres), adductor longus (assists), adductor brevis (assists when in

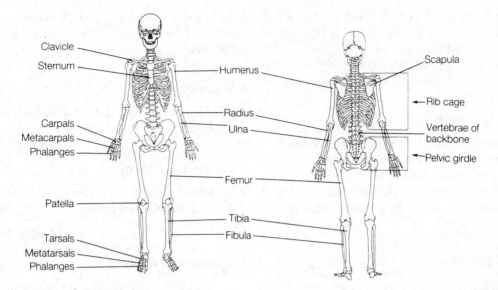

Figure 12.27 The major bones of the body

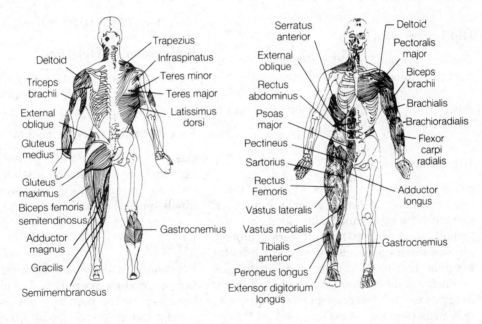

Figure 12.28 The major muscle groups of the body

standing position), adductor magnus (flexion and inward rotation when upper fibres contract alone) and gracilis (when knee is extended).

Hip extension

Biceps femoris, semitendinosus, semimembranosus, gluteus maximus, gluteus medius (posterior fibres), gluteus minimus (posterior fibres), adductor brevis (if hip is already in flexed position it extends and adducts the hip) and adductor magnus (extension and outward rotation when lower fibres contract alone).

Hip adduction

Pectineus, adductor longus, adductor magnus (when whole muscle contracts), gracilis, adductor brevis (when in standing position, but if hip is in flexed position it extends and adducts the hip) and gluteus maximus (lower portion assists).

Hip abduction

Sartorius, rectus femoris, tensor fasciae latae, gluteus maximus (upper third), gluteus medius and gluteus minimus.

Hip inward rotation

Tensor fasciae, semitendinosus, gluteus medius (anterior fibres), gluteus minimus (anterior fibres), gracilis and adductor magnus (inward rotation and flexion when upper fibres contract alone).

Hip outward rotation

Sartorius, gluteus maximus, obturator externus, obturator internus, gemellus superior, gemellus inferior, quadratus femoris, piriformis, gluteus medius (posterior fibres), gluteus minimus (posterior fibres), adductor magnus (outward rotation and extension when lower fibres contract alone), adductor longus (assists), biceps femoris (assists) and pectineus (weak assistor).

MOVEMENTS OF THE KNEE

Knee flexion

Biceps femoris, sartorius, semitendinosus, semimembranosus, gracilis, popliteus, plantaris (weak assistor) and gastrocnemius (assists when plantar flexion occurs at the same time).

Knee extension

Rectus femoris, vastus lateralis, vastus intermedius and vastus medialis.

Knee inward rotation

This is only possible when the knee is flexed. The muscles involved are sartorius and semitendinosus.

Knee outward rotation

This is possible only when the knee is flexed. Biceps femoris is the main muscle involved.

MOVEMENTS OF THE FOOT AND ANKLE.

Foot flexion (dorsiflexion)

Tibialis anterior, extensor digitorum longus, extensor hallucis longus and peroneus tertius.

Foot extension (plantar flexion)

Gastrocnemius, soleus, peroneus longus, peroneus brevis, flexor digitorum longus (assists), flexor hallucis longus (assists) and tibialis posterior (assists).

Eversion

Eversion is usually accompanied by abduction to produce pronation. Peroneus longus, peroneus brevis, peroneus tertius and extensor digitorum longus are all involved.

Inversion

Inversion is usually accompanied by adduction to produce supination. The muscles responsible are tibialis anterior, tibialis posterior and flexor digitorum longus.

Foot supination

Tibialis anterior, extensor hallucis longus, tibialis posterior, flexor digitorum longus (assists) and flexor hallucis longus (assists).

Foot pronation

Extensor digitorum longus, peroneus tertius, peroneus longus and peroneus brevis.

MOVEMENTS OF THE SHOULDER JOINT (INCLUDING THE HUMERUS)

Shoulder flexion

Biceps brachii, deltoid (anterior portion and anterior fibres of middle portion), pectoralis major (clavicular portion), subscapularis (assists) and coracobrachialis (assists).

Shoulder extension

Deltoid (posterior fibres of middle portion assist), deltoid (posterior portion), pectoralis major (sternal portion), latissimus dorsi, teres major, teres minor and triceps brachii (assists).

Shoulder abduction

Deltoid (middle portion), deltoid (anterior portion assists), pectoralis major (clavicular portion abducts humerus when above horizontal), pectoralis minor, supraspinatus, subscapularis (assists) and biceps brachii (assists).

Shoulder adduction

Pectoralis major (sternal portion), latissimus dorsi, teres major, deltoid (posterior portion assists) and triceps brachii (assists).

Horizontal flexion

Deltoid (anterior portion), pectoralis major, coracobrachialis, deltoid (anterior fibres of middle portion assist) and biceps brachii (assists).

Horizontal extension

Deltoid (posterior portion), teres minor and infraspinatus.

Inward rotation

Subscapularis, pectoralis major (clavicular portion), teres major and deltoid (anterior portion assists).

Outward rotation

Teres minor, deltoid (posterior portion assists) and biceps brachii (assists).

MOVEMENTS OF THE SCAPULA

Various muscles are involved, including trapezius, rhomboid major, rhomboid minor, levator scapulae, pectoralis minor and serratus anterior.

MOVEMENTS OF THE ELBOW

Elbow flexion

Biceps brachii, brachialis, brachoradialis, coracobrachialis, flexor carpi radialis (assists) and flexor digitorum sublimis (assists).

Elbow extension

Triceps brachii and anconeus.

Supination

Supinator (forearm supination) and biceps brachii (when triceps brachii contract at the same time to prevent elbow flexion).

Pronation

Pronator teres and pronator quadratus (forearm pronation).

MOVEMENTS OF THE WRIST AND HAND

Wrist flexion

Flexor carpi radialis, flexor digitorum sublimis, flexor carpi ulnaris and palmaris longus (assists).

Wrist extension

Extensor carpi radialis longus, extensor carpi radialis brevis, extensor carpi ulnaris and extensor digitorum.

Supination

Biceps brachii (when triceps contract at the same time to prevent elbow flexion).

Abduction

Flexor carpi radialis, extensor carpi radialis longus and extensor carpi radialis brevis.

Adduction

Extensor carpi ulnaris and flexor carpi ulnaris.

MOVEMENTS OF THE TRUNK

Flexion

Rectus abdominis, external obliques (when both sides contract) and internal oblique (when both sides contract).

Extension

Intertransversarii (when both sides contract together), interspinales, multifidus (when both sides contract together), semispinalis thoracis (when both sides contract together), semispinalis cervicis (when both sides contract together) and psoas (hyperextension of the lumbar region).

Lateral flexion

Quadratus lumborum (when only one side contracts), rectus abdominis (when only one side contracts), external obliques (towards the opposite side if one side contracts alone), intertransversarii (when only one side contracts), multifidus (towards the opposite side when only one side contracts), semispinalis thoracis (towards the opposite side when only one side contracts) and semispinalis cervicis (towards the opposite side when only one side contracts).

Rotation

External obliques (towards the opposite side if one side contracts alone), internal oblique (towards the same side if one side contracts alone), multifidus (towards the opposite side when only one side contracts), semispinalis thoracis (towards the opposite side when only one side contracts) and semispinalis cervicis (towards the opposite side when only one side contracts).

REFERENCES AND RECOMMENDED READING

Abernethy, P., Wilson, G. and Logan, P. (1995). Strength and power assessments: Issues, controversies and challenges. *Sports Medicine*, **19** (6), 401–417.

McArdle, W.D., Katch, F.I. and Katch, V.L. (1996). *Exercise Physiology: Energy Nutrition and Human Performance* (4th ed.). London: Williams and Wilkins.

Wilmore, J.H. and Costill, D.L. (1994). *Physiology of Sport and Exercise*. Champaign, IL: Human Kinetics.

2020 VISION

Our understanding of the role exercise can play in public health has developed considerably over the last 20 years to a point where Morris (1994) can suggest that physical activity may be 'the best public health buy' in the UK and a Surgeon General's report can be published in the USA on the relationship between active living and health. What will happen over the next 20 years is an important question for, by encouraging a debate about the future patterns of physical activity now, we can start to develop strategies to overcome potential problems and identify ways of maximising opportunities. We also believe that attempting to predict the future of any area of health provision can only aid long-term planning and help health professionals identify their training needs to meet the long-term demands of their patients and employers. In articulating our view of the future we have attempted, where possible, to extrapolate from current trends and the research that we have presented in the preceding 12 chapters. However, we have also based some of our ideas on our professional experience (or perhaps more accurately on our 'gut feelings'). We found writing this section very enjoyable and thought-provoking and would encourage readers to attempt a similar exercise in relation to physical activity or another area of health provision. With these comments in mind we make 20 predictions, which we hope will help you think about the agenda for exercise promotion in the year 2020.

THE BAD NEWS

1. Opportunities for active living will continue to be *designed* out of daily life by architects and town planners. Lifts will be easier to find in public buildings than staircases, which will continue to be uncarpeted and devoid of art work, mirrors or murals. Despite continued concern over the pollution caused by cars, out-of-town shopping and leisure facilities will develop without serious provision for cycle or pedestrian access.

2. Just as the car has reduced the need for active transport so information technology will reduce the number of journeys made. So, instead of being sedentary behind a steering wheel, people will stay at home and be sedentary in front of a computer screen. In addition, the lack of contact with people in the workplace will lead to an increase in depression and anxiety within the pop-ulation and the incidence of repetitive strain injury and back pain will increase.

3. A new generation of virtual sports and sedentary computer games will begin to replace the major team games, such as football, in the affection of schoolchildren and adolescents. A number of these virtual sports will form national governing bodies and apply to the European Sports Council for recognition. Once accepted, they will begin to lobby for entry to the Olympic Games. Traditionalists will become concerned about how

sports such as rugby can compete against virtual sports, which were designed specifically to capture the imagination of children and to maximise their enjoyment.

4. Children won't walk to school any more because they will hardly ever go to school. Interactive CD-ROMs and the Internet will make learning a home-based activity. Teachers will work with children only once a week, in a group setting. The concept of the virtual school and the virtual campus will be enthusiastically supported by government as a means of cutting costs (i.e. the number of teachers) and ensuring national standards of provision. Whilst a number of subject areas (e.g. mathematics and foreign languages) will embrace these changes to the benefit of pupils, others, notably physical education, will struggle to adapt.

5. Although research into the link between genetics and health problems such as CHD has progressed it will not lead to any quick or simple fixes. For most people healthy living will still be the best investment for a good quality of life.

6. Inequalities between men and women and young and old in terms of exercise participation will reduce, because men and young people alike will take less exercise!

7. Obesity will become a fashion statement – whether as a result of market forces or a greater tolerance of diversity is hotly disputed by sociologists. However, the number of specialist shops catering for size 20 and above will increase considerably and a number of officially overfat men and women will become supermodels.

8. Sports shops will no longer sell equipment and kit but fashion accessories that are damaged by sweat.

9. The London Marathon will be abandoned because of declining numbers.

10. Bigger and better sports stadiums will be built for 100 000 people to sit down and watch 22 people be active. At the same time the number of open spaces for active recreation will be reduced by 40%, largely due to the growth of virtual schools (see point 4) and the resultant sale of school playing fields to property developers. While in the past these developers were forced through 'planning gain' to provide local communities with recreation facilities (e.g. swimming pools), city councils will now require them to link local communities to the World Wide Super Web.

THE GOOD NEWS

1. Exercise physiologists will have identified how little exercise people need to do to remain healthy. The 'jogging boom' of the 1980s appears to have been misguided, with commentators pointing out that a 'walking boom' might have been more sustainable and would lead to greater adherence and long-term public health benefit.

2. Exercise psychologists will have a greater insight into the determinants of partcipation in physical activity and will have designed methods to identify those most at risk from drop-out. Inevitably these questionnaire and interview formats can be downloaded from the Internet and sent directly to patients' portable computers.

3. Exercise biomechanics will have made a significant contribution to exercising safely by isolating those movements which can lead to exercise-related injury. There will be a revolution in both trainers and sports surface design, both of which will become 'smart' and respond to the demands placed upon them.

4. Exercise therapists and scientists will become valued members of both primary healthcare and hospital teams. Patients will be as familiar with being referred to these new professional groups as they are to physiotherapists.

5. Health professionals will have developed innovative and exciting methods of using information technology to promote physical activity. Campaigns and program development will be sponsored by the leading software companies.

6. The millennium will lead to a change in cultural attitudes, prompting a greater understanding of holistic approaches to health and the importance of health-promoting behaviours. Historians will comment, with some surprise, on the unhelpful comments of politicians who in the 1990s attacked health promotion as being part of the 'nanny state', when it is clear that the key message was one of individual responsibility and taking control of one's own health.

7. The Healthy Living Centres established as a result of the Labour party's legislation on The People's Lottery (1997) will be shown by randomised controlled trials to have significantly improved the health of the communities they serve.

8. A 'womaned' mission to Mars will be made possible by the work of exercise scientists, who overcome the problem of astronauts losing bone density through lack of weight-bearing activity by designing exercise machines that mimic the effect of jogging in a weightless environment. Video footage of astronauts working out in space will start a mini-exercise boom with children, who for a short period of time will see exercise as 'hip'. Progressive physical educators will capitalise on this to explain how performance in the new virtual reality sports can be improved through exercise and its positive effect on precompetition anxiety.

9. Exercise science will become a mandatory module on all medical degree courses. As a result newly qualified GPs will no longer say 'you need to get some more exercise' without also saying how this can be achieved.

10. The new government will set targets for increasing the levels of physical activity amongst the population and commit substantial financial resources to the programme. The new Prime Minister will state that 'Just as we have stopped the nation smoking so we must stop it being sedentary and get the country moving' as she jogs toward parliament for Prime Minister's Question Time!

Whilst we freely admit that scientists don't always make the best astrologers we hope that our predictions will help you develop your own vision of the future. We may disagree on the specifics but we trust that no one will underestimate the challenge that faces us all in helping people live physically active lives in the new millennium. We trust that this book has provided you with some of the information, skills and enthusiasm to begin, or continue your work in helping your patients lead active and healthy lives.

REFERENCE

Morris, J.N. (1994). The role of exercise in the prevention on coronary heart disease: Today's best buy in public health. *Medicine and Science in Sport and Exercise*, **26**, 807–813.

INDEX